# EYECARE
# PRACTICE
# TOOL KIT

# EYECARE PRACTICE TOOL KIT

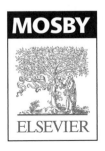

MOSBY

ELSEVIER

11830 Westline Industrial Drive
St. Louis, Missouri 63146

EYECARE PRACTICE TOOL KIT
**Copyright © 2007 by Mosby, Inc., an affiliate of Elsevier Inc.**

ISBN-13: 978-0-323-03941-3
ISBN-10: 0-323-03941-3

---

**Notice**

Knowledge and best practice in this field are constantly changing. As new research and experience broaden our knowledge, changes in practice, treatment and drug therapy may become necessary or appropriate. Readers are advised to check the most current information provided (1) on procedures featured or (2) by the manufacturer of each product to be administered, to verify the recommended dose or formula, the method and duration of administration, and contraindications. It is the responsibility of the practitioner, relying on their own experience and knowledge of the patient, to make diagnoses, to determine dosages and the best treatment for each individual patient, and to take all appropriate safety precautions. To the fullest extent of the law, neither the Publisher nor the Editor assumes any liability for any injury and/or damage to persons or property arising out or related to any use of the material contained in this book.

---

ISBN-13: 978-0-323-03941-3
ISBN-10: 0-323-03941-3

*Publishing Director:* Linda L. Duncan
*Senior Editor:* Kathy Falk
*Senior Developmental Editor:* Christie M. Hart
*Publishing Services Manager:* Julie Eddy
*Associate Project Manager:* Laura Kudowitz
*Senior Book Designer:* Julia Dummitt

Working together to grow
libraries in developing countries

www.elsevier.com | www.bookaid.org | www.sabre.org

ELSEVIER   BOOK AID International   Sabre Foundation

Printed in the United States of America

Last digit is the print number: 9 8 7 6 5 4 3 2 1

# Editorial Board

# How to Use this Book/CD-ROM Package

Congratulations on your selection of the *Eyecare Practice Tool Kit* to enhance your patient communications, practice administration, and management of your practice. Developed by optometrists who share your daily concerns and experiences in optometric practice, the *Eyecare Practice Tool Kit* offers you a vehicle to help ensure patient satisfaction.

Optometry school prepared us to be competent practitioners, but never prepared us to practice optometry in a marketplace with increased competition and complex insurance systems. Today's patients exercise their right to know all options available to them in terms of optometric treatment, and they seek out optometrists in whom they can have faith and confidence. Thus, the optometrist is judged by the patient both for the quality of service provided and for the ability to communicate clearly. It is very difficult for patients to gauge how much we know or how well we did in school; but they can judge how well we communicate and how much we seem to care.

Incorporating the *Eyecare Practice Tool Kit* into the daily practice of optometry will help you communicate in a clear, consistent manner that will enhance patient satisfaction. Let's face it: the bottom line is directly related to how well we educate our patients on treatment needs, as well as how well the patient accepts our recommendations.

### Where to Begin

One of the easiest ways to incorporate the documents included in the *Eyecare Practice Tool Kit* into your practice is to browse the table of contents in the book. You may want to note those documents that you feel will be used most often in your practice.

All the documents are easy to find on the CD-ROM. After installing the *Eyecare Practice Tool Kit on* your computer, it will run seamlessly in Microsoft Word—no need to learn a new program! However, to familiarize yourself with the contents more quickly, it might be best to begin with the printed manual.

### Customized Patient Education Made Easy!

Documents desired can be checked on a master page, the patient's name entered, and a customized, printed package, including practice information, will be printed for the patient to take home and read.

**Remember:** *Any document can be altered to reflect more accurately the philosophy and environment of your practice. ALL documents have been designed to be altered in whatever way suits YOUR needs.*

The *Eyecare Practice Tool Kit* is divided into five sections:

- Part 1: *Patient Handouts* contains descriptions of diseases, education, and treatment protocols that can be used as handouts to patients.
- Part 2: *Letters and Forms* contains those forms and letters useful in the administration of an optometric practice. This section is devoted to documents primarily used by office staff to expedite intraoffice communication, insurance claims processing, patient information, and referrals. Forms useful for a low vision, binocular vision, refractive surgery, or contact lens practice are all included.
- Part 3: *Practice Administration and Sample Contracts* contains sample contracts, staff evaluations, employment agreements, and partnership agreements.
- Part 4: *Office Manual Section* contains everything you need to develop your own office manual. Sample language for office policies, personnel policies, and job descriptions are all there; pick and choose as you wish.
- Part 5: *Office Policies and Procedures for Handling Managed Care Patients* contains sample office policies and procedures for handling patients with managed care health plans.
- Part 6: *Folletos Para Pacientes* is a Spanish translation of Part 1. It contains Spanish versions of the descriptions of diseases, education, and treatment protocols that can be used as handouts to Spanish-speaking patients.

We suggest a staff meeting to acquaint the entire team with the documents contained in the *Eyecare Practice Tool Kit*. Take this opportunity to determine the best documents to use and how to alter them.

# Preface

The *Eyecare Practice Tool Kit* was created with today's busy practitioner in mind. We look at it as the perfect practice communication tool. It was created by three optometrists, all with successful private practices, who felt a need to communicate more effectively with patients and who had experienced a general dissatisfaction with all the pre-printed patient education pamphlets that were then available. No matter how well the patient handouts were written, they were not suitable because they:
- Did not fit their individual practice philosophies
- Were not well written
- Had to be purchased in expensive bulk lots, creating cost and inventory issues
- Did not allow the text to be modified easily as materials and techniques changed
- Used lay terminology and "spoke down" to the patient
- Did not cover enough topics

Many optometrists are excellent communicators, but they usually communicate verbally and they like to communicate *once*. If there is a need to explain something more than once, productivity is lost. Because of the nature of these explanations and the unease patients feel when discussing potential loss of vision, many patients tend to remember only two things an optometrist tells them: "Welcome to our office" and "Thank you for coming."

There was an obvious need to put into writing the issues specifically relating to ocular treatment for that particular patient so that no one would have to spend additional time repeating things to the patient or family. In a written form, the patient information would be available for the patient to review later, to show a spouse, and to begin to become comfortable with the anticipated treatment. Using excellent patient education handouts means that the optometrist will receive fewer notes from the staff asking him or her to call the patient to explain again something that had been discussed in the office.

Patient handouts are included for most of the common conditions and treatments. They were created over time, with changes made along the way, in an attempt to cover all the bases. Ideally, a patient will read the patient handout and will not have additional questions. Letters to insurance carriers, referral letters, and front office organizational forms also are included. Everything has been streamlined as much as possible in an effort to make the forms useful for multiple related situations, in English as well as Spanish.

The creators of these patient handouts and in-office forms and letters have used every form at one time or another. The authors are big fans of having the ability to change, update, and edit any and all forms. Anything included can be easily and neatly rewritten when and where needed.

As far as use of the forms, letters, and handouts go, an optometrist will not use every one every day, but he or she will use some every day. Many topics lend themselves to use of more than one related patient education form, to be placed together in a patient information package. The patient may feel for the first time that he or she truly understands how everything the optometrist does works together to produce a final excellent result. We are confident that as soon as you begin incorporating this customizable CD-ROM into your daily practice, you will not want to work without it again. We hope that your practice will thrive with this high-quality new practice management tool. It is yours to change, to customize, or to add your practice name or letterhead.

**We especially thank the following people and organizations for their help in compiling the information needed to create this manual:**

**The University of California School of Optometry, Southern California College of Optometry, Brookside Optometry, Bay Area Retina Associates Medical Group, Family Eyecare Associates, Woodcrest Vision Clinic, Kensington Optometry, Sun City Vision Center, Dr. Wayne DeCroupet, the College of Optometrists in Vision Development, the American Optometric Association, and Vision West, Inc. and Hariett Stein (10E. Lee Street #2405, Baltimore, Maryland 21202).**

Many of you will discover that you have additional forms or materials that would be helpful to your colleagues. If you wish to share them for possible use in the next edition, please send your submissions to:

> Lawrence Thal, OD, MBA, FAAO
> University of California, School of Optometry
> 302 Minor Hall #2020
> Berkeley, CA 94720-2020

or electronically to: LarryThal@berkeley.edu

I would like to thank David G. Kirschen, OD, PhD, and Peter G. Shaw-McMinn, OD, for their assistance in compiling this material.

Enjoy, and please let us know how we can make the *Eyecare Practice Tool Kit* better in the future!

**Lawrence S. Thal, OD, MBA, FAAO**

# Contents

### LOW VISION

### REFRACTIVE SURGERY

# PART 3—PRACTICE ADMINISTRATION AND SAMPLE CONTRACTS

# PART 4—OFFICE MANUAL

# PART 5—OFFICE POLICIES AND PROCEDURES FOR HANDLING MANAGED CARE PATIENTS

# PART 6—FOLLETOS PARA PACIENCIA

# Part 1

# Patient Handouts

# Accommodative Disorder

## (Handout to accompany report to school nurse or other professionals)

### Definition
Accommodative disorder is a nonpresbyopic, nonrefractive, sensory and neuromuscular anomaly of the visual system. It can be characterized by inadequate accommodative accuracy, reduced facility and flexibility, reduced amplitude of accommodation, or the inability to sustain accommodation.

### Symptoms
The symptoms and signs associated with an accommodative dysfunction are related to prolonged, visually demanding, near-centered tasks, including the following:

1. Asthenopia (eye strain)
2. Transient blurred vision
3. Photophobia
4. Abnormal fatigue
5. Headaches
6. Difficulty sustaining near visual function
7. Dizziness
8. Abnormal postural adaptation/abnormal working distance
9. Orbital pain

### Diagnostic Factors
Accommodative dysfunctions are characterized by one or more of the following diagnostic findings:

1. Low accommodative amplitude relative to age
2. Reduced accommodative facility at near and/or far
3. Reduced ranges of relative accommodation
4. Abnormal lag of accommodation
5. Unstable accommodative findings

NOTE: Additional testing may be appropriate as part of the differential diagnostic workup for accommodative dysfunction to rule out other concurrent medical conditions and differentiate associated visual conditions.

### Therapeutic Considerations

#### A. Management
The doctor of optometry determines appropriate diagnostic and therapeutic modalities and frequency of evaluation and follow-up on the basis of the urgency and nature of the patient's condition and unique needs. The management of the case and duration of the treatment are affected by the following factors:

1. The severity of symptoms and diagnostic factors, including onset and duration of the problem
2. Implications of the patient's general health and associated visual condition
3. Extent of visual demands placed on the individual
4. Patient compliance
5. Prior interventions

#### B. Treatment
A number of cases are successfully managed by prescription of therapeutic lenses and/or prisms. However, accommodative dysfunctions may also require orthoptics/vision therapy. Optometric vision therapy usually incorporates the prescription of specific treatments to achieve the following:

1. Normalize accommodative amplitude relative to age
2. Normalize the ability to sustain accommodation
3. Normalize relative ranges of accommodation
4. Normalize accommodative facility relative to age
5. Normalize accommodative/convergence relationship
6. Integrate accommodative function with information processing

#### Duration of Treatment
The following treatment ranges are provided as a guide for third-party claims processing and review purposes. Treatment duration will depend on the particular patient's condition and associated circumstances. When duration of treatment beyond these ranges is required, documentation of the medical necessity for additional treatment services may be warranted.

1. The most commonly encountered accommodative dysfunction usually requires 24 to 32 hours of office therapy.
2. Uncomplicated accommodative dysfunction characterized by only a transient loss of accommodative function typically requires up to 8 hours of office therapy.

*Continued*

## Accommodative Disorder—cont'd

3. Accommodative dysfunction complicated by:
   a. Reduced amplitude or facility for age: up to an additional 12 hours of office therapy.
   b. Accommodative/convergence abnormalities: up to an additional 16 hours of office therapy.
   c. Other diagnosed visual anomalies may require additional therapy.
   d. Associated conditions such as stroke, head trauma, or other systemic diseases may require substantially more office therapy.

### Follow-up Care

At the conclusion of the active treatment regimen, periodic follow-up evaluations should be provided at appropriate intervals. Therapeutic lenses may be prescribed at the conclusion of vision therapy for maintenance of long-term stability.

# Amblyopia

## Definition
Amblyopia describes poor vision attributable to improper visual development. During childhood, proper visual stimulus is required for good vision to develop. Amblyopia has three potential causes: out-of-focus vision, a turned eye, and visual deprivation. Out-of-focus vision results when one or both eyes have a substantial degree of myopia, hyperopia, or astigmatism. When a large asymmetry in focusing exists between the two eyes, the most out-of-focus eye can develop amblyopia. When one eye is turned inward or outward, the brain will suppress vision out of that eye to prevent double vision. However, the turned eye becomes amblyopic. For out-of-focus vision or an eye turn, glasses, eye patches, and sometimes dilating eye drops can strengthen the amblyopic eye when prescribed early. A less-common cause of amblyopia is visual deprivation, which may be caused by a congenital cataract or a congenitally droopy eyelid. Cataract surgery or eyelid surgery in these cases can minimize the development of amblyopia.

## Symptoms
The symptoms and signs associated with amblyopia include the following:
1. Reduced acuity in affected eye
2. Poor depth judgment
3. Head tilt/turn
4. Incoordination, reduced ability to direct and coordinate movement visually
5. Anisometropia
6. Strabismus

## Diagnostic Factors
Amblyopia is characterized by one or more of the following diagnostic findings:
1. Reduced acuity in the affected eye that does not normalize with the appropriate refractive prescription
2. Inability to maintain stable foveal fixation
3. Suppression of binocular vision
4. Spatial distortion
5. Reduced stereopsis
6. Reduced accommodative facility
7. Inaccurate ocular motor efficiency
8. Asymmetry in performance between the two eyes in the areas of ocular motor and visual information processing skills
    NOTE: Additional testing may be appropriate as part of the differential diagnostic workup for amblyopia to rule out other concurrent medical conditions and differentiate associated visual conditions.

## Therapeutic Considerations
### A. Management
The doctor of optometry determines appropriate diagnostic and therapeutic modalities and frequency of evaluation and follow-up on the basis of the urgency and nature of the patient's condition and unique needs. The management of the case and duration of treatment are affected by the following factors:
1. The severity of symptoms and diagnostic factors, including onset and duration of the problem
2. Implications of the patient's general health and associated visual conditions
3. Extent of visual demands placed on the individual
4. Patient compliance
5. Prior interventions
6. Other associated anomalies such as anisometropia or strabismus

### B. Treatment
A small percentage of cases are successfully managed by prescription of therapeutic lenses and/or prisms. However, most amblyopia requires orthoptics/vision therapy. Optometric vision therapy usually incorporates the prescription of specific treatments to achieve the following:
1. Eliminate any anisometropia
2. Stabilize central foveal fixation
3. Normalize visual acuity
4. Normalize monocular skills, including oculomotor, accommodative, and reaction time
5. Minimize spatial distortion
6. Eliminate suppression
7. Eliminate any strabismus
8. Integrate visual function with appropriate and accurate motor response
9. Normalize binocular function

*Continued*

# Amblyopia—cont'd

**Duration of Treatment**

The following treatment ranges are provided as a guide for third-party claims processing and review purposes. Treatment duration will depend on the particular patient's condition and associated circumstances. When duration of treatment beyond these ranges is required, documentation of the medical necessity for additional treatment services may be warranted.

1. The most commonly encountered amblyopia usually requires 28 to 40 hours of office therapy.
2. Amblyopia complicated by:
   a. Associated visual adaptations (e.g., abnormal retinal correspondence, eccentric fixation, spatial distortion) require additional office therapy.
   b. Associated visual anomalies (e.g., strabismus, nystagmus, cataract) require additional office therapy.
   c. Associated conditions such as birth defects and strabismus surgery require substantially more office therapy.

## Follow-up Care

At the conclusion of the active treatment regimen, periodic follow-up evaluations should be provided at appropriate intervals. Therapeutic lenses may be prescribed at the conclusion of vision therapy for maintenance of long-term stability. Some cases may require additional therapy because of decompensation.

# The Amsler Grid

The Amsler grid was developed by Marc Amsler to allow patients to test their own central (reading) vision for early signs of retinal disease that may be treatable. The test consists of a grid of vertical and horizontal lines.

## Directions

1. Look through your reading glasses or bifocals.
2. Hold the grid approximately 12 inches from the eye.
3. Keep both eyes open and look at the dot in the center of the grid.
4. Cover the left eye. While looking at the dot, answer the following questions. Can you see all four corners of the grid? Are any of the lines blurry, wavy, distorted, bent, gray, or missing?
5. Repeat the previous step with the right eye.
6. If you note any changes in how you see the grid, call your optometrist.
7. We recommend you use the grid two to three times a week.
8. Place the grid in a convenient place to remind you to use it regularly (e.g., the refrigerator door or bathroom mirror).

You can use the grid below to take the test on your computer screen. Download the grid for use as a screen saver. Alternatively, download the black-on-white version for printing.

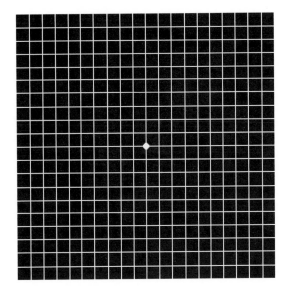

# Attention Deficit–Hyperactivity Disorder and Vision

Some children with learning difficulties exhibit specific behaviors of impulsivity, hyperactivity, and distractibility. A common term used to describe children who exhibit such behaviors is attention deficit–hyperactivity disorder (ADHD).

Undetected and untreated vision problems can elicit some of the same signs and symptoms commonly attributed to ADHD. Because of these similarities, some children with vision problems are mislabeled as having ADHD.

A recent study by researchers at the Children's Eye Center, University of San Diego, uncovered a relation between a common vision disorder, convergence insufficiency, and ADHD. The study "showed that children with convergence insufficiency are three times as likely to be diagnosed with ADHD than children without the disorder." Dr. Granet of the Children's Eye Center commented, "We don't know if convergence insufficiency makes ADHD worse or if convergence insufficiency is misdiagnosed as ADHD. What we do know is that more research must be done on this subject and that patients diagnosed with ADHD should also be evaluated for convergence insufficiency and treated accordingly."

This new research appears to support what many doctors have known for some time—a significant percentage of children with learning disabilities have some type of vision problem. One study found that 13% of children between 9 and 13 years of age have moderate to marked convergence insufficiency, and as many as one in four, or 25% of school-age children, may have a vision problem that can affect learning.

Vision problems can have a huge impact on academic performance and behavior in the classroom. Parents who suspect a vision problem may be contributing to their child's learning or behavior problems should arrange for a complete functional vision examination.

# Blepharitis

Acute infections of the eyelid—those that flare up with little or no warning—are irritating and can affect your vision. You may have symptoms such as itchy or burning eyes, blurred vision, gritty or granular sensations, or oily tears. These conditions are caused by either blepharitis, a medical term that means inflammation of the eyelid, or meibomianitis, inflammation of the oil-producing glands of the eye.

Blepharitis is usually caused by *Staphylococcus* bacteria that thrive in excess oil produced by the glands of the eyelid. Blepharitis sometimes accompanies outbreaks of acne. The inflammation may be worsened by tea or alcohol consumption and may become chronic. The essence of therapy is to prevent the infection from causing chronic symptoms or more serious problems.

Depending on the severity of your symptoms, we may prescribe any or all of the following therapies:

1. Warm or hot moist compresses applied to the eye.
2. Eyelid cleansing procedures. Although neither this nor hot compresses are a cure for infection, both actions help remove debris that has become trapped in the glands and eyelashes.
3. Manual expression of excess oil from the oil glands at the edges of the eyelids. Applying hot compresses before the expression usually helps the glands flow more freely and release trapped bacteria.
4. In more severe cases we may prescribe antibiotic eye drops. These may or may not be in combination with a corticosteroid, an antiinflammatory drug. Sometimes, instead of an antibiotic eye drop, antibiotic topical ointment is prescribed that should be applied along the edge of the eyelids. Oral antibiotics may also be used (a treatment usually reserved for special cases).

Blepharitis can recur or remain chronic if not treated completely. Eyelid hygiene procedures are important in removing the bacteria that remain trapped in your lashes or lid areas of your eyes.

## Directions for a Warm Soak of the Eyelids

1. Wash your hands thoroughly.
2. Moisten a clean washcloth with warm water.
3. Close the eyes and place the washcloth on the eyelid for approximately 5 minutes.
4. Repeat several times daily.

## Directions for an Eyelid Scrub

1. Wash your hands thoroughly.
2. Mix warm water and a small amount of shampoo that does not irritate the eye (e.g., baby shampoo).*
3. Close one eye and use a clean washcloth (a different one for each eye) to rub the shampoo mixture back and forth across the eyelashes and the edge of the eyelid.
4. Rinse with cool, clear water.
5. Repeat on the other eye.

If the eye becomes red or painful, consult an eye care professional immediately.

---

*Your doctor of optometry may also recommend commercially available lid scrubs.

# Branch Retinal Vein Occlusion

Branch retinal vein occlusion (BRVO) is a cause of painless vision loss in the upper, lower, or central field of vision. It may also occur with no symptoms. Occlusion occurs when blood flow in a vein is reduced or blocked.

When BRVO occurs, we look for associated conditions. If vision is affected, treatment with a laser may improve vision or reduce the risk of further vision loss. In most cases, we wait for spontaneous improvement. If vision is blurred, treatment is guided by techniques that have been tested in national controlled clinical trials.

In BRVO, an artery crossing over the retinal vein at the point of obstruction is usually present. This can pinch the vein, like stepping on a garden hose, thereby cutting off blood flow. The area of the retina that drained through this vein may become congested or swollen. Areas of the retina may bleed or die. Sometimes the obstruction is reversible, and sometimes it is irreversible.

The leading cause of blurred vision in BRVO is macular edema, in which swelling of the central retina is caused when blood cannot flow through the blocked vein, allowing water to leak into the retina.

## Causes

The most common cause of BRVO is arteriolosclerosis. However, it may be more likely to occur in people with a history of hypertension, diabetes, glaucoma, ocular inflammation, or carotid artery disease. BRVO may occur in hyperviscosity syndromes, in which the blood is too thick. The conditions associated with BRVO are detected by complete ocular and general examinations and laboratory or blood tests. If a systemic condition is found, treatment reduces risk for the other eye.

## Visual Loss: Proliferation and Macular Edema

At its worst, BRVO can rarely cause closure of vessels in the macula and nonfunction. Areas of retina with poor blood flow may sometimes allow new vessels to grow on the back surface of the vitreous gel. When these vessels grow, they are fragile. They can break, bleed, and fill the eye with blood. Symptoms of floaters or cobwebs may be present.

Macular edema is the most common cause of vision loss in BRVO. Cystlike spaces form within the retina, causing swelling and potentially reversible visual loss.

## Treatment

Laser is a light focused to a pin point. It can dry swollen retinal tissues or burn retinal tissue that has new vessels. Laser treatment for macular edema is brief. A grid pattern of laser is used if vision is 20/40 or worse for 2 to 3 months with cystoid macular edema. Laser therapy is a simple outpatient procedure performed in the office. Treatment occasionally must be repeated if swelling is still present 3 months after the initial laser treatment.

An alternative treatment for macular edema instead of, or in addition to, laser is the injection of triamcinolone in the vitreous. This is also performed in the office.

Surgery on the obstructed vein and the overlying artery to relieve the blockage with a vitrectomy shows some promise.

If new vessels grow, scatter laser photocoagulation indirectly treats these vessels, reducing the risk of bleeding.

## Prognosis

Many BRVOs are asymptomatic. If vision is affected, laser treatment for macular edema increases the chances of vision improvement by more than 60%. An injection of a steroid may help patients for whom laser alone does not help. If vitreous bleeding occurs, scatter laser reduces the chance of severe visual loss in more than 85% of patients. The blood usually clears spontaneously.

# Cataract

A cataract is an opaque film or cloudiness that occurs in the lens within the eye. It may consist of varying size opacities and/or water vacuoles. In general, it is an alteration in the normal lens tissue that reduces its normal high degree of transparency. This, in turn, interferes with the degree and quality of light reaching the retina.

## Symptoms

Symptoms of cataract include blurred vision at far and near, poor night vision, glare sensitivity, need for more light to see indoors, distorted lights when viewing at night, and halos around lights.

## Risk Factors

Risk factors include radiation (sunlight and treatments), smoking, alcohol, medications, and genetics. The main cause of cataract is sunlight radiation. The sunlight tans the lens inside our eye much like it tans our skin. Whereas we get new skin cells on an average of every 26 days, the lenses inside our eyes have to last our entire lives. The energy in the sunlight, particularly ultraviolet radiation, causes the formation of unstable molecules called free radicals. These free radicals change the lens tissue, causing distortion and darkening.

Cataracts can be directly or indirectly affected by medications and diseases. Many medications cause the opening of the eye to enlarge, allowing more harmful light into the eye. Examples are antidepressants, antihistamines, amphetamines, nitroglycerin, and beta-blockers. Other drugs, such as steroids and tamoxifen, can cause cataracts. Some drugs, like diuretics (water pills), cause the tissue to be photosensitized, which results in increased sensitivity to sunlight. Medical conditions such as diabetes, hypertension, rheumatoid arthritis, and other connective diseases are commonly associated with cataracts.

## Treatment

Treatment includes eyeglasses, contact lenses, and surgery. New technologies in eyeglasses and contact lenses allow better vision. Ultraviolet radiation filters, nonglare technology, and the correction of higher-order aberrations with wavefront technology can result in better vision through cataract changes. The best preventive treatment for the progression of cataracts is polarized sunglasses with the addition of an antireflection coating on the backs of the lenses.

Cataracts are generally not surgically removed until vision cannot be improved to reasonable levels with eyeglasses or contact lenses. The decision for having surgery usually depends on whether you can see well enough to do what you want to do. Phakoemulsification is a surgical technique used to allow small incisions sometimes not requiring any sutures. An artificial lens is implanted that may provide excellent vision without the need for strong glasses or contact lenses. Prognosis for good vision is excellent.

Cataracts tend to progress at a slow pace and, as a rule, can be monitored on a yearly basis. At the appropriate time we can recommend the best surgeon for your particular type of cataract.

For the near future we should monitor your eye health status and cataract development on a regular basis.

# Lenses for Patients with Developing Cataracts

Our doctors and staff are pleased to be able to provide you the latest technology in eyeglasses. Summarized below are new improvements in technology and the benefits available to you.

During the course of your examination we discovered that you are showing cataract changes. Today's lens technology allows us to prescribe glasses that will slow the development of your cataracts as well as improve your remaining vision. You may recall from the explanation given by the doctor that the lens inside the eye tends to become cloudier with age. This prevents the lens from properly focusing light on the retina at the back of the eye, resulting in a loss of vision. The clouding results from chemical changes within the lens. Ultraviolet (UV) light and visible light can cause the lens to "tan," much like tanning your skin. We replace our skin cells every 26 days, but the lens inside the eye must last throughout our lives.

## Sun Lenses

The lens technology we have prescribed for you will block 100% of the most damaging light in the atmosphere. The tint recommended for you will block from 60% to 85% of the visible light necessary to see during daylight hours. Some tints are prescribed to allow normal color perception, and others are designed to increase contrast. The appropriate tint depends on the extent of your cataract changes and your personal needs. New lens technology also reduces the glare off surfaces such as roadways or reflections off water.

Lenses specifically designed to inhibit the progression of cataracts are manufactured from high-technology polymers, which are the least likely to break in case of an accident. The lens material is lighter, thinner, and the safest available.

## Indoor Lenses

The clouding of the lens of the eye causes less light to reach the retina. New lenses allow nearly 10% more light to enter the eye. Thinner lens designs also result in more light reaching your retina. Newer lenses eliminate irritating reflections and improve contrast with high-technology tints and coatings. The additional light, loss of glare, and improved contrast will allow you to read more comfortably and see better when driving at night.

These indoor lenses and sun lenses have properties that will provide you with better vision as well as protect you from the light rays contributing to the cataracts. Remember to wear your special sunglasses during all outdoor activities in the daylight. Try them on cloudy days and you may discover after a minute or so that you will adapt and see well with the sun lenses.

Our doctors and staff will continue to monitor new changes in lens technology that will benefit you. With today's new lens technology and adherence to your doctor's prescriptions, you can expect to see well the rest of your life. Thank you for the opportunity to provide you with your vision care. We look forward to seeing you in the future.

# Central Retinal Vein Occlusion

Central retinal vein occlusion (CRVO) is a cause of painless vision loss throughout the field of vision, often worst centrally. It may also occur with minimal symptoms. Blood flow in the main vein draining the retina is blocked or reduced. If vision is poor because of swelling of the central retina, give an injection or surgery may improve vision. If vision is severely affected, laser therapy to prevent painful glaucoma. Treatment guidelines have been developed by national controlled clinical trials to stop unwanted new blood vessels from growing in the eye.

## How the Eye Works

The eye works like a camera. The lens and cornea focus light rays into the back of the eye. The retina works like the photographic film in a camera. The macula is part of the central retina, with which we see fine details and color.

Arteries bring blood to the retina. Veins take blood away from the retina. The main vessel that leads from the retina through the optic nerve to the heart is the central retinal vein.

## Obstruction of the Central Retinal Vein

In CRVO an obstruction of the central retinal vein in the optic nerve is usually present. The vein may be pinched, as when stepping on a garden hose, thereby cutting off the flow. The retina may bleed, die, or become congested and swollen. A leading cause of blurred vision in CRVO is macular edema. In some cases we treat this to improve vision, especially if vision at presentation is poor.

If vision has dropped to 20/200, there is up to a 20% chance of improving to 20/100 or better without treatment. Only 6% of patients improve by three lines on the visual activity chart. If vision is good to begin with, it often stays good. If the vision is fair, it may worsen in 47% of patients.

## Causes of Central Retinal Vein Occlusion

The cause of CRVO is usually unknown. It is more likely to occur in people with a history of hypertension, diabetes, glaucoma, ocular inflammation, or carotid artery disease. It may also occur in hyperviscosity syndromes, in which the blood is too thick. The conditions associated with CRVO are detected with complete ocular and general examinations and laboratory or blood tests. Their treatment may reduce risks of vein occlusion in the other eye.

## Neovascular Glaucoma

The worst complication of CRVO is growth of new blood vessels in the drain for fluid inside the eye, or anterior chamber angle. If the retina has lost blood flow and vision is quite poor, the retina produces a chemical that calls for vessels to grow, which can cause painful glaucoma.

Eyes with severe CRVO should be monitored every month for 6 months, then every 3 months thereafter. If new vessels are found, laser treatment may stop this vessel growth, control intraocular pressure, and prevent pain in the eye.

## Retinal Neovascularization

Rarely, new vessels grow from the surface of the retina. These new vessels may break, bleed, and fill the eye with blood. Retinal detachment is a late cause of vision loss. Laser treatment with focused intense light may cause the blood vessels to disappear and preserve some vision. If the eye fills with blood, surgery is occasionally indicated to restore some vision. However, reading vision is generally poor.

## Macular Edema

Swelling of the retina is a common cause of vision loss in CRVO. In eyes that still have blood flow to the macula, intravitreal steroids may lead to visual improvement, but not in all cases. More than one injection may be needed. In others, vitrectomy with radical optic neurotomy may be indicated. Not everyone with CRVO and macular edema is a candidate for treatment with intravitreal steroid injection or radical optic neurotomy. Ask your doctor for details.

## Conclusion

CRVO is a significant cause of vision loss and discomfort. Frequent follow-up is often required. We are able to help improve vision in some eyes, and appropriate laser treatment may prevent severe glaucoma.

# Central Serous Chorioretinopathy

Central serous chorioretinopathy (CSC) is a cause of painless vision loss in the central field of vision. Distortion, a central blind or gray spot, and color vision changes may be present, and objects may look smaller. In some people the onset of symptoms may be accompanied or preceded by migrainelike headaches.

In most cases we wait for spontaneous improvement, with the majority of patients (80% to 90%) returning to 20/25 or better vision.

Patients with classic CSC have a 40% to 50% risk of recurrence in the same eye. If vision is affected, treatment with laser may improve vision or reduce the risk of further vision loss.

## How the Eye Works

The eye works like a camera. The lens and cornea focus light rays. The retina works like the photographic film in a camera.

The retina is transparent. The layer beneath it, the retinal pigment epithelium (RPE), gives an orange color to the inside of the eye. Beneath this is the choroid, a layer of blood vessels thought to be the source of fluid under the retina in CSC.

## Fluid under the Central Retina

The hallmark of CSC is fluid under the central retina. This is seen as a leak from one or more spots on a fluorescein angiogram. RPE detachments and multiple leaking spots may also be present. The other eye will be affected in up to 20% of patients at some point.

## Who Gets Central Serous Chorioretinopathy?

Traditionally, CSC has been thought of as a disease affecting young 20- to 45-year-old men. It has recently been diagnosed with increasing frequency among patients older than 50 years. In this age group, the male to female ratio diminishes to 2:1 from the 10:1 ratio seen in younger patients. CSC is uncommon among African Americans but is frequent in whites, Hispanics, and Asians.

## Causes

The exact cause of CSC is highly controversial. An imbalance appears to exist in the amount of fluid that enters the subretinal space and the RPE's ability to remove it. This results in a net accumulation of fluid beneath the retina.

Systemic associations of CSC includes organ transplantation, exogenous steroid use, endogenous hypercortisolism (Cushing's syndrome), systemic hypertension, systemic lupus erythematosus, pregnancy, and use of some medications.

Finally, type A personalities and major stressful events may be associated with CSC, presumably because of elevated blood cortisol and epinephrine levels.

## Laser Treatment for Central Serous Chorioretinopathy

Laser photocoagulation is the application of a bright light to the area of leakage to seal the leak spot found on the fluorescein angiogram. Laser treatment shortens the course of the disease and decreases the risk of recurrence for CSC, but it does not appear to improve the final visual prognosis.

Laser photocoagulation should be considered under the following circumstances:
1. Persistence of a serous detachment for more than 3 to 4 months
2. Recurrence in a eye with visual deficit from previous CSC
3. Presence of visual deficits in the opposite eye from previous episodes of CSC
4. Occupational or other patient need requiring prompt recovery of vision, such as with police officers or pilots

Laser treatment may be considered in recurrent episodes of serous detachment with a leak located more than 300 μm from the center of the fovea. Each case must be approached individually.

Rarely patients develop choroidal neovascularization at the site of leakage and laser treatment. If laser treatment is performed close to the center of vision, a small blind spot may be present that usually fades. Despite treatment and reattachment of the retina, vision may not return to normal.

## Prognosis

The prognosis for visual recovery in CSC is generally good. The leaks usually close spontaneously and the detachment resolves over a period of weeks to months. Most patients (more than 90%) will retain vision of 20/30 or better in the affected eye. However, some patients may still note some mild changes in vision such as decreased contrast, mild distortion, and decreased night vision.

# Chalazia and Styes

Your eyelids are quite important. They protect your eyes from approaching objects and irritating particles in the air. When you blink, your eyelids help remove foreign objects and distribute tears, which lubricate your eyes. But sometimes your eyelids can have problems and need care. Two common conditions that affect your eyelids are chalazia and styes.

A **chalazion** results from a blockage of one or more of the small oil-producing glands (meibomian glands) found in the upper and lower eyelids. These blockages trap the oil produced by the glands and cause a lump on the eyelid that is usually about the size of a pea.

These are usually relatively painless, although in some cases you may appear to have a black eye. If the chalazion becomes infected, the eyelid can become swollen, inflamed, and more painful.

**Styes** are often confused with chalazia. Styes are infections or abscesses of an eyelid gland near an eyelash root or follicle. They generally occur nearer to the edge, or margin, of the eyelid than do chalazia, where they form a red, sore lump similar to a boil or pimple.

In some cases, both chalazia and styes may come to a head and drain on their own without treatment. However, in most instances they do not.

A chalazion may be treated by applying hot compresses and/or antibiotic eye drops.* In some cases, steroid drugs may be injected into or adjacent to the site of the chalazion. A chalazion may also be treated by surgical incision and drainage when necessary. Sometimes oral medications are prescribed.

Styes may also be treated with hot compresses.* Frequently, antibiotic and/or steroid eye drops or ointments may be needed.

Chalazia and styes most often respond well to treatment. If left untreated, however, they can be uncomfortable and unattractive and can lead to other problems. Chalazia and styes may recur. If this happens too frequently, your doctor of optometry may recommend additional tests to determine if other health problems may be contributing to their development.

## Directions for Application of Hot Compresses

1. Wash your hands thoroughly.
2. Moisten a clean washcloth with hot water.*
3. Close your eyes and place the washcloth on the eyelid for approximately 10 to 15 minutes.
4. Remoisten the washcloth as necessary to keep it hot.
5. Repeat at least four times a day.

---

*Caution: Be careful that hot water does not cause burns.

# Computer Glasses

More than 100 million Americans use computers every day at work, and 70% of them have vision problems. Computer use puts a great demand on our eyes. The doctor has completed an examination designed to reveal problems that can limit your performance when using a computer. He has determined that you can benefit from wearing glasses designed specifically for computer use.

## Focused for the Computer

Glasses designed for the computer have many special features. The prescription will focus your eyes to allow minimal effort when trying to see at computer distances. Focusing your eyes for the computer allows the muscles inside your eyes to relax, reducing the possibility of eye strain and fatigue.

## Nonglare Lenses

The lenses prescribed for you are nonglare lenses. Glare is a constant cause of visual disturbance when using computers. Reflections off the surfaces of your lenses can result in loss of nearly 10% of light. This loss of light entering your eye will decrease the contrast of the figures and letters. Loss of contrast can especially be a problem with those who have developing cataracts or macular degeneration. Reflections from the back of the spectacle lenses can also enter directly into the eye, causing irritating glare and degradation of the optical images. This glare is particularly noticeable in very nearsighted (myopic) individuals. The nonglare lens allows more light to the retina and reduces these reflections.

## High-Tech Lens Material

Today's technology allows lenses to be made from many different materials. Your lenses are composed of polycarbonate, the same material used in the aerospace industry and in compact disks. The benefit of this material is that it is nearly unbreakable. Polycarbonate is the safest lens material and is known as the most break-proof lens fabricated. The lens comes with a high-tech, scratch-resistant coating that allows it to last longer than other lenses.

## Thin and Light

Besides being breakage resistant, your lenses are also the thinnest and lightest available. This lower weight allows your glasses to maintain the proper adjustment so all measurements remain in the correct place, allowing you the best vision.

## High-Tech Lens Design

The doctor prescribed the lens design that allows you the most use of your vision while using the computer. The design may take several forms. New technology has provided designs specific to computer users. The new high-tech designs allow for normal head postures, relaxing the neck and shoulder muscles. Musculoskeletal symptoms are often the result of improper head postures caused by poor lens design or measurements. The computer glasses manufactured for you are designed to give you maximal vision and maximal comfort.

These glasses have been custom fit to your particular needs. No one else will probably get the same benefits from them as you. As your eyes change in the future, we will alter your computer glasses to ensure that you have comfort and are able to maximize your performance. If you have any questions, please give us a call. Remember our theme and our mission are to "provide you with good vision for the rest of your life."

(Reprinted from *Diagnosing and Treating Computer-Related Vision Problems*, Sheedy and Shaw-McMinn)

# Computer Vision Syndrome

## Eye Breaks

- Refocus eyes away from the monitor to across the room for 5 seconds every 15 minutes of monitor viewing. Look at objects that are varying distances from your computer.
- Perform several rapid and quick blinks to the eyes several times to rewet and refocus during this eye break. Application of artificial tears or rewetting drops for contact lens wearers at this time would be beneficial.

## Workstation Adjustments

- Ambient lighting should be available. Avoid harsh brightness changes from the computer monitor to the room.
- Minimize screen glare by repositioning the computer monitor or source of light to avoid glare and light reflections or consider an antiglare screen.
- Place the monitor directly in front of you, not off to one side. Adjust monitor sharpness, contrast (adjust to individual comfort), brightness (match room brightness), distance (20 inches to 26 inches), and viewing angle (approximately 15 degrees from eyes to monitor center).
- A larger monitor with higher resolution and refresh rate (70 Hz or higher) than your current monitor may also be helpful.
- Adjust your chair so that both feet touch the ground with knees approximately 90 degrees to the floor and elbows approximately 90 degrees to the keyboard. Allow for comfortable thigh support.
- Exercise when sitting with various stretches and joint rotation. Standing up and moving about is also helpful to keep your blood circulating.

# Computer Vision Syndrome: Treatment Sheet

Computer vision syndrome (CVS) is a complex optical and musculoskeletal disorder related to near work during computer use. The most common symptoms of CVS include the following:

- Headache
- Loss of focus, blurred vision
- Double vision
- Dry, burning, tired eyes
- Muscular strain
- Excessive tears
- General fatigue
- Excessive blinking/squinting
- Overall stress
- Neck or shoulder strain/pain

Some individuals react with more difficulty when focusing on characters on a computer screen as opposed to reading printed material on paper.

Treatment is varied and complex, with different solutions for different needs. For optimal patient comfort and performance, a specific computer correction is usually necessary. Your optometrist will assess your optical needs. A wide variety of lens styles are available, ranging from single-vision computer lenses to progressive-add bifocals, which can aid in achieving proper focus. Many different lens materials and treatments are also available (e.g., tints and antireflective coatings) to assist with comfort.

Your doctor will be testing your eyes to help find which solution works best for you. Some of these tests might include the following:

- Detailed refraction: a measurement of your visual system's focusing power needs.
- Binocular vision testing: an evaluation of your eyes' efficiency in working together at different distances.
- Dynamic retinoscopy: an evaluation of your eyes' focusing system function for near tasks.
- Tear assessment: an evaluation of your tear quantity and quality.

Studies show that approximately three quarters of computer users have symptoms of CVS. The good news is that the eye and vision symptoms, as well as other problems of CVS, can usually be alleviated by good eye care and by changes in the work environment.

The doctor has prescribed the following treatment for you at this time:

❑ Enhancement of tears
❑ Artificial tears (eye drops or gel)
❑ Antiinflammatory eye drops
❑ Punctal occlusion
❑ Computer glasses (with special computer lenses)
❑ Vision therapy (specific eye exercises that enhance focusing)
❑ Eye breaks
❑ Workstation adjustments

**Medications prescribed**                                    **Dosage and Frequency**

_____                            _____

_____                            _____

## Your Follow-up Visit

Date: _____            Dr.: _____

Time: _____            Phone: _____

# Conjunctivitis

**Conjunctivitis**, commonly known as **pink eye**, is an infection of the thin membrane that lines the inside of the eyelids and the white part of the eye. The three most common types of conjunctivitis are viral, bacterial, and allergic. Each requires different treatments. With the exception of the allergic type, conjunctivitis is typically contagious.

The viral type is often associated with a cold or sore throat. Bacteria such as *Staphylococcus* and *Streptococcus* often cause bacterial conjunctivitis. The severity of the infection depends on the type of bacteria involved. The allergic type occurs more frequently among those with allergic conditions. When related to allergies, the symptoms are often seasonal. Allergic conjunctivitis may also be caused by intolerance to substances such as cosmetics, perfume, or drugs.

## Symptoms
- Watery discharge
- Irritation or gritty feeling
- Itching
- Swollen eyelids
- Swelling of the conjunctiva
- Redness
- Tearing
- Mucous discharge that may cause the lids to stick together, especially after sleeping

## Diagnosis
Conjunctivitis is diagnosed during an eye examination with a biomicroscope. In some cases cultures are taken to determine the type of bacteria causing the infection.

## Treatment
Conjunctivitis requires medical attention. The appropriate treatment depends on the cause of the problem. Eye drops are prescribed in addition to nonsteroidal antiinflammatory medications, antihistamines, cool compresses, and artificial tears. Sometimes an oral antibiotic or ointment is used to treat the condition. Like the common cold, viral conjunctivitis has no cure; however, the symptoms can be relieved. Viral conjunctivitis usually resolves within 3 weeks.

To avoid spreading infection, take the following simple steps:
- Disinfect surfaces such as doorknobs and counters with diluted bleach solution
- Do not swim (some bacteria can be spread in the water)
- Avoid touching the face
- Wash hands frequently
- Do not share towels or washcloths
- Do not reuse handkerchiefs (tissues are best)
- Avoid shaking hands

# Allergic Conjunctivitis

Your eye doctor has given you the following prescription: _____

Eye drops have been prescribed to alleviate the symptoms of allergic conjunctivitis. An allergen has irritated the thin clear mucous membrane that lines the inside of your eyelids and the white part of your eye, called the *conjunctiva*. Symptoms vary from person to person. More than 22 million people in the United States suffer from the most common eye allergy: allergic conjunctivitis.

## What Is an Allergic Response?

An allergic response is an overreaction of the body's immune system to foreign substances known as allergens, which the body wrongly perceives as a potential threat. When the eye comes into contact with certain allergens, an allergic response can result. Plant pollens, animal dander, dust mites, mold spores, grass and ragweed, cosmetics and perfumes, skin medicines, and air pollution often cause allergies. Our eyes have millions of *mast cells* that release chemicals, causing the symptoms.

Common symptoms of allergic conjunctivitis include the following:

- Itchy eyes and eyelids
- Watery eyes
- Dilated vessels in the conjunctiva
- Burning sensation around the eyes
- Redness around the eyes
- Swollen eyelids
- Blurred vision
- Sensation of fullness in the eyes or eyelid
- Sensation of foreign body in the eye
- An urge to rub the eyes
- Lid twitches
- Dry eyes
- Long strings of mucus in the corner of the eye
- Floaters in the tears

The drops prescribed will alleviate the symptoms caused by the release of these chemicals and block the mast cells from releasing more.

Two types of allergic conjunctivitis exist, seasonal and perennial. The former is the more common of the two, occurring in the majority of people who have this condition. It is associated with seasonal allergies that commonly occur during the spring and summer months and is usually caused by exposure to airborne allergens, such as grass and plant pollens. Perennial allergic conjunctivitis persists throughout the year and is generally triggered by indoor allergens such as animal dander, dust mites, and mold spores.

Your doctor will evaluate the success of the eye drops and advise you regarding future use. If symptoms seem to worsen, call the office immediately.

# Convergence Insufficiency

## (Handout to accompany school nurse or other professionals)

### Definition

Convergence insufficiency is a sensory and neuromuscular anomaly of the binocular vision system characterized by an inability to converge or sustain convergence. Convergence occurs when eyes are turned inward so that lines of sight are directed on an object of regard.

### Symptoms

The symptoms and signs associated with convergence insufficiency are related to prolonged, visually demanding, near-centered tasks, including the following:

1. Diplopia (double vision)
2. Asthenopia (eye strain)
3. Transient blurred vision
4. Difficulty sustaining near visual function
5. Abnormal fatigue
6. Headache
7. Orbital pain
8. Abnormal postural adaptation

### Diagnostic Factors

Convergence insufficiency is characterized by one or more of the following diagnostic findings:

1. High exophoria at near
2. Tight accommodative-convergence/accommodation ratio
3. Receded near point of convergence
4. Low fusional vergence ranges and/or facility
5. Exofixation disparity with steep forced vergence slope

NOTE: Additional testing may be appropriate as part of the differential diagnostic workup for convergence insufficiency to rule out other concurrent medical conditions and to differentiate associated visual conditions.

### Therapeutic Considerations

#### A. Management

The doctor of optometry determines appropriate diagnostic and therapeutic modalities and frequency of evaluation and follow-up on the basis of the urgency and nature of the patient's condition and unique needs. The management of the case and duration of treatment are affected by the following:

1. The severity of symptoms and diagnostic factors, including onset and duration of the problem
2. Implications of patient's general health and associated visual conditions
3. Extent of visual demands placed on the individual
4. Patient compliance
5. Prior interventions

#### B. Treatment

A small percentage of cases are successfully managed by prescription of therapeutic prisms and lenses. However, most convergence insufficiencies require orthoptics and/or vision therapy. Optometric vision therapy usually incorporates the prescription of specific treatments to accomplish the following:

1. Normalize the near point of convergence
2. Normalize fusional vergence ranges and facility
3. Eliminate suppression
4. Normalize associated deficiencies in ocular motor control and accommodation
5. Normalize accommodative/convergence relation
6. Normalize depth judgments and/or stereopsis
7. Integrate binocular function with information processing

#### Duration of Treatment

The following treatment ranges are provided as a guide for third-party claims processing and review purposes. Treatment duration will depend on the particular patient's condition and associated circumstances. When duration of treatment beyond these ranges is required, documentation of the medical necessity for additional treatment services may be warranted.

1. The most commonly encountered convergence insufficiency usually requires 24 to 32 hours of office therapy.
2. Uncomplicated convergence insufficiency characterized by only a remote near point of convergence usually requires up to 12 hours of office therapy.

*Continued*

## Convergence Insufficiency—cont'd

3. Convergence insufficiency complicated by:
   a. Restricted fusional ranges usually require up to an additional 12 hours of office therapy.
   b. Suppression usually requires up to an additional 6 hours of office therapy.
   c. An accommodative element usually requires up to an additional 12 hours of office therapy.
   d. Other diagnosed visual anomalies may require additional office therapy.
   e. Associated conditions such as stroke, head trauma, or other systemic conditions may require substantially more office therapy.

### Follow-up Care

At the conclusion of the active treatment regimen, periodic follow-up evaluations should be provided at appropriate intervals. Therapeutic lenses may be prescribed at the conclusion of vision therapy for maintenance of long-term stability.

# Cool Soaks

Cool soaks are useful to relieve ocular itching, lid swelling, and discomfort caused by allergic reactions.

1. Use tap water. Run the tap for approximately 2 minutes to avoid still-standing water that may contain sediment from the pipes. You do not need to use distilled or purified drinking water.
2. Use cool (room temperature) tap water. You should not use refrigerated ice water.
3. Soak a clean washcloth in the water. Close both eyes and lay the washcloth over both closed eyes or as directed: _____
4. Leave the washcloth over your eyes until it warms up, then resoak in the cool water.
5. Attempt to maintain a consistently cool temperature when soaking.
6. Soak for a total of 5 minutes or as directed: _____
7. Soak three times a day or as directed: _____

# Corneal Abrasion

A corneal abrasion is an injury to the front surface of the eye. The injury can occur when a foreign object gets in the eye, when the cornea becomes scratched, or even from rubbing the eyes too hard. The cornea is very sensitive. Depending on the location and depth of the injury, an abrasion can be quite painful and even sight threatening, resulting in permanent visual impairment.

Treatment is important to prevent infection within the injured cornea. The medication that the doctor prescribes will help heal the cornea and prevent infection. Be sure to follow the doctor's instructions so that the cornea heals properly.

Small abrasions can heal within 24 hours but more severe abrasions can take up to several weeks to heal. This injury can be treated in different ways. The doctor will probably prescribe eye drops and/or ointment. You may need to wear a special contact lens overnight or longer to help with healing. Sometimes a patch may need to be worn on the eye overnight.

The doctor has prescribed the following treatment for you:

**Medications/Treatments Prescribed**                    **Dosage/Frequency**

_____                    _____

_____                    _____

Special instructions (follow the instructions that your doctor has checked):
❏ Fill the prescription today and begin medication as soon as possible.
❏ Apply eye drops, then close your eye. With one finger, apply mild pressure to the inner corner of the eye. Keep pressure on this area for 90 seconds. This will help the drop stay within the eye.
❏ Stay indoors and rest your eyes for the first 24 hours. Sunlight will be irritating. If you must go outdoors, wear sunglasses.
❏ You should notice some improvement in your condition within 24 hours. If the condition worsens, call your doctor's office immediately at one of the following phone numbers:
Office: _____ Emergency after-hours: _____

## Instructions for Contact Lens Wearers
❏ OK to wear your contact lenses.
❏ Do not wear your contact lenses until _____

## Your Follow-up Visit

Date: _____          Dr.: _____

Time: _____          Phone: _____

# Diabetic Retinopathy

Diabetes is a condition that can interfere with the body's ability to use and store sugar. Diabetes can also, over time, weaken and cause changes in the small blood vessels that nourish the eye's light-sensitive retina at the back of the eye where images are focused. When this condition occurs, it is called diabetic retinopathy. These changes may include leaking of blood, development of brushlike branches of the vessels, and enlargement of certain portions of these vessels. Diabetic retinopathy can seriously affect vision and, if left untreated, cause blindness.

Because this disease can cause blindness, early diagnosis and treatment are essential. We recommend having your eyes examined at least annually if you are a diabetic or if you have a family history of diabetes.

To detect diabetic retinopathy, we look inside your eyes with an instrument called an ophthalmoscope, which lights and magnifies the retinal blood vessels in your eyes. The interior of your eyes may also be photographed to provide more information.

The beginning stages of diabetic retinopathy may cause blurriness in your central or peripheral (side) vision, or they may produce no visual symptoms at all. It mainly depends on where the blood vessel changes are taking place in your eye's retina. As diabetic retinopathy progresses you may notice a cloudiness in your vision, blind spots, or floaters, which are usually caused by blood leaking from abnormal new vessels that block light from reaching the retina.

In the advanced stages, connective scar tissue forms in association with new blood vessel growth, causing additional distortion and blurriness. Over time, this tissue can shrink and detach the retina by pulling it toward the center of the eye.

Once diabetic retinopathy has been diagnosed, laser and other surgical treatments can be used to reduce the progression of this disease and decrease the risk of vision loss.

If you have vision loss from diabetic retinopathy, we may prescribe special vision aids to help maximize your vision. Some of the optical aids available include telescopic lenses for distance vision, microscopic lenses, magnifying glasses, and electronic magnifiers for close work.

Not every diabetic patient develops retinopathy, but the chances of getting it increase after having diabetes for several years. Evidence also suggests that factors such as pregnancy, high blood pressure, and smoking may cause diabetic eye disease to develop or worsen.

As a diabetic or a person at risk for diabetes, you should take steps to help prevent the development of diabetic retinopathy, including the following:

- Take your prescribed medication as instructed.
- Follow a proper diet.
- Exercise regularly.
- Have your eyes examined regularly.

By following these recommendations, chances are good that you can enjoy a lifetime of good vision and health.

# Drugs That Cause Problems with the Eyes

If you are taking any of the following classes of drugs, you could eventually have problems with your eyes. Talk to your eye doctor about ways you can prevent losing vision when taking these medications. These medications can contribute to the development of cataracts, macular degeneration, and glaucoma or cause irritating symptoms.

Antihistamines
Antidepressants
Heart/blood pressure agents
Oral contraceptives
Antibiotics
Antifungals
Antimalarials
Tranquilizers
Sulfa drugs
Isotretinoin

Corticosteroids
Oral diabetic agents
Nonsteroidal antiinflammatories
Allopurinol
Statins
Cancer drugs
Erectile dysfunction agents
Tetracycline
Amphetamines
Antipsychotic agents

Some of these drugs can cause tissue damage.

Tissue damage occurs when high-energy light rays are absorbed by the body, which change its structure. In the most extreme cases, DNA is altered and cancerous tissue grows. The most common change in eye tissue is cataract, which occurs from the lens inside the eye absorbing the sun's rays. Some of the drugs mentioned above cause the pupils of the eyes to dilate, resulting in more than the normal amount of light to entering the eye and causing damage.

In individuals taking these medications, 100% ultraviolet-absorbing eyeglasses are necessary to protect the eyes both indoors and outdoors. The need for protection during or after a variety of medications is crucial to maintaining good vision. Visible light also has energy and can cause damage, so dark sun lenses will be necessary to protect the vision. Sun lenses that are polarized will reduce uncomfortable glare when driving or from reflections off water. Lenses that change in the sunlight will also provide protection except when the windshield of a car prevents them from darkening. The effects of cataracts and macular degeneration are increased by the need for time for the lenses to change to different light conditions. Nonglare technology can be used on the backs of the lenses to prevent reflections going directly into the eyes.

## Consult Your Eye Doctor

When taking medications, consult your eye doctor about the best way to protect your eyes. Your eye doctor is dedicated to providing good vision for the rest of your life.

# Drusens

Drusens are seen through the transparent retina as little yellow spots. They are essentially waste products of retinal metabolism that are present because certain structures surrounding the retina have developed a reduced capacity to process metabolic debris. This seems to be, for the most part, a normal process of growing older.

Drusens generally develop in later years; however, exceptions exist. Drusens may or may not be related to a vision problem. However, they bear close watching because they can be related to some vision loss.

The visual effect, if any, can be appreciated and demonstrated on the Amsler grid.

The first indication that drusens may present a problem is when you note a distortion in the grid pattern. The grid should appear perfect, with all the lines straight and parallel. If you note any distortion, voids, or wavy lines, notify us immediately.

Remember, for the most part drusens are a normal change of growing older and probably will not develop into a problem. However, caution dictates that one should not leave such matters to chance.

## Using the Amsler Grid

1. If reading glasses are customarily worn, wear them.
2. Test one eye at a time while closing the other.
3. Look (concentrate) at the central dot and note the surrounding grid pattern. If the pattern is perfect, you have completed the test. If it is not perfect, mark the area of imperfection and notify us.

This daily test only takes a few seconds to administer.

# Dry Eye

The natural tears that your eyes produce are composed of three layers: the outer oily layer, the middle watery layer, and the inner mucous layer.

Dry eye is the term used to describe eyes that do not produce enough tears or that produce tears without the proper chemical composition in any of these layers. Dry eye is most often a result of the eyes' natural aging process. Most people's eyes tend to become drier as they age, but the degree of dryness varies, with some people having more problems than others. In addition to age, dry eye can result from the following:

- Problems with normal blinking
- Certain medications such as antihistamines, oral contraceptives, and antidepressants
- Environmental factors such as a dry climate and exposure to wind
- General health problems such as arthritis or Sjögren's disease
- Chemical or thermal burns to the eye

Dry eye symptoms are often different in different people, but the following are commonly experienced by those whose tear production is inadequate:

- Irritated, scratchy, dry, or uncomfortable eyes
- Redness of the eyes
- A burning sensation of the eyes
- A feeling of a foreign body in the eye
- Blurred vision
- Excessive watering as the eyes try to comfort an overly dry eye
- Eyes that seem to have lost the normal clear, glassy luster

If untreated, dry eye can be more than just irritating or uncomfortable. Excessive dry eye can damage eye tissue and possibly scar the cornea, the transparent front covering of the eye, impairing vision. Contact lens wear may be more difficult because of the possibility of increased irritation and a greater chance of eye infection.

If you have the symptoms of dry eye, your optometrist can perform dry eye tests with diagnostic instruments to give a highly magnified view and special dyes to evaluate the quality, amount, and distribution of tears. Your optometrist will also need to know about your everyday activities, general health, medications you are taking, and environmental factors that may be causing your symptoms.

In most cases dry eye cannot be cured, but your eyes' sensitivity can be lessened and treatment prescribed so that your eyes remain healthy and your vision is not affected. Possible treatments include the following:

- Frequent blinking to spread tears over the eye, especially when using a steady focus for an extended period
- Changing environmental factors, such as avoiding wind and dust and increasing the level of humidity
- Using artificial tear solutions
- Using moisturizing ointment, especially at bedtime
- Administering cyclosporine immunomodulator drops

Other forms of treatment include the following:

- Insertion of small plugs in the corners of the eyes to slow drainage and loss of tears
- In rare cases, surgery

Whatever treatment is prescribed, you must follow your doctor of optometry's instructions carefully. Dry eye does not go away, but by working together, you and your doctor can keep your eyes healthy and protect your vision.

## Treatment

The doctor has prescribed the following treatment for you.

**Artificial Tears**

_____

_____

**Dosage and Frequency**

_____

_____

## Special Instructions

After applying the drops, close your eye and, with one finger, apply mild pressure to the inner corner of the eye. Keep pressure on this area for 90 seconds. This will help the drop stay within the eye.

## Additional Treatment

The doctor is considering the following additional treatments, depending on the results of the artificial tears.

❑ Medication     ❑ Nutritional supplements     ❑ Punctal occlusion

## Your Follow-up Visit

Date: _____     Dr.: _____

Time: _____     Phone: _____

# Eight Reasons Why You Should Purchase Your Eyewear from Us

### 1. Fast Service
We have our own optical laboratory and full-time opticians so that your eyeglasses can be made fast. Most prescriptions are ready in 2 days, and many can be ready the same day.

### 2. 1-Year Warranty
All eyeglasses carry a 1-year guarantee against breakage at no additional charge. If your eyeglasses break for any reason, return the broken parts and they will be repaired or replaced free.

### 3. 15-Day Exchange Privilege
After getting your new eyeglasses, if you decide you do not like the frames, you can exchange them for other frames. If new lenses are required, a small laboratory regrinding fee will be charged. The regrinding fee varies with the type of lens used; check with the receptionist.

### 4. Huge Selection of Frame Styles
Our dispensary has more than 3,000 frames in stock, several times that of the average office. Our frame stylists will help you find the perfect size, shape, and color in your price range.

### 5. Competitive Price Guarantee
If you find the same frames priced less within 90 days of your purchase, bring in written confirmation and we will gladly refund the difference.

### 6. All Plastic Lenses Have Scratch-Resistant Coating at No Extra Charge
This factory-applied coating makes plastic lenses tough. They are guaranteed for 1 year not to scratch, or the lenses will be replaced free (only one replacement pair per year).

### 7. We Stand Behind Our Prescription
Our doctors are available to review your prescription needs at no charge if you have any difficulties. We want you to love your eyewear!

### 8. Emergency Repairs and Free Adjustments
Our office is open 6 days a week to best serve our loyal patients. Bring your eyewear in for repairs and free adjustments and cleaning to keep your frames looking good and feeling comfortable.

# Epiretinal Membrane

Macular pucker, or epiretinal membrane (ERM), is a common disorder of the central retina that leads to symptoms of distortion and central blur. An ERM is excessive scar tissue on the surface of the retina. Most eyes with ERM are without symptoms.

## How an Epiretinal Membrane Develops

The vitreous shrinks as we get older and finally separates from the retina. As it peels away from the retina, it roughs up the surface of the macula. In response, the retina sends out reparative cells to smooth over its surface, like a scab forming over a scraped knee. However, the scar tissue may develop into a permanent structure that does not peel away. If it affects the central retina, it will affect central vision. Most eyes do not require surgery. If vision is poor enough, vitrectomy with membrane peeling may improve vision in 75% to 90% of patients. Surgery can be performed when vision is 20/50 to 20/70 or worse.

The ERM may appear transparent or as a dense, white plaque. It may wrinkle the retina or induce swelling of the macula or central retina. Fluorescein angiography may be performed to assess the possible causes of the membrane and determine specific characteristics. If left untreated, an ERM does not cause blindness. However, once central vision is significantly affected, it rarely spontaneously improves. Fine reading vision may worsen.

If the ERM is the result of previous retinal detachment, central vision may be limited by prior macular detachment. Macular degeneration, cataract, or a preexisting ocular pathologic condition may also limit final visual acuity after surgery.

## Vitrectomy for Epiretinal Membrane

Vitrectomy is the surgical removal of the gel in the eye, or vitreous. A bent needle or pick is used to elevate an edge of the ERM, and microforceps then peel the scar tissue away from the retina. The gel is replaced with clear sterile saline. This is an outpatient procedure that usually takes 35 to 60 minutes. Surgery is most often performed under local anesthesia but can be done under general anesthesia as well. You may go home the same day as surgery.

After vitrectomy, you may feel the self-absorbing sutures for approximately 4 weeks. Eyeglasses may be prescribed approximately 3 months after surgery to obtain the best acuity. Vitrectomy with membrane peeling can lead to visual improvement in 75% to 90% of eyes with enough distortion and blur to warrant surgery. The average postoperative acuity is halfway between preoperative vision and 20/20. Vision improves in approximately 3 months but may continue improving for a year after surgery.

Postoperative vision may not be perfect, but 90% of eyes that undergo this surgery have a decrease in distortion. Eyes that have had a prior retinal detachment in the macula are less likely to have return of fine vision.

## Complications of Vitreous Surgery

Any time surgery is performed, rare complications may occur. Risks of this surgery include bleeding, infection, retinal tear, and retinal detachment. All these events are quite rare and are listed not to scare you away from surgery, but to let you know that any time you have surgery complications are possible.

More commonly, cataract may advance at a faster pace after vitrectomy. Vision may improve 3 months after vitrectomy, then blur from cataract. This generally takes months to years and will respond to surgery.

# Eye Drops and Ointment

## Eye Drop Instillation

1. Wash your hands thoroughly.
2. Read the label and make sure that you are instilling the correct drops.
3. Shake well if directed to do so. Some medications are in suspension and need to be shaken to ensure the correct dosage.
4. Stand in front of a mirror, looking directly forward with the head tipped slightly back.
5. Gently pull the lower lid down with one hand while squeezing 1 to 2 drops from the bottle with the other hand. To avoid contamination, do not allow the dropper to touch the eye or face. Instilling the drops toward the outer corner of the eye is usually easier.
6. After instillation, close the eye gently for 2 minutes or press firmly on the inner corner of the upper and lower lids for 1 minute. Either technique will enhance the result.

## Ointment Application to Lid Margins

1. Wash your hands thoroughly.
2. Check the label to verify correct medication and instructions.
3. Apply ¼ to ½ inch of ointment on the tip of the index finger. With the eye closed, apply along the lid margins at the lash line. Cover both the upper and lower lids from inner to outer corner.
4. Alternate technique: squeeze ¼ to ½ inch of ointment onto a cotton-tipped applicator. While looking directly in the mirror, apply along the lid margins at the lash line of both the upper and lower lids.

## Ointment Application Inside Lower Lid

1. Wash your hands thoroughly.
2. Check the label to verify correct medication and instructions.
3. Look directly into a mirror and tilt head down slightly. Gently pull lower lid down and squeeze about ½ inch of ointment inside the lower lid. Twist tube to separate ointment from tube. Because of the risk of contamination, avoid touching the lid or the eye with the tube.
4. Alternate technique: squeeze ½ inch of ointment onto the index finger and transfer to the inside of the lower lid.

**Medications Prescribed**                                  **Frequency and Duration**

_____                  _____

_____                  _____

## Your Follow-up Visit

Date: _____            Dr.: _____

Time: _____            Phone: _____

# Eyelid Problems

The doctor has prescribed the following treatment for you.

## Warm Compresses

1. Wash your hands thoroughly.
2. Dampen a clean, folded, or rolled washcloth with warm water, or warm it in the microwave on medium for 20 seconds. Make sure the washcloth is warm and not hot.
3. Keeping the eyes closed and the washcloth folded/rolled, apply the washcloth to one or both eyelids. Application of some pressure to the upper lids is acceptable during this process.
4. Apply _____ time(s) a day.
5. Continue for     ❑ 2 weeks     ❑ 1 month     ❑ continuous     ❑ other _____

## Eyelid Scrubs

1. Wash your hands thoroughly.
2. ❑ Use commercially prepared eyelid cleanser pads in sealed packets.
   ❑ Mix a small amount of baby shampoo with warm water and saturate a make-up remover pad with the solution.
3. Close the eyelid and run the cleanser pad back and forth across the upper eyelashes and edge of the eyelid (approximately 15 times). Scrub lower lid by pulling it away from the eye. Avoid getting cleanser into the eye. Repeat for the other eye with a different pad.
4. Rinse excess solution with clear water.
5. Perform _____ time(s) a day.
6. Continue for ❑ 2 weeks ❑ 1 month ❑ continuous ❑ other _____

**Medications Prescribed**                                   **Frequency and Duration**

_____            _____

_____            _____

## Special Instructions

_____

_____

_____

## Your Follow-up Visit

Date: _____            Dr.: _____

Time: _____            Phone: _____

# Eyelid Problems: Treatment Sheet

The eyelids perform many important functions, including protecting and lubricating the eye, producing oil secretions, and helping drain away tears. The following conditions are usually not serious and can often be easily treated. However, if left untreated, they can be uncomfortable, unattractive, and lead to more serious problems. Eyelid problems can affect the upper or lower eyelid in one or both eyes. Your doctor has checked the box(es) that describe(s) your condition.

## ❏ Blepharitis

Blepharitis is a chronic or long-term inflammation of the eyelid margins (the edges of the eyelids) often caused by bacteria around the lashes and outer tissues of the eye.

Symptoms can include swelling of the lid margin, irritation, sensitivity to light, itching, burning, redness along the lid margin, and redness of the eyeball itself. A crust or roughness along the lid margin and possibly dandruff on the lashes are present. This can be worse in the morning upon awakening. Patients who wear contact lenses will often have these symptoms to a greater degree because the lenses will seem dry.

### Treatment

In most cases, good eyelid hygiene and daily cleaning of the eyelid margins will control blepharitis. Eyelid hygiene is particularly important when awakening because bacteria builds up during the night. In more severe cases, eyelid hygiene and medication may be combined for good control. In cases in which the conjunctiva (the front surface of the eye) is affected, the doctor may prescribe additional treatment.

## ❏ Chalazion

A chalazion results from a blockage of one or more of the small oil-producing glands found in the upper and lower eyelids. Symptoms are inflammation and swelling in the form of a round lump within the eyelid that may or may not be painful. If the chalazion becomes infected, the eyelid can become swollen, inflamed, and more painful.

### Treatment

A chalazion may be treated by applying warm compresses. At times this condition may require additional treatments that your doctor will prescribe.

## ❏ Stye

A stye is a bacterial infection of one of the eyelid glands near the lid margins at the base of the lashes. It forms a red, sore lump similar to a boil, causing pain and inflammation.

### Treatment

Styes are usually treated with warm compresses. Antibiotic and/or steroid eye drops or ointments may also be needed.

# Eyelid Massage

During your examination today, the doctor found excess oil in the oil-secreting glands of your eyelids. Too much oil disrupts the normal function of the tear film, and excess oil can become hardened and back up in the glands, causing additional dry eye problems as well as possible chronically plugged, enlarged glands (chalazion). Massage of the eyelids helps restore a normal flow of oil and will help prevent backing up of the glands.

1. Use a clean washcloth folded in half.
2. Use warm, not hot, water. Allow the tap to run for 2 minutes. Do not use still-standing water, which may have sediment from the pipes. You do not need to use distilled or purified drinking water.
3. Soak the folded edge of the washcloth in the warm water and wring out the excess. Then close your eyes and lay the washcloth on your eyelids for approximately 30 seconds. Then resoak the cloth to maintain the warmth. Do this soaking for approximately 2 minutes.
4. After soaking with the cloth, massage the upper eyelids with the edge of the cloth while your eyes are closed. When doing the lower eyelids, look up slightly before beginning the massage. When massaging, go from side to side with the cloth, with each back and forth motion counting as one time. Massage both lower and upper eyelids approximately 20 times each. Avoid the center part of your eye or any other part while your eyes are open.
5. Massage your eyelids twice a day or as directed:

   _____

6. Use artificial tears as recommended:

   _____

Please contact us if you have any questions or problems.

## Your Follow-up Visit

Date: _____        Dr.: _____

Time: _____        Phone: _____

# Eyelid Scrubs

During your examination today, the doctor found crusts on your eyelashes that must be removed. If these crusts are not removed, the bacteria in the crusts can irritate your eyes. They may cause chronic infections (conjunctivitis, keratitis, blepharitis) or possibly partial loss of eyelashes or scarred eyelids.

1. Use cotton balls or a washcloth folded in half.
2. Make a solution of either:
   a. ½ teaspoon salt to 1 quart of water, *or*
   b. 1:4 mixture of baby shampoo to water
3. Use room temperature water. Allow the tap to run for 2 minutes. Do not use still-standing water, which may have sediment from the pipes. You do not need to use distilled or purified drinking water.
4. Use one cotton ball per eye, soaking the ball in the solution and squeezing out the excess, or soak the folded edge of the washcloth in the solution.
5. Gently scrub the upper eyelids and eyelashes with your eyes closed. When scrubbing the lower lids and lashes, look up slightly before scrubbing. When scrubbing, go from side to side with either the cotton ball or washcloth, with each back and forth counting as one time. Scrub both upper and lower eyelids approximately 20 times each. Avoid scrubbing the center part of your eye or any other part while your eyes are open. Either solution may sting somewhat if it gets into your eyes.
6. Throw away the cotton ball when you are done with one eye and use a new cotton ball for the other eye. If you need to use a second ball on the same eye, use a fresh one. Do not resoak a previously used ball in the same solution, or rinse out the washcloth and resoak when scrubbing the other lids.
7. When you have finished one scrubbing session, throw the solution away and do not save it. Make a fresh solution every time you scrub your lashes and lids.
8. Scrub your eyelids twice a day or as directed _____.

   Please contact us if you have any questions or problems.

## Your Follow-up Visit

Date: _____        Dr.: _____

Time: _____        Phone: _____

# Floaters and Flashes

## Floaters

The small specks, "bugs," or clouds that you may sometimes see moving in your field of vision are called floaters. They are frequently visible when looking at a plain background, such as a blank wall or blue sky. These visual phenomena have been described for centuries; the ancient Romans called them *muscae volitantes*, or "flying flies," because they can appear like small flies moving around in the air. Floaters are actually tiny clumps of gel or cellular debris within the vitreous, the clear, jellylike fluid that fills the inside cavity of the eye. Although these objects appear to be in front of the eye, they are actually floating in the fluid inside the eye and cast their shadows on the retina (the light-sensing inner layer of the eye). Moving your eyes back and forth and up and down creates currents within the vitreous capable of moving the floater outside your direct line of vision.

## Causes

The vitreous gel degenerates in middle age, often forming microscopic clumps or strands within the eye. Vitreous shrinkage or condensation is called posterior vitreous detachment* and is a common cause of floaters. It also occurs frequently in nearsighted people or in those who have undergone cataract operations or YAG laser surgery. Occasionally, floaters result from inflammation within the eye or from crystal-like deposits that form in the vitreous gel. The appearance of floaters, whether in the form of little dots, circles, lines, clouds, or cobwebs, may be alarming, especially if they develop suddenly. However, they are usually nothing to be concerned about and simply result from the normal aging process.

## Are Floaters Serious?

The vitreous covers the retinal surface. Occasionally the retina is torn when degenerating vitreous gel pulls away. This causes a small amount of bleeding in the eye, which may appear as a group of new floaters. A torn retina can be serious if it develops into a retinal detachment. Any sudden onset of many new floaters or flashes of light should be promptly evaluated by your eye doctor. Additional symptoms, especially loss of peripheral or side vision, require repeat ophthalmic examination.

## Flashing Lights

When the vitreous gel, which fills the inside of the eye, rubs or pulls on the retina, it sometimes produces the illusion of flashing lights or lightning streaks. You may have experienced this; it is usually not cause for worry. On rare occasions, however, light flashes accompany a large number of new floaters and even a partial loss or shadowing of side vision. When this happens, prompt examination by an eye doctor is important to determine if a torn retina or retinal detachment has occurred.

Flashes of light that appear as jagged lines or "heat waves," often lasting 10 to 20 minutes and present in both eyes, are likely to be migraine caused by a spasm of blood vessels in the brain. If a headache follows, it is called a migraine headache. However, these jagged lines or "heat waves" commonly occur without a subsequent headache. In this case, the light flashes are referred to as ophthalmic migraine, or migraine without headache.

---

*Complete separation of the vitreous takes approximately 6 to 8 weeks and represents the period of greatest risk. Therefore the health of your retinas should be checked again in 8 weeks. In the meantime check your field of vision every day and report immediately if you note any reduction in your peripheral (side) vision, poorer straight-ahead vision, or an increase in flashes or floaters.

# Glaucoma

Glaucoma is an eye disease in which the passages that allow fluid in the eye to drain become clogged or blocked. This results in the amount of fluid in the eye building up and causing increased pressure inside the eye. This increased pressure damages the optic nerve, which connects the eye to the brain. The optic nerve is the main carrier of vision information to the brain. Damage to it results in less information sent to the brain and a loss of vision.

The exact cause of glaucoma is not known and it cannot currently be prevented. It is one of the leading causes of blindness in the United States. But, if detected at an early stage and treated promptly, glaucoma can usually be controlled with little or no further vision loss. Regular optometric examinations are therefore important. People of all ages can develop glaucoma, but it most frequently occurs in the following populations:

- Those older than 40 years
- Those with a family history of glaucoma
- Those who are very nearsighted
- Diabetics
- Blacks

Of the different types of glaucoma, primary open-angle glaucoma often develops gradually and painlessly without warning signs or symptoms. This type of glaucoma is more common among blacks than whites. It can cause damage and lead to blindness more quickly in blacks, making regular eye examinations, including tests for glaucoma, particularly important for blacks older than 35 years. Another type, acute-angle closure glaucoma, may be accompanied by the following symptoms:

- Blurred vision
- A loss of side vision
- Appearance of colored rings around lights
- Pain or redness in the eyes

Regular eye examinations are an important means of detecting glaucoma in its early stages and include the following:

- Tonometry: a simple and painless measurement of the pressure in the eye
- Ophthalmoscopy: an examination of the back of the eye to observe the health of the optic nerve
- Visual field test: a check for the development of abnormal blind spots

Glaucoma can usually be treated effectively by eye drops or other medicines. In some cases surgery may be necessary. Unfortunately, any loss of vision from glaucoma usually cannot be restored. But, early detection, prompt treatment, and regular monitoring can enable you to continue living in much the same way as you have always lived.

Protect your eye health and your vision; be sure to visit your doctor of optometry regularly.

# Headaches, The Eyes, and Vision

Headaches are a common symptom associated with the eyes and vision. They can be related to allergies, muscle strain, strained vision, glare, migraines, and eye disease.

## Allergies

The eyes are surrounded by several sinus cavities, which may become congested from colds or allergies. The tissue that lines the eyes is the same as that lining the sinuses. Your doctor will be able to recognize the signs of allergies in your eyes. People with headaches caused by allergies often wake up with them. Nearly 50% of the general population has allergies.

## Muscle Strain

The eyes are controlled by six muscles on the outside and additional muscles inside. The outside muscles control eye movements and coordination. Difficulty using the eyes together often causes headaches, particularly during near tasks such as computer work. The muscles inside the eyes are used for focusing. A computer user changes focus an estimated 10,000 times during a 6-hour day. Our eyes were not made for this. Problems focusing commonly result in headaches and blurred vision.

## Strained Vision

Many individuals can see well enough to get by but may notice a slight blur, or image overlapping the clear image. Even small amounts of astigmatism can result in strained vision, making discrimination between the numbers 8, 3, and 5 difficult. Other times a person may simply be trying to read print that is too small or of poor contrast. Trying to decipher poor handwriting can result in headaches. The clearer the image, the more comfortable your vision will be.

## Glare

Four types of glare make seeing comfortably difficult. Uncomfortable glare is caused by everyday bright light—outdoors even on cloudy days, indoors with overhead fluorescent lights. Disabling glare is caused by excessive light, as from a window on a bright day. Blinding glare comes from shiny surfaces such as computer screens, glass, metal, water, snow, or concrete. Distracting glare comes from reflections from eyeglass lenses without nonglare technology. Each of these can cause squinting, eye strain, and headaches.

## Migraines

Severe headaches are often thought to be migraine headaches by the general public. True migraine headaches are actually caused by the dilation of blood vessels in the brain. Usually the blood vessels constrict first, causing the vision part of the brain to get less oxygen and resulting in a strange vision phenomena. After approximately 20 to 30 minutes, the brain calls for more oxygen, dilating the blood vessels and causing the headache. Migraine headaches run in families.

## Eye Disease

Many eye diseases may cause headache and discomfort. One type of glaucoma, conjunctivitis, iritis, and other inflammations of the eye can result in headaches. They are often associated with symptoms such as blurred vision, haloes around lights, and extreme sensitivity to light.

Your eye doctor will use several examination techniques to rule out vision and the eyes as a cause of your headaches. Treatment may include lenses, eye drops, oral medications, nonglare technology, eye exercises, or changes in the environment.

# Iritis

Iritis is inflammation predominantly located in the iris, which is the colored part of the eye. The iris controls the size of the pupil, the opening that allows light into the back of the eye. It is located behind the cornea and just in front of the focusing lens of the eye.

## Symptoms
- Pain
- Light sensitivity
- Red eye
- Tearing
- Blurred vision
- Floaters
- Small pupil

Iritis is often associated with an infection or disease of another part of the body, including ankylosing spondylitis, reactive arthritis (Reiter's syndrome), psoriatic arthritis, irritable bowel disease, Crohn's disease, multiple sclerosis (HLA B15), sarcoidosis, systemic lupus erythematosus, Lyme disease, juvenile idiopathic arthritis, "cat scratch" disease, toxoplasmosis, toxocariasis, presumed ocular histoplasmosis syndrome, Whipple's disease, valley fever, tuberculosis, leptospirosis, Rocky Mountain spotted fever, and others. Patients known to have these disorders should be examined for chronic mild iritis on a regular basis.

## Diagnosis
Iritis is diagnosed during an eye exam with a biomicroscope. Because iritis is associated with other diseases, blood tests, skin tests, and x-rays may be used to determine the cause of the inflammation.

When the iris is inflamed, white blood cells are shed into the anterior chamber of the eye where they can be observed on biomicroscopic examination to be floating in the convection currents of the aqueous humor. These cells can be counted and form the basis for rating the degree of inflammation. This is measured on a scale of 1 to 4, with 4 being the most cells.

## Treatment
Initial treatment is through the use of topical corticosteroids. If adhesion is anticipated, then a dilating drop is used to relax the ciliary body to prevent the iris from adhering to the lens in a closed position. Iritis that is stubborn, recurrent, or chronic may require systemic treatment through the use of oral steroids or other immunomodulating drugs.

Some of the consequences to the lack of treatment or under treatment are epiretinal membrane formation, cystoid macular edema, cataracts, glaucoma, detached retina, vitreous hemorrhage, and vascularization of the retina. Uveitis is the third leading cause of preventable blindness in the developed world.

# Jump Ductions

## Purpose

The purpose of this exercise is to improve your ability to change the focus of your eyes (accommodation) smoothly and quickly over a wide range of distances. This exercise will also help you improve your convergence.

## Equipment

Postage stamp with fine detail, a window, and a clock with a second hand.

## Set-up

Place the postage stamp on a clear window. Pick out a distant target with fine detail that you can see clearly. A street sign or license plate will make a good target.

## Procedure 1

Stand as close as you can to the stamp, keeping all its detail clear and single. Jump your gaze (fixation) from the stamp to the distant target and get it clear and single. Quickly return your fixation back to the stamp and once again concentrate on getting it clear and single. *Do not change your fixation until the target you are looking at is perfectly clear and single.*

Note the time that it takes you to make 20 cycles from distance to near (40 fixation jumps). Do _____ sets of 20 cycles with a short rest period between each. Record your best daily effort and the distance you stood from the stamp.

Your goal is to be able to change your focus from distance to near and back smoothly and quickly while standing as close as possible to the near target.

## Procedure 2

Repeat procedure 1 through a special pair of glasses or clip-on lenses that will be supplied by your clinician. Record your best daily effort and distance from the near target as before.

# Keratoconus

Keratoconus is a progressive thinning of the cornea that, if not treated appropriately, will result in considerable vision loss from the irregular corneal shape this condition may cause. Perforation of the cornea and scarring may occur. Spectacle lenses can only improve vision marginally and do not afford any therapeutic effect. In other words, the keratoconus will continue to progress.

The most universally recognized and accepted treatment modality for keratoconus is the prescription of rigid, gas-permeable contact lenses. In the foreseeable future soft contact lenses will be available for treating keratoconus by using wavefront technology to correct higher-order aberrations.

Rigid contact lenses tend to reshape the keratoconus to a more reasonable or normal shape, thus enabling the patient to achieve normal or near normal vision. Because the cornea is soft tissue, this effect is only achieved while wearing the contact lenses, which is why the lenses should be worn as prescribed.

Keratoconus represents one of the most difficult contact lens fitting challenges. It requires a great deal of patience and perseverance for both patient and doctor. Continued monitoring on a regular basis is essential because keratoconus requires a lifetime of support and care. It should not be taken lightly. You should be seen at least every 6 months to make changes when necessary to ensure the maintenance of corneal health. Properly fitted contact lenses tend to reduce the progression of the cone and afford a greater degree of comfort.

The majority of keratoconus patients can maintain their contact lens–corrected vision throughout life with acceptable levels of comfort.

The only other alternative is corneal transplantation, which, for obvious reasons, is reserved as a treatment of last resort.

# Keratoconus: Treatment Sheet

Keratoconus (KC) is a condition of the cornea, the "clear window" on the front surface of the eye. The cornea is normally round or spherical shape. With KC, the cornea bulges, distorts, and assumes more of a cone shape, causing distorted or blurred vision. KC can occur in one or both eyes.

In the early stages, eyeglasses are usually successful in correcting the vision. However, as the disease advances, vision is not adequately corrected and requires rigid contact lenses to aid in flattening the corneal surface and providing optimal visual correction. Your doctor is a specialist at designing a custom contact lens that fits the shape of the cornea.

Contact lens fitting can be difficult in patients with KC, requiring frequent follow-up visits to monitor the corneal health and make adjustments to the design of the contact lenses. The goal is to fit the lenses to maximize comfort, vision, and eye health. For the greatest success, patients will also be required to use eye drops and adhere to a wearing schedule prescribed by the doctor.

When good vision can no longer be attained with contact lenses or when intolerance to the contact lens develops, corneal transplantation may be recommended. This is only necessary in approximately 10% of patients with KC and carries a success rate of greater than 90%.

The doctor has prescribed the following treatment for you at this time.

❑ Cold compresses, applied daily.
❑ Lubrication drops to rewet the surface of your eyes.
❑ Topical medication (eye drops) to relieve the symptoms of itching.
❑ Therapeutic management of contact lenses to improve the quality of vision.
❑ Consultation with a corneal surgeon.

**Medications Prescribed**                     **Dosage and Frequency**

_____              _____

**Lubrication Drops Prescribed**               **Dosage and Frequency**

_____              _____

## Special Instructions

Do not rub your eyes because this may be one of the factors contributing to the worsening of the condition.

## Your Follow-up Visit

Date: _____       Dr.: _____

Time: _____       Phone: _____

# Lattice Degeneration

Lattice degeneration is a common peripheral retinal degeneration characterized by oval or linear patches of retinal thinning. Atrophic retinal holes and tractional retinal tears may complicate lattice degeneration and increase the risk of retinal detachment. Patients with lattice degeneration are typically asymptomatic, and the lesions are usually an incidental finding of dilated exam.

The acute onset of floaters, flashes of light, peripheral field loss, or central vision loss may indicate the presence of retinal tear or retinal detachment, which are complications of lattice lesions. Patients with lattice degeneration should be examined on an annual basis.

The eye works like a camera. The lens and cornea focus light rays. The retina works like the photographic film in a camera. The hollow center of the eye is filled with a gel called vitreous. When this shrinks, it may pull and tear the retina.

Lattice degeneration is characterized by oval or linear patches of atrophic retina with a reddish base and is usually located within the front portion of the retina. Fine vision is in the macula.

## Thinning of the Retina

Lesions may be isolated or multifocal, variable in dimension, and usually oriented concentric or slightly oblique to the front edge of the retina. Condensed vitreous at the margins of the lattice lesions appears as vitreous opacities and represents regions of increased vitreoretinal adhesion. The vitreous over lattice is liquid. Sclerosed vessels appear as crisscrossing, fine, white lines that account for the term lattice degeneration.

Lattice lesions appear to be caused by dropout of peripheral retinal capillaries, which leads to thinning of all retinal layers. The thinning may become so profound that a full-thickness retinal hole forms at the lattice lesion.

The best and most often used examination to detect lattice degeneration is indirect ophthalmoscopy with pushing on the eye or scleral depression to see it on edge.

## Who Has Lattice Degeneration?

Lattice degeneration affects approximately 10% of the population, with 30% to 50% of those affected having it in both eyes. The prevalence peaks by the second decade and is minimally progressive. It may be more common in some families. It is more common in nearsighted eyes and correlates with increasing axial length, reaching 15% prevalence in the eyes with the greatest axial length. No reported infectious, trauma, gender, or racial differences exist in lattice degeneration.

## Clinical Course of Lattice Degeneration

Lattice lesions are believed to develop early in one's lifetime. Features such as crisscrossing sclerotic vessels, pigmentation, and atrophic retinal holes subsequently may develop over many years.

Retinal detachment is a rare complication of lattice degeneration (less than 1% of patients with lattice). But lattice is associated with as many as 40% of all retinal tear–associated detachments.

An acute posterior vitreous detachment complicated by retinal tear formation usually is signaled by new-onset floaters and/or flashes. Patients with these symptoms constitute a true ocular emergency and need urgent ophthalmic examination.

## Laser Treatment for Lattice Degeneration

The presence of uncomplicated lattice does not interfere with visual function and does not constitute a high risk for future development of retinal detachment. Prophylactic treatment is clearly indicated only in the context of specific circumstances.

Lattice degeneration complicated by tractional tears as the result of an acute posterior vitreous detachment represents a high-risk situation for future retinal detachment and is an urgent indication for laser retinopexy. Lattice and atrophic holes complicated by progressively increasing subretinal fluid represent an additional indication for surgical intervention. The presence of lattice lesions in the other eye of patients who have sustained retinal detachment in the first eye may be treated prophylactically. Subsequent retinal detachments may also occur as a result of lesions developing in healthy retina, so the protection is not absolute. If a cataract, lens implant, or strong family history of retinal detachment is present, preventative laser treatment may lessen the chance of retinal detachment. In the absence of the aforementioned features, definitive data does not yet exist to clearly indicate prophylactic laser treatment of lattice lesions.

## Lattice Degeneration Prognosis

Patients with significant lattice lesions, and those who have had prophylactic treatments, are always at increased risk compared with the population at large for vision loss caused by retinal detachment. These patients must have routine follow-up examinations. Be aware of the signs and symptoms of retinal and vitreous detachment and the necessity to seek urgent care when needed.

# Macular Degeneration

Macular degeneration is the leading cause of central vision loss among older people. It results from changes to the macula, a portion of the retina responsible for clear, sharp vision that is located on the inside back wall of the eye.

The macula is many times more sensitive than the rest of the retina; without a healthy macula, seeing detail or vivid color is not possible.

Macular degeneration has several causes. In one type, the tissue of the macula becomes thin and stops working well. This type is thought to be a part of the natural aging process in some people.

In another, fluids from newly formed blood vessels leak into the eye and cause vision loss. If detected early, this condition can be treated with laser therapy, but early detection and prompt treatment are vital in limiting damage.

Macular degeneration develops differently in each person, so the symptoms may vary. Some of the most common symptoms include the following:

- A gradual loss of ability to see objects clearly
- Distorted vision; objects appear to be the wrong size or shape, or straight lines appear wavy or crooked
- A gradual loss of clear color vision
- A dark or empty area appearing in the center of vision

These symptoms may also indicate other eye health problems, so if you are experiencing any of these, contact your doctor of optometry immediately.

In a comprehensive eye examination, your doctor will perform a variety of tests to determine if you have macular degeneration or another condition causing your symptoms.

Unfortunately, central vision damaged by macular degeneration cannot be restored. However, because macular degeneration does not damage side vision, low vision aids such as telescopic and microscopic special lenses, magnifying glasses, and electronic magnifiers for close work can be prescribed to help make the most of remaining vision. With adaptation, people with macular degeneration can often cope well and continue to do most things they were accustomed to doing.

Remember: early detection of macular degeneration is the most important factor in determining if you can be treated effectively. Use an Amsler Grid as directed by your optometrist and maintain a regular schedule of optometric examinations to help protect your vision.

# Monovision

Monovision is a compromise approach to satisfy visual needs. It compromises, to some degree, both distance and near vision. However, it does enable one to get by reasonably well for both far and near without the use of eyeglasses. Monovision seems to work best for social occasions, for general all-around situations, and for those patients doing light office work.

One area of concern is driving a motor vehicle, especially at times of low levels of illumination. For example, if light from an oncoming headlight were to strike the distance viewing eye so that it was occluded or partially obstructed, it might compromise distance vision because oncoming vehicles would be mostly viewed through the near vision eye. This is why we recommend a pair of eyeglasses be worn with contact lenses, or after monovision refractive surgery, enabling you to have binocular distance vision while driving. The eyeglasses would be corrected so that the near eye would now be focused for distance. With both eyes now focused normally for distance, compromise is not necessary.

Another area of concern for those patients who have been doing well for the most part with monovision, but have taken on added visual demands for near work, is visual discomfort or stress. This situation can also be remedied by wearing eyeglasses that correct the distance viewing eye, thereby focusing both eyes for near vision.

# No Perfect Pair

Our goal as eye care professionals is to provide every patient with the perfect pair of glasses. Unfortunately, in today's world, when you look at the range of patients' needs, it quickly becomes clear that no single pair of glasses can be ideal everywhere, all the time.

Each individual patient needs to see well in many different situations. They need good vision in bright sun and while driving at night. They need to see while playing tennis, working at a computer, and doing needlepoint. Patients also want to look the best they can in these situations and countless others.

One way to look at these needs is to remember that we change clothes at least once each day, and each time we select a specific look or function. You wear one set of clothes to clean the house, another to go to work, and yet another to play tennis or socialize. You can think of your "eyewear wardrobe" as being like your clothes closet, complete with options for work, leisure, and social occasions.

Glasses are often required for the following:

- Protection from the sun's damaging rays
- Comfort on the computer
- Sports
- Hobbies
- Social functions
- Safe night driving
- Comfortable reading
- Safety at work or while using power tools

Each pair of glasses the doctor prescribes for you has a specific function. The glasses you wear for working on the computer are not appropriate for playing sports. The sunglasses you use for driving during the day should not be used for watching movies in a darkened theater. One frame may be an excellent shape for your face and will look good in the office, and another may be a sport frame perfect for jogging and tennis.

Today, the average person requires glasses to prevent damage to the eyes from the sun, glasses for seeing indoors and at night, and computer glasses. Many would ideally have additional pairs depending on their desired appearance and recreational needs.

## Consult Your Eye Doctor and Optician

Your eye doctor will determine what is best to improve the quality of your life, allow you to perform at the highest level at work and play, and prevent the loss of vision. Your optician will provide a full range of eyewear that will make you look good and feel good.

# Ocular Hypertension

Ocular hypertension is a condition in which the pressure of fluids within the eye is higher than average. When the pressure within the eye is elevated to an extent that interferes with the normal physiology of the optic nerve, resulting in optic nerve damage, it is referred to as "glaucoma."

Many people can tolerate higher than average eye pressure without any optic nerve compromise. However, caution dictates that one should not leave such matters to enhance and should monitor eye pressures considered higher than average on a regular basis. Several tests are important to ensure the health of the optic nerve regarding elevated pressure. To ensure the safety of your optic nerve tissue, we would like to see you again in _____ months to perform the following tests that have been checked.

❑ Visual field examination
❑ Dilated fundus examination
❑ Image of optic nerve (for comparative evaluation over time)
❑ Eye pressure test
   ❑ Morning
   ❑ Afternoon
❑ Retinal nerve fiber layer analysis
❑ Pachymetry
❑ Gonioscopy

# Orthokeratology

Orthokeratology (Ortho-K) is a nonsurgical approach to reduce myopia (nearsightedness). A series of rigid contact lenses are used to flatten the corneal curvature. Because two thirds of the total power of the eye can be explained by the corneal curvature, efforts have been made to alter the cornea to change the overall refractive status. Can corneal tissue be permanently altered by such nonsurgical means? The University of California School of Optometry at Berkeley and the University of California School of Medicine at San Diego both agreed, after substantial time and effort spent on the Ortho-K project, that no significant permanent improvement was noted regarding myopia reduction.

Myopia reduction was noted with the wearing of retainer lenses for a significant portion of time. However, with the permanent cessation of contact lens wear this effect was soon lost.

Many of our patients have had good success with Ortho-K, having qualified for employment that requires improvement in their uncorrected visual acuity or pursuing hobbies (e.g., mountain climbing requiring oxygen) or sports that make wearing eyeglasses or contact lenses impractical. Depending on your vision requirements and type of refractive error, your doctor of optometry can advise you regarding your chance of success with orthokeratology.

# Refractive Error

When considering all the variables that go into the total visual process it is, indeed, a miracle that we see as well as we do. The visual process is a highly complex one involving cerebral and perceptual aspects that are too involved to describe in one page.

The refractive power of the visual system is mostly attributed to the corneal curvature, with the transparent media and the eyeball length accounting for the remainder. If all these variables coincide nicely so that all light focuses sharply on the retina, one is said to have perfect vision for distance viewing, or *emmetropia*. This definition does not consider perceptual, integrative, or binocular vision aspects that, if not in harmony with the refractive state, can result in discomfort, perceptual problems, and reading difficulties.

If light focuses prematurely in front of the retina, the condition is referred to as *myopia*, or nearsightedness, because near objects are seen more clearly than distant objects. The majority of myopia cases develop before the age of 25 years.

If light passes through the media as if the retina were not there and hypothetically focuses behind the retina, the condition is referred to as *hyperopia*, or farsightedness, because vision is more adaptable for distance viewing. Farsighted people involuntarily and continually maintain a focusing effort to keep vision clear. A farsighted person will not necessarily have clear distance vision and blurred or fuzzy near vision because these factors can be altered by focusing ability as well as the degree or magnitude of the farsightedness.

Another refractive condition is referred to as *astigmatism*. In this condition, all the light does not focus on the retina. The portion that does not may focus in front of the retina or behind it. The degree of disparity or difference is related to the amount of the astigmatism, which is the result of the cornea not being perfectly spherical (like a marble) but shaped more like a spoon.

Approximately 20% of what causes blur in the typical eye is from higher-order aberrations. Until recently these could not be measured and corrected by eyeglasses or contact lenses. Even people who have no refractive error (emmetropes) can have many higher-order aberrations. The effect is usually poor night vision, particularly when driving. Correcting the aberration gives the individual "high-definition" vision similar to high-definition televisions.

Reduction in function is something that is most appreciated or recognized as we grow older. In youth one might be able to run a 4-minute mile, but when one reaches the age of 40 years, a 6- or 7-minute mile is about all that can be achieved. A similar process occurs in the visual process. We refer to this reduction in function or reduced ability to alter or adjust the visual system for clear near vision as *presbyopia*.

Near-point asthenopia is a condition that is not necessarily related to a specific refractive error but may be associated with any of them. These patients seem to have difficulty handling near work tasks, such as reading, and note a significant degree of stress. Because this condition is not related to presbyopia and is often managed or treated in a similar fashion, a different category is required. This problem is one in which the balance between focusing and turning of the eyes is not in perfect harmony. Appropriate reading lenses (as in presbyopia) generally restore the balance. However, on occasion the eyes may require visual training exercises to restore harmony.

# Reading Glasses Comparison

People have many different alternatives when choosing how they would like their prescriptions filled for reading and close work. Each of the choices has advantages and disadvantages. This sheet compares each option to allow you to make an informed decision to fill your personal needs.

## Reading Glasses Only

Reading glasses are focused just for the reading distance or close distance (from 6 to 20 inches). When using these glasses for reading, doing close work, crafts, hobbies, or your job, things will be clear. The disadvantage of this type of glasses is that any time you have to look at a distance farther than 20 inches and see clearly, you must take your glasses off. You have the inconvenience of putting them on and taking them off. You also need to consider a strong frame because they will get much more abuse than if they were left on continuously.

## Half Eyes

This type of glasses has the same prescription as the reading glasses except they are only half the vertical height of normal glasses. This enables you to do your close work yet look over the top of them to see at a greater distance. One of the disadvantages of this system is again that you need a durable frame because your glasses are taken on and off so often.

## Bifocals

This is a system in which you have two focuses: far and near. This enables you to read and do close work; then when you look far away, you can see clearly without taking your glasses off. The biggest advantage of bifocal lenses is the convenience of not having to take glasses on and off constantly.

## Trifocals

This lens system has three focuses: far, for viewing something like a clock on a far wall; reading, for objects 6 to 12 inches away; and the intermediate or in-between range, such as soup cans on a shelf or the dashboard of your car.

## Invisible Progressive Multifocals

This lens system is the next extension beyond the trifocal. It has the advantage of not having any lines and has a continuous range of clear vision from far to intermediate to near. We have printed information and videos on multifocals in the office that discuss some of the advantages and disadvantages. Also, we have some samples of each type lens for you to see. Please take your time and decide what system works best for you.

## Bifocal Contact Lenses

This alternative has merit for individuals who perform minimal close work, such as homemakers or sales clerks, in which the person is not spending several hours at a time reading or studying, for example.

## Monovision

This system works with one eye focused for distance and the other eye focused for near. This can be done with any type of contact lens or refractive surgery.

# Reading and Writing

Everyone must visualize what is meant by the words we read and write. Sometimes people with learning-related vision problems can see the words, but they cannot understand what they mean. If you had that problem, would you find reading and writing easy?

Reading and writing are the two most common tasks people perform in school or at a desk job. Every time we read from a book, a sheet of paper, or a computer monitor, we are performing a visual task.

## How We Read

While we read, we need to aim two eyes at the same point simultaneously and accurately as well as the following:

- Focus both eyes to make the reading material clear
- Continue or sustain clear focus
- Move two eyes continually (as a coordinated team) across the line of print

When we move our eyes to the next line of print, we continue with the entire procedure.

## Reading Comprehension

To gain comprehension throughout the reading process, we are constantly taking in the visual information and decoding it from the written word into a mental image. Memory and visualization are also constantly used to relate the information to what is already known and help make sense of what is being read.

## How We Write

Writing is similar but almost works in the reverse order to reading. We start with an image in our minds and code it into words. At the same time, we control the movement of the pencil while continually working to keep the written material making sense. Throughout all this, we focus our eyes and move them together just as in the reading process.

Complicated visual procedures are involved in both reading and writing. A problem with any or all of the visual parts of the processes described will present difficulties in some way with reading and/or writing.

Sometimes a visual difficulty that affects reading and writing is easy to recognize; other times it can be quite subtle to detect. Optometrists are able to evaluate all parts of the visual process and, if necessary, prescribe lenses and vision therapy to improve reading and writing skills.

# Retinal Detachment

Retinal detachment occurs when the two layers of the retina become separated from each other and from the wall of the eye. The retina is like the film in a camera. Nerve cells in the retina detect light entering the eye and convert it into nerve signals to the brain.

Once the two layers of the retina, the sensory retina and the retinal pigment epithelium, lose contact with each other, the retina stops working properly because the eye cannot process what it sees. This causes vision loss in the affected area of the retina. Detachment always results in some vision loss, including severe loss or blindness.

## Symptoms

Retinal detachment may occur without warning. Symptoms include floaters in your field of vision and flashes of light or sparks when you move your eyes or head. Floaters and flashes do not always indicate retinal detachment, but they may be a warning sign and should be evaluated. If a flashing light occurs and does not go away within minutes, you should be examined immediately. The first sign of detachment may be a shadow or curtain effect across part of your visual field that does not go away, or new and sudden vision loss that gets worse over time.

Retinal detachment affects peripheral (side) vision first. Vision loss tends to get worse over time as more of the retina becomes detached, sometimes within a few hours or days. Once the detachment spreads to the center of the retina, vision loss becomes severe or even total. Surgery is needed to repair the detached retina to prevent permanent vision loss.

## Diagnosis

Retinal detachment is diagnosed by medical history and an examination of the eyes. If you have symptoms of retinal detachment, your doctor will examine your retina by using ophthalmoscopy. Ophthalmoscopy is a test that allows a doctor to see inside the back of the eye with a magnifying instrument with a light source. This test enables the doctor to see tears, holes, or detachment of the retina. Pictures may be taken to document the appearance of the retina.

## Treatment

Retinal detachment almost always demands urgent care. Without treatment, vision loss from retinal detachment can progress from minor to severe or total within a few hours or days. If discovered within 24 to 48 hours, comparatively simple laser surgery may restore good vision. If allowed to progress, the surgical techniques become much more difficult and the recuperation time longer, with a greater chance for permanent loss of vision.

# Retinitis Pigmentosa

Retinitis pigmentosa (RP) is one of a group of diseases that affect the retina of the eye. Approximately 400,000 Americans are affected by RP and other RP-like inherited forms of retinal degeneration.

Some of the most common symptoms of RP include night blindness and loss of peripheral (side) vision.

Symptoms of RP often appear for the first time during childhood or adolescence. Stumbling over objects that seem to be in plain sight and clumsiness may be the first indications of a problem. The symptoms of RP generally worsen over a period of years. Although some patients with RP and advancing age may become blind, most will retain at least some vision and are classified as legally blind. Each individual case differs.

RP develops inside the pigmented layer of the retina. The retina is a delicate layer of cells that acts like the film in a camera. It picks up a picture and transmits it to the brain, where "seeing" actually occurs. Two types of cells in the retina that participate in sending visual messages to the brain are the rods and cones. The rod-shaped cells are mostly used to help you see "out of the corners of your eyes" (peripheral vision) and at night. The cone-shaped cells enable you to distinguish colors, see during the day, and help you see with your central vision.

When RP begins, the rod-shaped cells begin to lose their ability to function. As a result, people with this condition frequently have trouble seeing at night or in areas of dim light. Poor or decreased night vision alone is not necessarily an indicator of RP, however.

"Tunnel vision" is also a symptom of RP. The field of vision gradually narrows, giving the effect of constantly looking through a tunnel.

As RP progresses to an advanced stage, you may also have difficulty reading, distinguishing colors, and seeing distant objects clearly. This is caused by the deterioration of the cone-shaped cells.

Your optometrist may be able to help you in maximizing your remaining vision by prescribing special low vision aids. Some of the optical aids available include telescopic lenses for distance vision, microscopic lenses, magnifying glasses, electronic magnifiers, night vision scopes, special filters, and field enhancers.

Unfortunately, although extensive research is being conducted, no treatment is available at this time to reverse the course of RP. However, early counseling by your optometrist can help you successfully adjust your lifestyle and career goals to this visual impairment. Potential problems can also be identified and forestalled by determining appropriate aids, training, and other job modifications in your chosen career field. When RP is diagnosed early, you can often take full advantage of educational and career guidance.

# Strabismus and Amblyopia

Strabismus is the condition in which a person is unable to align both eyes simultaneously under normal visual conditions (sometimes appearing as being "cross eyed"). The fovea of each eye is used for distinct vision. When they do not point at an object at the same time, one eye "turns" in relation to the other. This turning may be in, out, up, down, or in any combination of directions. This turning also may be constant, in which an eye turns all the time, or it may be intermittent. It may also alternate so that either eye turns. Besides the obvious turning of an eye, the individual has reduced binocular function and stereopsis (depth perception) and may develop reduced vision in one eye (amblyopia).

Strabismus has many different causes. The specific treatment depends on the specific type and cause. Strabismus can be treated at any age. Some factors favor younger patients, and compliance and motivation are more favorable with adults. Treatment typically consists of prescription lenses and prisms and a program of vision therapy. In certain patients surgery may be recommended in conjunction with vision therapy. Surgery may cosmetically straighten the eyes but does not typically improve visual function. The prognosis for optimal outcome in these cases is enhanced through presurgical and postsurgical vision therapy. Whether constant or intermittent, strabismus always requires treatment. It rarely goes away by itself, and children do not outgrow it.

Amblyopia, more commonly known as "lazy eye," is a condition manifested by reduced vision not correctable by glasses or contact lenses. It is not attributable to any apparent structural or pathologic condition. It may be related to strabismus because a turned eye generally loses vision to some extent from disuse. Many patients with amblyopia may be unaware of the condition until they undergo a vision screening or a comprehensive vision examination. Amblyopia has many causes, and the treatment depends on the cause. In general, the treatment consists of the use of lenses and prisms in conjunction with a vision therapy program. Patching of the nonamblyopic eye is of limited value unless it is part of an active vision therapy program.

For many years amblyopia was thought only to be amenable to treatment during the critical period, up to age 7 or 8 years. Current research has conclusively demonstrated that effective treatment can take place at any age, but the length of the treatment period increases dramatically the longer the condition has existed before treatment. Research has demonstrated that patients with amblyopia are more likely to sustain injuries resulting in the loss of their good eye than individuals with two good eyes. Early childhood examinations are therefore essential.

# Strabismus

## (Handout to accompany school nurse and other professionals)

### Definition

Strabismus is a sensory and neuromuscular anomaly of binocular integration resulting in the failure to maintain bifoveal alignment manifesting in a divergent (exotropia) or convergent (esotropia) deviation of the nonfixating eye.

### Symptoms

The symptoms and signs associated with strabismus include the following:

1. Occasional or constant eye turn
2. Diplopia
3. Poor depth perception
4. Head tilt/turn
5. Closing or covering one eye

### Diagnostic Factors

Strabismus is characterized by one or more of the following diagnostic findings:

1. Manifest angle of eye deviation
2. Deficient vergence abilities, reduced ranges of fusion with poor depth perception/stereopsis
3. Diplopia
4. Sensory adaptations (e.g., suppression, amblyopia, abnormal retinal correspondence)

NOTE: Additional testing may be appropriate as part of the differential diagnostic workup for strabismus to rule out other concurrent medical conditions and differentiate associated visual conditions.

### Therapeutic Considerations

#### A. Management

The doctor of optometry determines appropriate diagnostic and therapeutic modalities and frequency of evaluation and follow-up on the basis of the urgency and nature of the patient's condition and unique needs. The management of the case and duration of treatment would be affected by the following factors:

1. The severity of symptoms and diagnostic factors, including onset and duration of the problem
2. Implications of patient's general health and associated visual conditions
3. Extent of visual demands placed on the individual
4. Patient compliance
5. Prior interventions

#### B. Treatment

A small percentage of cases are successfully managed by prescription of therapeutic lenses or prisms. However, most patients with strabismus require orthoptics and/or vision therapy. Optometric vision therapy usually incorporates the prescription of specific treatments to achieve the following:

1. Normalize ocular motor control
2. Normalize spatial localization skills
3. Normalize accommodative abilities
4. Eliminate sensory adaptations
5. Establish fusion response at all distances and in all fields of movement
6. Normalize accommodative/convergence relation
7. Integrate oculomotor function with information processing

#### Duration of Treatment

The following treatment ranges are provided as a guide for third-party claims processing and review purposes. Treatment duration will depend on the particular patient's condition and associated circumstances. When duration of treatment beyond these ranges is required, documentation of the medical necessity for additional treatment services may be warranted.

### Exotropia

1. The most commonly encountered intermittent exotropia usually requires 36 to 48 hours of office therapy.
2. The most commonly encountered constant exotropia usually requires 50 to 64 hours of office therapy.
3. Exotropia complicated by:
   a. Associated visual adaptations (e.g., amblyopia, abnormal retinal correspondence) require additional office therapy.
   b. Associated visual anomalies (e.g., cyclotropia, hypertropia) require additional office therapy.
   c. Associated conditions such as stroke, head trauma, and strabismus surgery require substantially more office therapy.

*Continued*

## Strabismus—cont'd

### Esotropia

1. The most commonly encountered intermittent esotropia usually requires 40 to 52 hours of office therapy.
2. The most commonly encountered constant esotropia usually requires 60 to 75 hours of office therapy.
3. Esotropia complicated by:
    a. Associated visual adaptations (e.g., suppression, amblyopia, abnormal retinal correspondence) require additional office therapy.
    b. Associated visual anomalies (e.g., cyclotropia, hypertropia) require additional office therapy.
    c. Associated conditions such as stroke, head trauma, and strabismus surgery require substantially more office therapy.

### Follow-up Care

At the conclusion of the active treatment regimen, periodic follow-up evaluations should be provided at appropriate intervals. Therapeutic lenses may be prescribed at the conclusion of vision therapy for maintenance of long-term stability. Some cases may require additional therapy because of decompensation.

# Subconjunctival Hemorrhage

A subconjunctival hemorrhage occurs on the surface of the eye. It is caused by a rupture of a small blood vessel under the conjunctiva, the transparent outermost protective covering of the eye. This allows blood to spread under this tissue, often causing a dramatic presentation. However, in the majority of patients it is of no consequence but may take several weeks to completely resolve or be reabsorbed into the vascular system.

Generally, physical exertion, straining, coughing, or sneezing may be responsible for a rupture of a small blood vessel under the subconjunctival area; however, frequently no cause can be identified.

The standard recommended treatment is to apply cold compresses several times per day for 2 days to reduce any additional blood flow into the area followed by warm compresses to facilitate reabsorption.

If subconjunctival hemorrhages reoccur two or more times in a year, vascular system disease must be ruled out.

# Systemic Disease and Your Eyes

Many diseases in other parts of the body can result in problems with your eyes. Patients with certain systemic diseases should see their eye doctor on a regular basis to ensure that no vision loss occurs. Likewise, during the course of an eye examination, your eye doctor can often detect changes in the structure of your eyes that indicate a possible systemic disease. An eye doctor can typically detect signs of 400 diseases occurring in other parts of the body, including the following:

Diabetes
High blood pressure
High cholesterol
Heart disease
Arteriosclerosis
Leukemia
Stroke
Myasthenia gravis

Anemia
Multiple sclerosis
Autoimmune diseases
Arthritis
Toxoplasmosis
Histoplasmosis
Rosacea
Cancer

Because most eye disorders are painless and change gradually, you may not be aware of them until vision loss occurs. At that point it may be too late to recover the lost vision. An example of this is glaucoma or macular degeneration.

Your eye doctor can see signs of systemic disease in many ways by examining your eyes. By looking inside your eyes at the retina, he or she may observe new fragile blood vessels growing, as in diabetes. In hypertension, the arteries first become narrow, then hemorrhage and show leakages called exudates that eventually develop into optic nerve edema, which may indicate that a person is near death. Heart disease can cause a unique hemorrhage called a Roth spot. Plaque in a retinal artery may signal an increased risk for stroke. Scars in the retina may indicate a fungal disease or parasitic disease. Nearly any disease that can affect blood vessels may be seen inside the eye. Inside the eye is the one place your doctor can see the tiny blood vessels magnified several times without cutting open the skin.

Arthritis can be associated with inflammation of the white part of the eye, the sclera, or the colored part of the eye, the iris. High cholesterol can be detected by looking for a white ring on the back of the clear lens on the front of your eye, the cornea, or yellow deposits of cholesterol on the skin on your eyelids called xanthelasma. Your eye doctor can see the tiny blood vessels inside the eye filling up with cholesterol. If they are getting filled up, you run the risk of the heart vessels becoming clogged, causing a heart attack, or your carotid vessels becoming clogged, causing a stroke.

Nerve disorders such as multiple sclerosis may affect the optic nerve or the nerves leading to the eye muscles, eyelids, and face. Rosacea may affect the tears and the front of the eye, causing irritation. Melanoma and other cancers can metastasize from the eye or to the eye.

Regular eye examinations with your eye doctor can minimize the loss of vision from systemic disease. Your eye doctor may also detect signs of a disease you did not know you had.

# Vision Therapy for Adults

Many people think that vision therapy is only for children. This could not be further from the truth. Adults have as much need for this type of vision care as children do. Vision therapy is often more effective for adults because they are usually more motivated to improve their visual abilities, whereas children may not understand that they have a problem or how that problem may affect their interests or future.

Many people have visual problems sustaining near-centered work (reading, writing, and computer use), and they are not limited to children in school. When people have trouble using both eyes together or cannot focus for great lengths of time, they do not tend to grow out of these problems. Children with visual problems often become adults with visual problems.

Adults will figure out many ways to compensate for their visual problems so that they can continue with any strenuous visual work they need to do. Often, adults come home from work extremely tired when all they did was sit at a desk and do paperwork. Some people will feel as if they had just run a 10-K race! Children, on the other hand, tend to avoid tasks that are difficult or make them feel inadequate.

The right doctor can help reduce the strain of near work as well as work with any other kinds of visual problems. The proper lenses along with vision therapy make a tremendous difference in an adult's ability to function at work or play, just as with children of school age.

# Warm Soaks

Warm soaks help resolve eye infections by speeding up blood supply to the affected area.

1. Use tap water. Run the tap for approximately 2 minutes to avoid still-standing water that may contain sediment from the pipes. You do not need to use distilled or purified drinking water.
2. Use warm, not hot, water. Hot water can damage the delicate skin of the eyelids.
3. Soak a clean washcloth in the warm tap water. Close both eyes and lay the cloth over both eyes or as directed: _____
4. Leave the cloth over your eyes until it has cooled down and lost its warmth. Then resoak it in the warm water. You will probably need to resoak the cloth every 30 seconds.
5. Attempt to maintain a consistently warm temperature when soaking.
6. Soak for a total of 5 minutes or as directed: _____

   Soak three times a day or as directed: _____

# What is Vision Therapy?

Vision therapy is defined as the following:
- A progressive program of vision "exercises" or procedures
- Performed under doctor supervision
- Individualized to fit the visual needs of each patient
- Generally conducted in the office in once- or twice-weekly sessions of 30 minutes to an hour
- Sometimes supplemented with procedures done at home between office visits ("homework")
- Prescribed to help patients develop or improve fundamental visual skills and abilities
- Prescribed to improve visual comfort, ease, and efficiency
- Prescribed to change how a patient processes or interprets visual information

## Not Just Eye Exercise

Unlike other forms of exercise, the goal of vision therapy is not to strengthen eye muscles. Your eye muscles are already incredibly strong. Vision therapy should not be confused with any self-directed program of eye exercises that has been marketed to the public. Vision therapy is supervised by vision care professionals, and many types of specialized and medical equipment can be used, such as the following:
- Therapeutic lenses (regulated medical devices)
- Prisms (regulated medical devices)
- Filters
- Occluders or patches
- Electronic targets with timing mechanisms
- Computer software
- Balance boards

The first step in any vision therapy program is a comprehensive vision examination. After a thorough evaluation, a qualified vision care professional can advise you regarding whether you are a good candidate for vision therapy and whether vision therapy is appropriate treatment for you.

Vision therapy is sometimes referred to as visual therapy or vision training.

# Family Medical History and Risk

If you or a blood relative has a history of the following disorders, you are at risk of losing your sight. Talk to your eye doctor about how you can prevent the loss of vision caused by such medical conditions.

### Medical and Ocular Diseases: A Personal and Family History

In the medical history, specific questions about current or past personal, medical, or ophthalmic diseases may also be of value in prescribing eyeglass enhancements wisely to help promote healthy sight. The family history is an extension of this. In an individual with a strong family history of vision-threatening ocular disorders (e.g., cataract and macular degeneration), special care must be taken to minimize the risk of the patient developing similar problems. This same caution holds true for patients with beginning cataracts or those with retinal abnormalities such as drusens, which might progress to the more serious macular degeneration. Also important in the medical history are other diseases that might have ocular implications, such as diabetes, autoimmune disorders, cancer, and circulatory disease. Early detection, and treatment when indicated, are essential to maintain both good health and good sight over a lifetime.

You run a greater risk for vision loss if you or a blood relative have:

| | |
|---|---|
| Diabetes | Eczema or psoriasis |
| High blood pressure | Thyroid disease |
| Leukemia | Hypoglycemia |
| Anemia | Autoimmune disease |
| Multiple sclerosis | Glaucoma |
| Arthritis | Cataract |
| Migraines | Macular degeneration |
| Heart disease | Amblyopia |
| High cholesterol | Eye muscle disorder |
| Epilepsy | Allergy or asthma |

### Protecting Your Eyes

- Wear sunglasses that protect you from ultraviolet radiation.
- Wear a brimmed hat to reduce direct sunlight.
- Eat a diet rich in fruits and leafy green vegetables.
- Watch blood pressure and limit saturated fats and cholesterol.
- Limit alcohol intake.
- Most importantly, **stop smoking**.

| APPOINTMENT SCHEDULE | M  T  W  TH  F  S | MO. | DAY | YR. |
|---|---|---|---|---|

| ROOM 1 | ROOM 2 |
|---|---|

| | ROOM 1 | | | ROOM 2 |
|---|---|---|---|---|
| **8** | 00 | | **8** | 00 |
| | 15 | | | 15 |
| | 30 | | | 30 |
| | 45 | | | 45 |
| **9** | 00 | | **9** | 00 |
| | 15 | | | 15 |
| | 30 | | | 30 |
| | 45 | | | 45 |
| **10** | 00 | | **10** | 00 |
| | 15 | | | 15 |
| | 30 | | | 30 |
| | 45 | | | 45 |
| **11** | 00 | | **11** | 00 |
| | 15 | | | 15 |
| | 30 | | | 30 |
| | 45 | | | 45 |
| **12** | 00 | | **12** | 00 |
| | 15 | | | 15 |
| | 30 | | | 30 |
| | 45 | | | 45 |
| **1** | 00 | | **1** | 00 |
| | 15 | | | 15 |
| | 30 | | | 30 |
| | 45 | | | 45 |
| **2** | 00 | | **2** | 00 |
| | 15 | | | 15 |
| | 30 | | | 30 |
| | 45 | | | 45 |
| **3** | 00 | | **3** | 00 |
| | 15 | | | 15 |
| | 30 | | | 30 |
| | 45 | | | 45 |
| **4** | 00 | | **4** | 00 |
| | 15 | | | 15 |
| | 30 | | | 30 |
| | 45 | | | 45 |
| **5** | 00 | | **5** | 00 |
| | 15 | | | 15 |
| | 30 | | | 30 |
| | 45 | | | 45 |
| **6** | 00 | | **6** | 00 |
| | 15 | | | 15 |
| | 30 | | | 30 |
| | 45 | | | 45 |
| **7** | 00 | | **7** | 00 |
| | 15 | | | 15 |
| | 30 | | | 30 |
| | 45 | | | 45 |
| **8** | 00 | | **8** | 00 |
| | 15 | | | 15 |
| | 30 | | | 30 |
| | 45 | | | 45 |

## AUTHORIZATION FOR RELEASE OF IDENTIFYING HEALTH INFORMATION

Patient Name _____ DOB _____

Address _____

Phone Number _____

I authorize _____ to release my health

information to: _____

Information to be released:     □ Copy of completed records

□ Copy of spectacle RX

□ Copy of contact lens RX

Comments:

It is completely your decision to sign this authorization form. We cannot refuse to treat you if you choose not to sign this authorization.

If you sign this authorization, you can revoke it later. The only exception to your right to revoke is if we have already acted in reliance upon this authorization. If you want to revoke your authorization, send us a written note telling us that your authorization is revoked. Send this note to the person listed at the top of this form.

I HAVE READ AND UNDERSTAND THIS FORM. I AM SIGNING IT VOLUNTARILY. I AUTHORIZE THE DISCLOSURE OF MY HEALTH INFORMATION AS DESCRIBED IN THIS FORM.

Patient Signature _____ Date _____

**Billing Statement**

## Statement of Services

**Please return this form to the receptionist**

### PATIENT INFORMATION

PATIENT ☐M ☐F DATE

ADDRESS

CITY　　STATE　　ZIP

PHONE　　DATE OF BIRTH

EMPLOYED BY

INSURANCE CARRIER　POLICY NO.　GROUP NO.

POLICY HOLDER　RELATION TO INSURED　MEDICAL/MEDICAID NO.

OCCURRENCE RELATED TO
☐Accident ☐Indust. ☐Preg. ☐Other　DATE OF OCCURRENCE

DATES FROM:　TO:　OK TO RETURN TO WORK

NEXT APPT. ON: DAY　DATE　TIME ☐AM ☐PM

☐Office Visit ☐Exam ☐Post Op Treat ☐Other

I Hereby Authorize Payment Directly To The Below Named Doctor of the Group Insurance Benefits Otherwise Payable To Me.

SIGNATURE INSURED PERSON

### ATTENDING DOCTOR'S STATEMENT

| CODE | SERVICE | FEE |
|---|---|---|
| 101 | Vision Analysis & Diagnosis .................. | $ |
| 102 | Consultation & Prescription. ................ | |
| 104 | Professional Prescription Services ......... | |
| 105 | Progress Evaluation ........ | |
| 601 | Multifocal and/or Presbyopic Services ...... | |
| 602 | Tonometry ................. | |
| 604 | Color Vision ............. | |
| 606 | Visual Fields ............ | |
| 610 | Depth Perception ......... | |
| 301 | Supplemental Visual Training Evaluations ...... | |
| 301.1 | Visual Skills ............ | |

Doctor's Signature

### Explanation of Service

| CODE | SERVICE | FEE |
|---|---|---|
| 301 | Supplemental Visual Training Evaluation ...... | |
| 301.1 | Visual Skills ............ | |
| 301.3 | Developmental Vision ...... | $ |
| 302 | Visual Training Consultation & Workshop..... | |
| 303 | Visual Training Therapy ...... | |
| 201 | Supplemental Contact Lens Evaluation........ | |
| 701 | Office Visit ............. | |
| 702 | Vision Screening ......... | |
| 800 | Replacements/Repairs ...... | |
| 801 | Frame Adjustments ........ | |
| 811 | Contact Lens Modification .... | |

| | | |
|---|---|---|
| Professional Prescription Services | | |
| Frames | | |
| Lenses | | |
| | Total | $ |
| | | $ |

### ACCOUNT INFORMATION

| PREV. BALANCE | TODAY'S CHARGES | PAYMENTS | | NEW BALANCE |
|---|---|---|---|---|
| | | ☐Cash ☐Check | | |

# Pre-Collection Statement

Dear _____:


Our records show that you have an outstanding balance of $ _____ as of _____.
The current amounts due include the following:

Professional Services

_____  $ _____

_____  $ _____

_____  $ _____

Materials and Contact Lenses

_____  $ _____

_____  $ _____

Total  $ _____


Please return your check for the full amount due in the enclosed self-addressed envelope. Payment of less than the full amount due may be possible if a payment plan is approved by our office.

Thank you for your prompt attention to this matter. We look forward to continuing to provide you the very best vision care possible.



Sincerely,

Dr._____

# Collection Call Planning Form

Name of Patient                                    Telephone No.

1. Basic Information (see Pre-Collection Statement)
   • Date of visits
   • Treatment rendered
   • Amount due

2. Previous Collection Steps (see Collection Letter)
   • Bills (dates)
   • Calls (dates)
   • What happened with previous collection attempts?

3. Past Payment Record
   • How often has patient been past due?
   • How long has this patient been a patient in our office?
   • What is the payment history with other family members? (confidential)

4. Prepare Fact-Finding Questions
   • What are patient's reasons for not paying?
   • What can we do to help bring account up to date?

5. Payment Plan
   • What payments are acceptable?
   • Dates payments must be received: _____

Prepare an Opening Statement
   • Identify yourself and our office
   • Give the reason for calling
   • Strategic pause
Speak to the Correct Person (responsible party)

# Collection Letter

Dear _____:

During the past _____ months our office staff has contacted you several times regarding your outstanding balance of $_____. As you are aware, extending credit to you or failing to collect amounts due us for services provided will increase fees for other patients. I hope you agree that is not fair.

    If there is some misunderstanding about the service our office provided, please contact me directly. Otherwise please pay your bill by return mail. Another envelope is enclosed for your convenience. Thank you.

    If you were not happy with the services we provided, I need to know that. However, I am sure you understand that doctors, lawyers, and other professionals give their time and expertise and charge fees accordingly for these professional services. For that fee, they do the best job they can for their patients or clients. They do not and cannot promise success. Nor is their fee contingent on this success.

    The next step is one we both want to avoid: turning your account over to a collection agency.

Sincerely yours,

Dr. _____ and Staff

# Consent to Payment

Patient: _____  Date: _____

Account No: _____

    I consent to authorize the indicated eyecare services to be performed. I understand that at any time I may terminate or postpone the proposed treatment. I have been informed of treatment alternatives that relate to my eye condition(s), their respective advantages and disadvantages, the substantial risks, and consequences of limited or delayed treatment or nontreatment. I have been informed of the costs of the treatment and alternative treatment. I have been informed of financial arrangements available to me. All questions have been answered to my satisfaction, and I have read and understand the above directions and cautions.

Payment in full will be rendered at each appointment for treatment completed at that appointment. I will pay by ❑ Master Card ❑ VISA ❑ Cash ❑ Personal check at each appointment.

Payments are to be made for $_____ per month for _____ months.

Payment is due no later than the _____ day of the month.

Postdated checks or authorization of credit card for the balance of $_____ is to be paid by _____ and the remaining balance of $_____ to be paid by _____.

Coupon booklet: Payments to be received by the _____ day of the month for _____ months.

Monthly payment will be $_____.

    The estimate of fees for services is guaranteed for 90 days. If treatment is not begun within 90 days of the estimate date, cost of treatment could vary. Once treatment has begun, changes in the anticipated treatment plan may be required, depending on ocular conditions encountered. I will be informed if this occurs and given the option of continuing treatment, changing treatment, or canceling treatment.

    If my balance becomes 60 days or more overdue, the office reserves the right to interrupt or discontinue treatment and/or send my account to an attorney for collection. In the event that my account is sent for collection, I will be responsible for all costs and fees incurred, including reasonable attorney's fees. If payment is not made within 30 days, my account will be charged at an interest rate of 1.5% per month. State regulations and standard-of-care legal options require that I be given treatment options, listed procedures, total fees for the procedures, and indicated financial arrangements. This is for the mutual protection of both the patient and the doctor.

_____     _____

Financial Coordinator's Signature            Date

# Financial Arrangements

Our goal in discussing financial arrangements relative to your vision needs includes informing you of the following:
- Treatment alternatives
- Advantages and disadvantages of treatment alternatives
- Consequences and/or risks of limited, treatment delayed treatment and/or nontreatment

We will discuss with you the costs of the treatments and any alternative treatments. We will gladly answer your questions until you are completely satisfied.

## Vision Insurance

We are happy to assist you in receiving your maximum vision insurance benefits. Vision insurance is a contract between your employer, who selects your coverage limits, and the insurance company. You (the subscriber) will receive the vision benefits as defined within this plan. Insurance payments received by this office will be credited to your account or refunded to you in the case of an overpayment. We cannot guarantee insurance carrier payments on any insurance reimbursement estimates this office generates. You are responsible for all fees (charges) that your insurance company has not paid, for whatever reason, within a 60-day period from when treatment is begun. You will be expected to pay the full amount due.

Our office will accept assignment of vision insurance benefits directly to our office. Please bring your vision plan benefits booklet to our office to allow our staff to make a reasonable estimate of what the insurance company will pay for a given procedure. For an exact statement of benefits, a predetermination of benefits form can be sent to the insurance company. This process requires a vision insurance form with your section of the form completed to be used to request a predetermination of benefits from your insurance carrier. The insurance carrier will return the form stating its payment and your co-payment responsibility. You may need to bring in a completed insurance form for **each** appointment at which **new** treatment is begun.

## Payment Options

In addition to accepting payments directly from your insurance carrier, financial arrangements need to be made for your co-payment. The co-payment is the difference between the treatment costs and the insurance payment. We offer a 5% courtesy discount for full payment before beginning treatment. Our financial coordinator can discuss monthly payment arrangements such as postdated checks, credit card authorization, and coupon booklets.

## Fee Guarantees and Nonpayment Procedures

We are obligated by state regulations to be certain you understand your vision treatment needs, appropriate treatment and options, fees involved, and financial arrangements. This is for the mutual protection of both you and us.

The estimated fees we provide for services are guaranteed for 90 days. If treatment is not begun within 90 days of the estimate date, cost of treatment could vary. Once treatment has begun, changes in the anticipated treatment plan may be required, depending on conditions encountered. You will be informed if this occurs and given the option of continuing treatment, changing treatment, or canceling treatment.

If your balance becomes 60 days or more overdue, our office reserves the right to interrupt or discontinue treatment and/or send your account to a collection agency. In the event that your account is sent for collection, you will be responsible for all costs and fees incurred, including reasonable attorney's fees. If payment is not made within 30 days, your account will be charged at an interest rate of 1.5% per month.

# Budget Plan Receipt

Date: _____          Name: _____

**PLEASE READ THIS AGREEMENT CAREFULLY**

**EXTENDED PAYMENT PLAN**
AMOUNT OF ACCOUNT    _____
BUDGET PLAN CHARGE  _____
                    TOTAL _____
DOWNPAYMENT _____
BALANCE DUE _____

**PENALTY CHARGE — $3.00 FOR EACH LATE PAYMENT**

**Payment as Follows per Month        Payment Starts**

$ _____ by the 18th          _____
for _____ months

**PAYMENTS ARE DUE ON ABOVE DATES WITHOUT NOTICE**

If no payment has been made within 30 days of agreed date, this plan becomes **VOID**. A finance charge of 1.5% per month (18% annually) will be charged on all unpaid balances. Collection then will be through _____.
I have read and understand the above agreement. I will make my payments in the full amount and on the date shown.


_____          _____
Signed                                     Witness

## AMBLYOPIA TREATMENT FLOW SHEET

Patient's Name: _____ Date of Birth: _____
Cycloplegic Ret:    OD_____    OS_____    Date:_____
Rx:                 OD_____    OS_____    Date:_____
Rx:                 OD_____    OS_____    Date:_____

Diagnosis:    1) Amblyopia: OD/OS/none 2) Strabismus: OD/OS/none 3) Correspondence: NRC/ARC
              4) Fixation OD: central/steady eccentric/unsteady eccentric
                 Fixation OS: central/steady eccentric/unsteady eccentric

The following is a chronological time sheet to monitor the visual function of the patient.

| Date | Single Symbol Acuity | | Linear Visual Acuity | | SS/linear | Contrast Sensitivity | | | Fixation | | Comments | Patching |
|---|---|---|---|---|---|---|---|---|---|---|---|---|
| | OD VA | OS VA | OD VA | OS VA | Chart Used | OD/CS | OS/CS | Chart Used | OD | OS | | |
| | | | | | | | | | | | | |
| | | | | | | | | | | | | |
| | | | | | | | | | | | | |
| | | | | | | | | | | | | |
| | | | | | | | | | | | | |
| | | | | | | | | | | | | |
| | | | | | | | | | | | | |
| | | | | | | | | | | | | |
| | | | | | | | | | | | | |
| | | | | | | | | | | | | |

## Binocular Vision Evaluation

Date: _____                          Managing Doctor: _____

Patient: _____          D.O.B: _____          Age: ___ yrs ___ ms  Grade: ___

| Visual Acuity: sc/cc | Single Letter | Linear | Snellen | Other |
|---|---|---|---|---|
| Both eyes open | | | | |
| Right eye | | | | |
| Left eye | | | | |

| Near V.A.: sc/cc | Single Letter | Linear | Snellen | Other |
|---|---|---|---|---|
| Both eyes open | | | | |
| Right eye | | | | |
| Left eye | | | | |

Contrast Sensitivity: Mr. Happy/Cambridge

| | | | |
|---|---|---|---|
| Both eyes open | | | |
| Right eye | | | |
| Left eye | | | |

Color Vision: Ishihara/F2/D15                Visual Fields: Monster/Conf/H30-2/FDT

| | | | |
|---|---|---|---|
| Both eyes open | | | |
| Right eye | | | |
| Left eye | | | |

| Retinoscopy: Dry | | Retinoscopy: Wet | |
|---|---|---|---|
| Right Eye | | Right Eye | |
| Left Eye | | Left Eye | |

| Refraction: Dry | | Refraction: Wet | |
|---|---|---|---|
| Right Eye | 20/ | Right Eye | 20/ |
| Left Eye | 20/ | Left Eye | 20/ |

| Balanced: | | Prescribed: | |
|---|---|---|---|
| Right Eye | 20/ | Right Eye | |
| Left Eye | 20/ | Left Eye | |

| Tracking and Integration: | Developmental Eye Movement |
|---|---|
| test | |
| Pursuits: | Vertical total: ___ secs ___ SD |
| Saccades: | Horizontal: ___ secs ___ SD |
| "Figure 8" | Ratio: |
| Head movements | Errors: |

Comments
_____

*Continued*

**Binocular Vision Evaluation—cont'd**

## Ocular Motility:

Head Posture:

Fixation:

Pursuits:        Horiz:                        Vertical:

Saccades:      Horiz:                        Vertical:

Versions:

A/V Pattern:

Ductions:

---

Cover Test: Distance (    ) sc cc

---

Cover Test: Near      (   ) sc cc

---

Binocular Vision, Fusion and Stereopsis

Convergence to near point:                Dipl: [   ]      Suppr: [        ]

Worth's Lights: Dots/Ped      Distance:      Dipl: [   ]      Suppr: [        ]
                              Near:          Dipl: [   ]      Suppr: [        ]

Vergence ranges: sc/cc        Distance: BIN              BOT:
                              Near: BIN                  BOT:

Reflex Fusion Test: 10 cycles      BIN: _____ secs      BOT: _____ secs

Stereopsis: _____ "arc

---

Accommodation

Near Point: cms    OD:_____    OS:_____    Fatigue [   ]

Flippers: (+/-_____) Bin:_____ cpm    OD:_____ cpm OS:_____ cpm

Lead/Lag: MEM/PRIO/Saladin

Potential add: Near: _____ DS        VDT:WD_____ cms _____ DS

---

Ocular Health: Gtts: Fluress, NaFl strip, Pcaine, 1% Cyclo, 2.5% Phenyl, 1% Trop, 0.5% Trop

Date:                    Time            IOP;

| Anterior | Right | Left | Posterior | Right | Left |
|----------|-------|------|-----------|-------|------|
| Adnexia/lids | | | O.N: Size/CD | | |
| Conj | | | O.N. Color | | |
| Cornea | | | Vasculature | | |
| Ant. Chamb | | | Foveal reflex | | |
| Lens | | | Mac. mound | | |
| Vitreous | | | Periphery | | |

Assessment:

Plan:

Comments

Binocular Vision Treatment Form

| VISUAL SKILLS/BINOCULAR VISION EVALUATION & TREATMENT | | |
|---|---|---|
| NAME | VISIT # | DATE |

PURPOSE OF VISIT

HISTORY (SYMPTOMS, SIGNS, HOME TRAININGS, NOTES, ETC.)

| TESTS/THERAPY | RESULTS |
|---|---|

IMPRESSIONS/EXPECTATIONS

| THERAPY/ADVICE | SPECIFIC INSTRUCTIONS/RATIONALES |
|---|---|

FUTURE TESTING/THERAPY

## Binocular Vision Treatment Letter

Thank you for your interest in our Binocular Vision Clinic and the services we provide. We look forward to seeing you and trust that we will be able to help you and your child with his/her visual difficulties.

Before you can start any treatment, you will be scheduled for a binocular vision evaluation. This evaluation consists of a complete assessment of the binocular vision system and is usually scheduled as two 90-minute visits.

**Before your visit, <u>please</u>:**                                                                                   **Checklist**

- Complete the Developmental History Form                                                           [ ]
- Complete the History Form                                                                                   [ ]
- Bring any previous or present glasses/contact lenses                                             [ ]
- Ask your doctor/therapist for a referral letter, if appropriate                                   [ ]
- Request a copy of previous eye exams, if appropriate                                             [ ]
- Bring copies of educational testing reports                                                            [ ]
- Most recent IEP (Individual Educational Plan)                                                       [ ]
- Recent Speech-Language report                                                                             [ ]
- Recent Occupational Therapy report                                                                     [ ]
- Current insurance information and authorization                                                    [ ]

Following the binocular vision evaluation, we will explain all our findings and discuss treatment options for focusing, eye coordination, and/or visual perceptual skills difficulties.

Since our clinic acts as a specialty clinic into which many doctors refer their patients, our appointment slots are in high demand. Whenever a patient fails to show for an appointment, another patient is deprived of early treatment.

**If you are unable to keep your appointment, please give 24 hours notice. No-show visits (missed appointments without 24 hours notifications) will be charged $_____.**

Many insurance companies will cover your initial Binocular Vision Evaluation (CPT code 92060). Please be sure to bring your vision insurance information so that we may be able to process it correctly.

Thank you again for the trust that you have placed in our clinic. We look forward to meeting you.

Sincerely,

Binocular Vision Treatment Policies
Policies for Visual Therapy and Visual Training Equipment

Visual therapy is a set program of specialized visual activities that are designed to enhance visual abilities and remediate visual dysfunction.

Your individually designed visual therapy will consist of blocks of visual therapy sessions combined with daily home vision sessions of 30 minutes. Each block of visual therapy consists of six visual therapy sessions. Most children with moderate visual dysfunction reach their goal after two blocks of therapy or 12 sessions.

We recommend that you keep your appointments on the same day and time each week until your treatment is completed.

### Financial Arrangements
The fee for one block of six sessions is $_____. You may secure your place on the therapy schedule with a deposit of $_____ prior to the first therapy session. Credit cards are accepted.

### Visual Training Equipment
During the course of visual therapy, we will be prescribing various procedures and activities as home exercises. Many exercises will require special equipment. A complete set of visual therapy equipment may be purchased through our clinic for $_____. A majority of this equipment will be useful as refresher exercises well after the completion of your therapy. If you choose to return the equipment, we will credit you $_____ toward further services. In the event that the equipment is lost, broken, or worn beyond usefulness, no credit will be extended.

### Canceled or Missed Appointments
Regular weekly appointments and daily home training sessions are important for a successful program. If you are unable to keep an appointment, please give us 24 hours notice. No-show visits (missed appointments without 24 hours notification) will be charged $_____. Inconsistent appointment attendance or two consecutively missed appointments without notice may result in dismissal.

### Insurance
Many insurance companies will cover your initial Binocular Vision Evaluation (CPT code 92060) and some of your visual therapy (Orthoptics CPT code 92065). We will be glad to help you complete any necessary forms.

If you have any questions regarding fees and scheduling, please call _____.

I have read and understand the policies for Visual Therapy and Visual Training Equipment.

Parent or Guardian's Signature: _____ Date: _____

# Binocular Vision Therapy Kit
# Visual Therapy Kit

**Visual Therapy Equipment**

During the course of your visual therapy, we will be prescribing various procedures and exercises as home vision therapy. Many of those exercises require special equipment. A complete set of visual therapy equipment is included in this visual therapy kit. As you become more proficient with the different exercises, we will exchange the content of the kit to higher-powered equipment.

A majority of this equipment will be useful for refresher exercises after the completion of your therapy. We therefore recommend that you store it in the plastic pockets within the folder that we have provided.

**Content:**

Handouts:

Binocular Vision and Visual Skills Clinic—Services and Fee Schedule Policies for Visual Therapy and Visual Training Equipment—Statement of Position: Visual Therapy —American Foundation for Vision Awareness Vision, Learning and Dyslexia, A Joint Organizational Policy Statement—American Academy of Optometry, American Optometric Association

Training Material:

The Accommodative Rock Card Series
Cards with words and letters
Hart chart for near and distance activities

Equipment:

Brock string with three colored beads for eye coordination exercises

Eye patch to be used with monocular focusing exercises

Fixation target on spatula for push-up exercises

Flipper lenses with lower power, for focusing exercises

Lifesaver cards

Loose prism of lower power, for eye coordination exercises

Random dot "Magic Eye" exercises for finetuning of eye coordination and focusing

Red/green filter glasses

Red pointer to be used with "lifesaver cards" and similar exercises

Sliding vectogram for horizontal and vertical eye coordination exercises

Tranaglyph panel for eye coordination exercises

Vertical filter bar to be used for antisupression reading exercises

## BINOCULAR VISION AND VISUAL SKILLS REPORT

## Clinical work copy

Name:                    Age:              Grade:                    Exam Date:
Date of Report:                            Managing Doctor:

Reason for exam and history: Signs and symptoms. General and ocular health. Previous intervention.

Refraction (cycloplegic) and visual acuity:

    Right eye:                    Without Rx: V.A: 20/              With Rx: V.A: 20/
    Left eye:                     Without Rx: V.A: 20/              With Rx: V.A: 20/

[Legend: X = within norms  X/- = Borderline  - = below norms, needs attention]

| | RESULTS | X | X/- | - | Comments |
|---|---|---|---|---|---|
| **Ocular posture** | | | | | |
| **Cover test:** **Without glasses** | Primary gaze (far): Primary gaze (near): Up gaze (near): | | | | |
| **Fixation:** | | | | | Steady |
| **Pursuits:** Following eye movements | | | | | Smooth |
| **Saccades:** Fixation eye movements | | | | | Accurate without head movement |
| **Versions/ductions:** | | | | | Full |
| **Near point convergence** | cms | | | | Expected: < 9 cm |
| **Convergence ranges @near** | | | | | Expected: 14/18/7 |
| **Divergence ranges @ near** | | | | | Expected: 11/19/10 |
| **Accommodation:** focusing ability/accuracy | OD      D OS      D | | | | Expected: 13D |
| **Accommodation:** focusing flexibility | Right:    cpm Left:    cpm Both:  cycles in 60 sec, | | | | Expected: 12 cpm  Expected: 8 cpm |
| **Stereopsis:** depth perception | "arc | | | | Randot Test |
| **Color vision** | Normal | | | | Ishihara |
| **Reading eye movements** Vertical time (sec): | sec within 1 standard deviation of normal | | | | Developmental eye movement test: Vertical: normal rapid automatic naming |
| Horizontal time (sec): | sec within 1 standard deviation of normal | | | | Horizontal: adequate oculo-motor and/or spatial planning |
| **Reflex fusion:** Converge (10 cycles) Diverge (10 cycles) | sec sec | | | | Expected: Converge < 25 sec Diverge < 25 sec |

*Continued*

## BINOCULAR VISION AND VISUAL SKILLS REPORT—cont'd

Eye Health (internal and external): Anterior ocular health is significant for trace peripheral corneal lipid deposits. Posterior ocular health is significant for a vitreal retinal tuft located in the peripheral superior temporal retina of the right eye. The arterial reflex of the retinal arteries is minimally larger than expected, indicating the beginning of atherosclerotic changes secondary to elevated blood lipid levels.

Other skills tested:

1.  TVAS (test of visual analysis skills): _____ grade level, indicating deficient/normal spatial planning skills.
2.  TAAS (test of auditory analysis skills): _____ grade, indicating deficient/normal phonemic awareness skills.
3.  Visagraph (eye tracking computer program): Average span of recognition and number of fixations slightly below grade norms. Regressions and average duration of fixation are above grade norms. Overall reading eye movement efficiency is at _____ grade level.

Recommendations:

1.  We released a prescription for:                for general use.
2.  We recommend vision therapy to expand accommodation and vergence ranges.
3.  We recommend a speech and language evaluation to further address the TAAS results.
4.  We recommend the patient's parent or guardian consult a pediatrician for lipid/blood work-up.
5.  We recommend a follow-up in 3 months to monitor the vitreal retinal tuft. We discussed the symptoms of retinal detachment and immediate return to the clinic if the patient experiences these symptoms.
6.  We recommend a line guide for reading and graph paper for math based on the TVAS results.
7.  We recommend continuing regular annual eye exams.

Please call us if there are any questions.

Sincerely,

**BINOCULAR VISION AND VISUAL SKILLS REPORT—cont'd**

**BUILDING BLOCKS OF VISION AND LEARNING**

Recommendations:

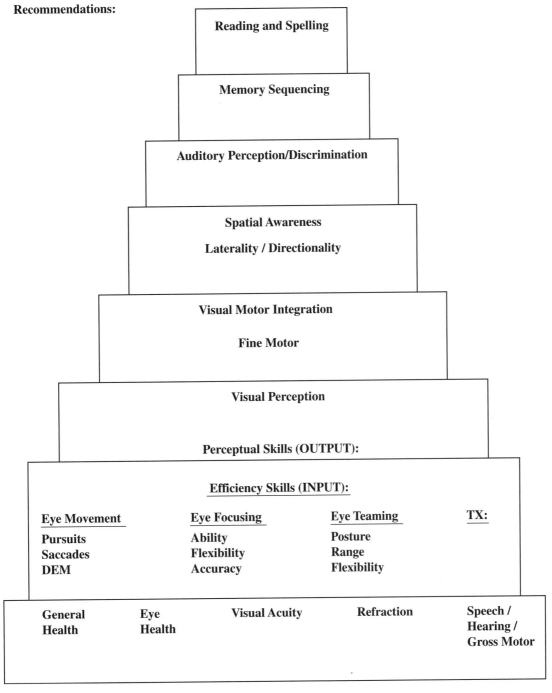

**Reading and Spelling**

**Memory Sequencing**

**Auditory Perception/Discrimination**

**Spatial Awareness**

**Laterality / Directionality**

**Visual Motor Integration**

**Fine Motor**

**Visual Perception**

Perceptual Skills (OUTPUT):

Efficiency Skills (INPUT):

| Eye Movement | Eye Focusing | Eye Teaming | TX: |
|---|---|---|---|
| Pursuits | Ability | Posture | |
| Saccades | Flexibility | Range | |
| DEM | Accuracy | Flexibility | |

| General Health | Eye Health | Visual Acuity | Refraction | Speech / Hearing / Gross Motor |
|---|---|---|---|---|

Reason For Evaluation:
CC:

## Binocular Vision Summary Sheet

Name: _____ DOB: _____ Date of Exam _____ PSA _____

CC: _____

Diagnosis: _____

        _____

Rx:    Dry: _____ Wet: _____ Given _____

| Tests | Initial Results | Goal | Today | Status/Comments |
|-------|-----------------|------|-------|-----------------|
| VA sc/cc @6 M | | | | |
| VA sc/cc @ _____cm | | | | |
| CT @ 6 M | | | | |
| CT @ ____ cm | | | | |
| NPA | | | | |
| NPC | | | | |
| Stereo_____ | | | | |
| RF BO/BI | | | | |
| PFV Distance | | | | |
| NFV Distance | | | | |
| PFV Near | | | | |
| NFV Near | | | | |
| NRA/PRA Thru_____ | | | | |
| Lead/Lag | | | | |
| Pursuits | | | | |
| Saccades | | | | |
| Flippers (+/–_____) | | | | |
|     Monocular | | | | |
|     Binocular | | | | |
| Color | | | | |
| Contrast Sensitivity | | | | |
| Pupils | | | | |
| EOM | | | | |

Ocular Health _____

Additional Testing/Training Results

Recommendations:

1. _____
2. _____
3. _____

| In-House Training: | At Home: | Next Week: |
|--------------------|----------|------------|
| 1. _____ | 1. _____ | 1. _____ |
| 2. _____ | 2. _____ | 2. _____ |
| 3. _____ | 3. _____ | 3. _____ |
| 4. _____ | 4. _____ | 4. _____ |
| 5. _____ | 5. _____ | 5. _____ |

## BINOCULAR VISION REPORT

Name _____    Exam Date(s) _____    DOB _____    Age: ___ yr ____ mo    Grade: _____

Significant History/Chief Complaint: _____

_____

| Eye Health | Pressure | Visual Field | Color | Contrast |
|---|---|---|---|---|
| __Normal  __Other | __Normal  __Other | __Normal  __Other | __Normal  __Other | __Normal  __Other |

Explanation: _____

| Visual Acuity | Without Lenses/With Current | | Refraction and Visual Acuity With Lenses | | |
|---|---|---|---|---|---|
| | **Distance** | **Near (_inches)** | **Dry/Wet** | **Distance** | **Near (_ inches)** |
| R | 20/ | 20/ | R | 20/ | 20/ |
| L | 20/ | 20/ | L | | 20/ |
| Both | 20/ | 20/ | Both | 20/ | 20/ |

| Visual Analysis | R | __Normal | __Nearsighted | __Farsighted | __Astigmatism |
|---|---|---|---|---|---|
| | L | __Normal | __Nearsighted | __Farsighted | __Astigmatism |

Vision Correction Recommendations

__None    __To help restore normal acuity    __To improve eye teaming and/or focusing skill

To be worn: ___Full Time    __Distance only    __Near only    __Classroom and near

| VISUAL SKILLS PROFILE (Norms) | Findings | -- | x | ++ | Comments/Recommendations |
|---|---|---|---|---|---|
| **EYE MOVEMENTS** | | | | | |
| **DUCTION**  RE/LE (FULL) | | | | | |
| **PURSUIT**  Horiz/Vert (4/4) | | | | | |
| **SACCADE**  Horiz/Vert (4/4) | | | | | |
| **DEM** | | | | | |
| Vertical | | | | | |
| Horizontal | | | | | |
| Ratio H/V | | | | | |
| **EYE TRACK (Visagraph)** | | | | | |
| Fixation & Regression / 100W | | | | | |
| Av. Recog. Span/Av. Fix. Dur | | | | | |
| Rate w/Compreh./% Comp | | | | | |
| Grade Equiv./% Regress. | | | | | |
| **EYE FOCUSING** | | | | | |
| **ABILITY** | | | | | |
| RE (15-1/4 Age) | | | | | |
| LE | | | | | |
| **FLEXIBILITY** | | | | | |
| +/-2.00 RE (12 cpm) | | | | | |
| LE (12 cpm) | | | | | |
| BOTH (8 cpm) | | | | | |
| **ACCURACY (MEM/x-cyl)** | | | | | |
| LE (+0.75/+1.00) | | | | | |
| RE | | | | | |
| Binoc. Xcyl(+0.50) | | | | | |
| **EYE TEAMING** | | | | | |
| DISTANCE POSITION (0-2XP) | | | | | |
| RANGE: Converge (7/15/8) | | | | | |
| NEAR POSITION (0-6 XP) | | | | | |
| RANGE: Converge (14/18/7) | | | | | |
| Diverge (11/19/10) | | | | | |
| **DEPTH PERCEPTION** (40") | | | | | |
| **FLEXIBILITY:** Converge (10 Cycles) | | | | | |
| Diverge (>25 sec) | | | | | |

Key    --: deficient/very weak    -: weak    x: borderline/average    +: strong    ++: adequate/very strong

*Continued*

## BINOCULAR VISION REPORT—cont'd

### Perceptual Skills Profile

| Category | Test | RS | AE | -- | - | x | + | ++ | Treatment |
|---|---|---|---|---|---|---|---|---|---|
| | | | % | | | | | | Recommendations |
| Visual | **1. TVPS** | | | | | | | | |
| Perception | Visual Discrimination | | | | | | | | |
| | Visual Memory | | | | | | | | |
| | Visual Spatial Relations | | | | | | | | |
| | Visual Form Constancy | | | | | | | | |
| | Visual Sequential Memory | | | | | | | | |
| | Visual Figure Ground | | | | | | | | |
| | Visual Closure | | | | | | | | |
| | **2. PMA** | | | | | | | | |
| | Perceptual Speed | | | | | | | | |
| | Spatial Relations | | | | | | | | |
| Visual | **3. VMI** | | | | | | | | |
| Motor | Berry-Buktenica | | | | | | | | |
| Integration | **4. Rosner TVAS** | | | | | | | | |
| | Test of Visual Analysis Skills | | | | | | | | |
| | **5. Wold Sentence Copy** | | | | | | | | |
| Fine Motor | **6. Frostig** | | | | | | | | |
| | **7. Groove Peg Board** | | | | | | | | |
| Spatial | **8. Gardner Reversal** | | | | | | | | |
| Awareness | Frequency | | | | | | | | |
| | I. Recall | | | | | | | | |
| | II. Recognition | | | | | | | | |
| | III. Matching | | | | | | | | |
| | **9. Jordon L/R Reversal** | | | | | | | | |
| | I. Letters/Numbers | | | | | | | | |
| | II. Words | | | | | | | | |
| | III. Sentence | | | | | | | | |
| | **10. Piaget R-L** | | | | | | | | |
| Auditory | **11. TAPS** | | | | | | | | |
| Perception | Digits Forward | | | | | | | | |
| | Digits Backward | | | | | | | | |
| | Sentence Memory | | | | | | | | |
| | Word Memory | | | | | | | | |
| | Discrimination | | | | | | | | |
| | **12. Rosner TAAS** | | | | | | | | |
| | Test of Auditory Analysis Skills | | | | | | | | |
| Memory | **13. Visual-Aural Digit Span** | | | | | | | | |
| Sequencing | Receptive-Expressive | | | | | | | | |
| | Organization | | | | | | | | |
| | VADS:        REO: | | | | | | | | |
| | Aural-Oral        Auditory-Verbal | | | | | | | | |
| | Visual-Oral        Visual-Verbal | | | | | | | | |
| | Aural-Written        Auditory-Motor | | | | | | | | |
| | Visual-Written        Visual-Motor | | | | | | | | |
| Reading and | **14. DDT: Dyslexia** | | | | | | | | |
| Spelling | Determination | | | | | | | | |
| Strategies | Decoding Level | | | | | | | | |
| | % Eidetic | | | | | | | | |
| | % Phonetic | | | | | | | | |

KEY:    --: Deficient/Very Weak        -: Weak/Borderline        X: Average        +: Strong/Adequate        ++: Very Strong

# DEVELOPMENTAL HISTORY FORM

Child's Name _____ Birthday _____/_____/_____ Age _____yr _____mo
Grade _____ School's Name and Address _____
Teacher's Name _____
Mother's Name _____ Occupation _____ Phone _____
Father's Name _____ Occupation _____ Phone _____
Mailing Address _____
Who referred you to this clinic? _____ Number of children in family _____

**I.**   Please state the major reason you would like your child examined:

_____
_____

**II.**   **Vision:**

| | Yes | No | Comments |
|---|---|---|---|
| 1. Headaches | | | |
| 2. Blurred distance vision | | | |
| 3. Blurred reading vision | | | |
| 4. Holds books closer than normal | | | |
| 5. Eyes hurt | | | |
| 6. Eyes tire | | | |
| 7. Double vision | | | |
| 8. Eye turn (crossed or wall-eyed) | | | |
| 9. Blinks excessively | | | |
| 10. Covers one eye while doing homework | | | |

**III.**   **School:**

| | | | |
|---|---|---|---|
| 1. Is your child having problems in school? | | | |
| 2. Does your child like the teacher? | | | |
| 3. Is the school satisfied with the child's performance? | | | |
| 4. Are you satisfied with the child's performance? | | | |
| 5. Do grades really show his or her ability? | | | |
| 6. Is there trouble completing written assignments? | | | |
| 7. Does your child lose his or her place while reading? | | | |
| 8. Does your child misread words that are known? | | | |

**IV.**   **Behaviors:** Please rate your child on the following items (place a number in the blank space to the left of the item that best describes his/her school or home behavior).

1—Always    2—Frequently    3—Occasionally    4—Rarely    5—Never    6—Unknown

| | | |
|---|---|---|
| _____ Hyperactive | _____ Poor ability to organize work | _____ Confusion following a series of verbal instructions |
| _____ Easily Distracted | _____ Indistinct speech | _____ Variable school performance (from hour to hour/day to day) |
| _____ Short attention span | _____ Awkward or clumsy | _____ Reverses letters, words, or numbers in reading |
| _____ Easily frustrated | _____ Poor peer group relationships | _____ Reverses letters, words, or numbers in writing |
| _____ Impulsive | _____ Behavior problems | _____ Shows confusion about right or left |
| _____ Easily fatigued | _____ Emotional problems | _____ Shows confusion about directional orientation |

**V.**   **Physical development:** At what age in years and months did your child:

speak words clearly_____ start to crawl _____ walk unaided _____

*Continued*

## DEVELOPMENTAL HISTORY FORM—cont'd

**Which phrase describes the child's physical maturity (please circle number)?**

1—Physically immature      2—Average physical      3—Advanced physical
    for age                     maturity for age           maturity for age

**VI.**     **School progress:** Rate your child's progress in the following subjects:

1—Below grade level          2—Grade level          3—Above grade level

_____ Reading        _____ Spelling        _____ Writing        _____ Arithmetic

_____ Art        _____ Physical education        _____ Other _____

What specific type(s) of work is your child having trouble with? _____

_____

Have other family members had difficulties learning any of the above subjects?     No _____     Yes _____
If yes, state relationship to child and subjects: _____

_____

Does your child have memory difficulties?      No_____      Yes _____   If so, what type of information?

_____

**VII.**     **General history:** Is there a history of pregnancy or birth complications?     No_____     Yes _____
    If yes, please explain: _____

Has there been any severe childhood illness, high fever, injury, or physical impairment?    No _____   Yes _____
If yes, please explain: _____

Has your child received a hearing test?     No _____    Yes _____   Date: _____
Has a hearing or speech deficiency been previously diagnosed?     No _____    Yes _____
If yes, please explain: _____

Has your child received a complete eye examination?    No _____    Yes _____    Date: _____
Has a visual problem been diagnosed?     No _____    Yes _____
If yes, please explain: _____

Does your child have any allergies?     No _____    Yes _____
If yes, please explain: _____

Is your child currently taking any medications or pills?     No _____    Yes _____
If yes, please list the medications, their purposes, and duration: _____

_____

Has your child previously taken medication for hyperactivity?     No _____    Yes _____

**VIII.**     **Therapy:** Has there been any previous therapy for learning difficulties or visual or speech problems?
No _____     Yes _____        If yes, please state the type of therapy, duration, and results: _____

_____

_____

_____

Signature: _____    Date: _____
Relationship to child: _____
Comments:

# BINOCULAR VISION REFERRAL FORM

DATE:

Referring Dr:    Name:                                          Phone:
Street:                                     City:              Zip:
Fax:                                        email:

Patient:         Name:                      Date of Birth:    /    /    Age:
Street:                                     City:              ZIP:
Home Phone:                                 Work Phone:
Cell Phone:                                 email:
If a minor, parent's name:                             Phone:
If different address:

TYPE OF SERVICES REQUESTED:

[   ] Binocular Vision Evaluation = Full and comprehensive evaluation, two 90-minute visits
[   ] Strabismus/Amblyopia/Nystagmus Evaluation = Full and comprehensive evaluation = two 90-minute visits
[   ] Head Injury or Stroke Evaluation = Neuro-optometric evaluation = two or three 90-minute visits
[   ] VDT Examination = one or two 90-minute visits
[   ] Sports Vision Evaluation = one or two 90-minute visits
[   ] Perceptual Skills Assessment = four to six visits depending on age and difficulties
[   ] Informal Reading Evaluation = 3 visits
[   ] Visual Therapy (Orthoptics) = Patient requires a binocular evaluation prior to start of therapy = 6
      sessions per block
[   ] Perceptual Training = Patient requires perceptual skills analysis prior to therapy = 6 sessions per block
[   ] Amblyopia management = Patient requires binocular vision evaluation prior to treatment = monthly and
      quarterly follow-up appointments for at least 18 months

Should your patient see a particular doctor?    [   ] No   [   ] Yes       If yes, please indicate whom

Specific information requested: (*A short written report will be sent to your office address.*)

Would you like to assist in treatment (if needed)
[   ] No                [   ] Yes. If yes, to what extent?

*Continued*

## BINOCULAR VISION REFERRAL FORM—cont'd

Patient's Name: _____

[  ]        Please ask patient to obtain/fill out patient questionnaire (adult or child)
[  ]        Please ask parent to obtain/fill out developmental form for children
[  ]        Please obtain BV patient information package

Patient's history and chief complaint:

Present glasses or C.L.s: Date:
OD:                                       OS:

Add:          Prism or IPD:

VA with Rx:    OD:             OS:          VA without Rx:    OD:           OS:

Most recent refraction:    OD:               VA: (dist.)        VA: (near)
Date:                     OS:               VA: (dist.)        VA: (near)

Binocular vision findings:

Oculomotor findings:

Ocular health findings:

Other pertinent information:

_____
Doctor Signature

## STRABISMUS EXAMINATION RECORD

| Name | | Examiner | Date |
|---|---|---|---|
| Address | | Recorder | Birth |
| City | Phone | Referred by | Report Rec'd |

## HISTORY

What is the main vision problem?

Has there ever been an eye-turn?          Is there now?          Age when first noticed?

How often and under what conditions does the eye turn?          Single object ever seen as two?

To what extent is the eye-turn apparent to others?          Any relative have eye-turn?

Any previous treatment?    Glasses?    Patching?    Exercises?    Surgery?

    Ages?

    Type?

    Results?

Other pertinent history?

## AMETROPIA AND GLASSES

| | | | | |
|---|---|---|---|---|
| a. Latest retinoscopy | RE | LE | Date | By |
| b. Latest subjective | RE | LE | Date | By |
| c. Present glasses (major lens) | RE | LE | Date | By |
| d. Other (e.g., prism or add) | RE | LE | Date | By |

## ACUITY

| | | | |
|---|---|---|---|
| Rx  a  b  c  d  (circle one) | RE | LE | Method |
| Rx  a  b  c  d  (circle one) | RE | LE | Method |

## CONFRONTATION

| | | | |
|---|---|---|---|
| Angle kappa and steadiness | RE | LE | Suggests |
| Hirschberg, primary gaze, Rx_____RE | | LE | Suggests |

Hirschberg, cardinal fields:

Observations and remarks: epicanthus, facial asymmetries, ptosis, torticollis, etc.

PP conv. (cm):          PD:

## OBJECTIVE COVER TEST

Rx_____at_____M.    Rx_____at_____M.    Rx_____at_____M.    Rx_____at_____M.

UNILATERAL Cover RE, LE moves:

    Cover LE, RE moves:

ALTERNATE    RE fixating:

    LE fixating:

UNILATERAL NEUTRALIZATION:

    LOOSE PRISM TEST:

[AC/A=_____$\Delta$/1.00D]

*Continued*

**STRABISMUS EXAMINATION RECORD—cont'd**

## ADDITIONAL TEST RESULTS

| Comitance | Monocular Fixation and Amblyopia |
|---|---|
| Retinal Correspondence (without bifixation) | Sensory and Motor Fusion, Suppression |

Other Results

## DIAGNOSIS

Oculomotor Deviation with following Rx: RE                  LE

| At____M: Magnitude     Direction | At____M: Magnitude     Direction |
|---|---|
| Laterality     Freq. of Squint | Laterality     Freq. of Squint |

Comitance

### Associated Conditions

| Monocular Fixation | Amblyopia |
|---|---|
| Retinal Correspondence | Suppression |
| Fusion | Ametropia |

Other Relevant Conditions

## IMPRESSIONS AND RECOMMENDATIONS

Impressions (including frequency of squint, cosmesis, and prognosis)

Recommendations

## VISUAL SKILLS RECORDING FORM

### D.E.M Recording Form

Name _____    DOB _____    Age _____    Grade _____

| ARTICULATION PRE-TEST | Y | N | | NUMBER KNOWLEDGE PRE-TEST | Y | N |

ARTICULATION PRE-TEST          Y    N          NUMBER KNOWLEDGE PRE-TEST          Y    N
/=substitution error                                    o=omission error
a=addition error                                        <or>=transposition error

| TEST A | | TEST B | | TEST C | | | | |
|---|---|---|---|---|---|---|---|---|
| 3 | 4 | 6 | 7 | 3 | 7 | 5 | 9 | 8 |
| 7 | 5 | 3 | 9 | 2 | 5 | 7 | 4 | 6 |
| 5 | 2 | 2 | 3 | 1 | 4 | 7 | 6 | 3 |
| 9 | 1 | 9 | 9 | 7 | 9 | 3 | 9 | 2 |
| 8 | 7 | 1 | 2 | 4 | 5 | 2 | 1 | 7 |
| 2 | 5 | 7 | 1 | 5 | 3 | 7 | 4 | 8 |
| 5 | 3 | 4 | 4 | 7 | 4 | 6 | 5 | 2 |
| 7 | 7 | 6 | 7 | 9 | 2 | 3 | 6 | 4 |
| 4 | 4 | 5 | 6 | 6 | 3 | 2 | 9 | 1 |
| 6 | 8 | 2 | 3 | 7 | 4 | 6 | 5 | 2 |
| 1 | 7 | 5 | 2 | 5 | 3 | 7 | 4 | 8 |
| 4 | 4 | 3 | 5 | 4 | 5 | 2 | 1 | 7 |
| 7 | 6 | 7 | 7 | 7 | 9 | 3 | 9 | 2 |
| 6 | 5 | 4 | 4 | 1 | 4 | 7 | 6 | 3 |
| 3 | 2 | 8 | 6 | 2 | 5 | 7 | 4 | 6 |
| 7 | 9 | 4 | 3 | 3 | 7 | 5 | 9 | 8 |
| 9 | 2 | 5 | 7 | | | | | |
| 3 | 3 | 2 | 5 | | | | | |
| 9 | 6 | 1 | 9 | | | | | |
| 2 | 4 | 7 | 8 | | | | | |

TIME: _____ sec

_____s errors          _____o errors

_____a errors          _____t errors

ADJUSTED TIME = TIME x $\dfrac{80}{(80-o+a)}$

ADJUSTED TIME = _____ sec.

TOTAL ERRORS (s+o+a+t) = _____

RATIO = $\dfrac{\text{HORIZONTAL ADJUSTED TIME}}{\text{VERTICAL ADJUSTED TIME}}$ = _____

TOTAL TIME: _____ sec

ADJUSTED TIME: _____ sec

ERRORS: _____

*Continued*

**VISUAL SKILLS RECORDING FORM—cont'd**

**DEVELOPMENTAL EYE MOVEMENT (D.E.M) TEST**

**NORMATIVE**

| AGE | VERTICAL TIME (seconds) MEAN (S.D.) | HORIZONTAL TIME (seconds) MEAN (S.D.) | ERRORS MEAN (S.D.) | RATIO (H/V) MEAN (S.D.) |
|---|---|---|---|---|
| 6.0-6.11 | 63.11 (16.59) | 98.26 (32.61) | 15.22 (11.49) | 1.58 (.45) |
| 7.0-7.11 | 54.83 (9.20) | 87.94 (28.18) | 12.50 (12.91) | 1.60 (.41) |
| 8.0-8.11 | 46.76 (7.89) | 57.73 (12.32) | 4.61 (6.91) | 1.24 (.18) |
| 9.0-9.11 | 42.33 (8.20) | 51.13 (13.30) | 2.17 (4.10) | 1.21 (.19) |
| 10.0-10.11 | 40.28 (7.43) | 47.64 (10.11) | 1.91 (2.68) | 1.19 (.17) |
| 11.0-11.11 | 37.14 (5.42) | 42.62 (7.61) | 1.68 (2.34) | 1.15 (.13) |
| 12.0-12.11 | 35.14 (5.87) | 39.35 (8.11) | 1.11 (1.17) | 1.12 (.10) |
| 13.0-13.11 | 33.75 (6.53) | 37.56 (7.23) | 1.61 (2.15) | 1.12 (.12) |

For completed analysis of the scores including standard scores, percentiles, grade norms, and case examples, please see the D.E.M. Examiners Manual.

## VISUAL ANALYSIS OF READING STRATEGIES AND SPELLING SKILLS
### Summary of Evaluation

Name:                    DOB:           Age:    Year    Months        Grade level:        Date of evaluation:

Known reading difficulties: [ ] phonem.awared [ ] phonics [ ] vocabulary [ ] fluency/speed [ ] comprehension

Visagraph:          Fixation: [ ] steady [ ] regular [ ] unsteady [ ] nystagmus
                    Saccades: [ ] accurate [ ] stair steps [ ] under-shoot [ ] over-shoot [ ] head movements
                    Number tracking: [ ] accurate [ ] stair steps [ ] normal returns [ ] overshoot [ ] undershoot [ ] head movements

                    Listening comprehension: (70% and better): [ ] below grade level [ ] at grade level [ ] above grade level

                    Silent reading comprehension: (70% and better): [ ] below grade level [ ] at grade level [ ] above grade level

                    Reading patterns: Consistent/variable/repeatable three times over two visits

                    Reading comprehension: Grade level with at least 70% comprehension: Grade level:

|  |  |  |  |
|---|---|---|---|
| Fixations: | [ ] below grade norms | [ ] at norms | [ ] better than grade norms |
| Regressions: | [ ] below grade norms | [ ] at norms | [ ] better than grade norms |
| Span of recognition: | [ ] below grade norms | [ ] at norms | [ ] better than grade norms |
| Duration of fixations: | [ ] below grade norms | [ ] at norms | [ ] better than grade norms |
| Reading rate: | [ ] below grade norms | [ ] at norms | [ ] better than grade norms |
| Correlation: | [ ] normal | [ ] below normal | |
| Comments: | | | |

Dyslexia Determination Test: DDT/ADT

|  |  |
|---|---|
| Sight-word recognition: | grade level |
| Use of phonic for higher grade level: | grade level [ ] yes [ ] no |
| Sight-word memory (eidetic) spelling: | % |
| Phonetic encoding = phonetic spelling | % |

Informal Reading Inventory:

Word list of sight-words (eidetic only):

|  |  |
|---|---|
| Independent (0–2 errors): | grade level |
| Instructional (3–4 errors): | grade level |
| Frustration (5+ errors): | grade level |

Word list of sight-words (allowing for phonetic decoding):

|  |  |
|---|---|
| Independent (0–2 errors): | grade level |
| Instructional (3–4 errors): | grade level |
| Frustration (5+ errors): | grade level |

Reading Comprehension:

|  |  |
|---|---|
| Independent (>80% correct): | grade level |
| Instructional (75% correct): | grade level |
| Frustration (<70% correct): | grade level |

Area of difficulty: [ ] main idea [ ] detail [ ] vocabulary [ ] cause-effect [ ] inference [ ] sequence

Listening Comprehension:

|  |  |
|---|---|
| Independent (>80% correct): | grade level |
| Instructional (75% correct): | grade level |
| Frustration (<70% correct): | grade level |

Area of difficulty: [ ] main idea [ ] detail [ ] vocabulary [ ] cause-effect [ ] inference [ ] sequence

Summary and Comments:

## Video Display Terminal Assessment

Dear Patient,

The vision and eye related problems that computer users experience can be caused by a vision problem and/or shortcomings in the VDT work environment. In most cases the problems can be resolved or lessened by proper care of the eyes and/or adjustment of the environment.

To best resolve your particular problems, we need to have information about your symptoms and about your work environment. This information is critical to give you the best care. **Please take a few moments to fill out the attached symptoms and environmental assessment and bring it with you to the examination.**

We look forward to assisting you with the problems you are experiencing at your computer.

Name _____        Date _____

**Video Display Terminal Assessment—cont'd**

**Symptom Assessment**

Please circle whether or not (Y or N) you experience each of the following symptoms. For each that you answer Y, please comment about the severity and frequency of occurrence.

Y   N     **Eye Strain**

          Comments:

Y   N     **Tired Eyes**

          Comments:

Y   N     **Irritated or Sore Eyes**

          Comments:

Y   N     **Dry Eyes**

          Comments:

Y   N     **Lighting or Glare Discomfort**

          Comments:

Y   N     **Blurred Vision**

          Comments:

Y   N     **Double Vision**

          Comments:

Y   N     **Neck or Shoulder Ache**

          Comments:

Y   N     **Back Ache**

          Comments:

Y   N     **Hand or Wrist Ache**

          Comments:

*Continued*

**Video Display Terminal Assessment—cont'd**

**Environmental Assessment**

## <u>Please use a measuring stick to provide the following measurements:</u>

_____      Height from floor to surface on which keyboard rests

_____      Height from floor to front edge of chair seat

_____      Distance from eyes to center of computer screen with usual posture

_____      Distance from eyes to reference documents

Are your eyes **higher** or **lower** (circle one) than the center of the computer screen?

_____      By how much?

## <u>Please make the following observations</u>

_____      Color of text characters

_____      Color of background on which text is displayed

Y   N      Are there bright lights (e.g., windows or overhead lights) in your field of view while looking at the computer?

Y   N      If so, shield your eyes from the bright lights. Does this make you feel more comfortable?

Y   N      Shield the screen (e.g., with a file folder) from the overhead lights or bright windows. Does this improve the screen visibility?

## <u>Please identify whether or not you have the following:</u>

Y   N      Adjustable chair

Y   N      Adjustable keyboard height

Y   N      Lower back support

Y   N      Document holder

Y   N      Anti-reflection screen (Is it **mesh** or **glass**?)

Y   N      Hood on the monitor

Y   N      Wrist rest

Y   N      Task lighting (e.g., desk lamp)

## CHRONOLOGICAL RECORD OF PATIENT CARE

Patient's Name _____

| DATE | SERVICE | DOCTOR | FEE | REC'T NO. |
|------|---------|--------|-----|-----------|
|  |  |  |  |  |
|  |  |  |  |  |
|  |  |  |  |  |
|  |  |  |  |  |
|  |  |  |  |  |
|  |  |  |  |  |
|  |  |  |  |  |
|  |  |  |  |  |
|  |  |  |  |  |
|  |  |  |  |  |
|  |  |  |  |  |
|  |  |  |  |  |
|  |  |  |  |  |
|  |  |  |  |  |
|  |  |  |  |  |
|  |  |  |  |  |
|  |  |  |  |  |
|  |  |  |  |  |
|  |  |  |  |  |
|  |  |  |  |  |
|  |  |  |  |  |
|  |  |  |  |  |
|  |  |  |  |  |

## PRESCRIPTION ORDER RECORD

Rx 1. PURPOSE　　　　　　　　　　　　　　DATE

|  | Sphere | Cylinder | Axis | Decenter In | Out | Prism | Base | P.D. |
|---|--------|----------|------|-------------|-----|-------|------|------|
| R |  |  |  |  |  |  |  | Dist. |
| L |  |  |  |  |  |  |  | Near |

|  | Add | Seg. Hgt. | Seg. Width | Seg. Dec. | Total Dec. | Size Box | Shape |
|---|-----|-----------|------------|-----------|------------|----------|-------|
| R |  |  |  |  |  |  |  |
| L |  |  |  |  |  |  |  |

| S.V. Type | Multi-focal | Base Curve |
|-----------|-------------|------------|
| Frame | Bridge　　Temple | Tint |

Rx 2. PURPOSE　　　　　　　　　　　　　　DATE

|  | Sphere | Cylinder | Axis | Decenter In | Out | Prism | Base | P.D. |
|---|--------|----------|------|-------------|-----|-------|------|------|
| R |  |  |  |  |  |  |  | Dist. |
| L |  |  |  |  |  |  |  | Near |

|  | Add | Seg. Hgt. | Seg. Width | Seg. Dec. | Total Dec. | Size Box | Shape |
|---|-----|-----------|------------|-----------|------------|----------|-------|
| R |  |  |  |  |  |  |  |
| L |  |  |  |  |  |  |  |

| S.V. Type | Multi-focal | Base Curve |
|-----------|-------------|------------|
| Frame | Bridge　　Temple | Tint |

**RIGHT EYE**

| Date | Clinician | Type/Lab | PCCR or Series | Diameter | Power | Color |
|------|-----------|----------|----------------|----------|-------|-------|
|  |  |  |  |  |  |  |
|  |  |  |  |  |  |  |
|  |  |  |  |  |  |  |
|  |  |  |  |  |  |  |
|  |  |  |  |  |  |  |
|  |  |  |  |  |  |  |
|  |  |  |  |  |  |  |

**LEFT EYE**

| Date | Clinician | Type/Lab | PCCR or Series | Diameter | Power | Color |
|------|-----------|----------|----------------|----------|-------|-------|
|  |  |  |  |  |  |  |
|  |  |  |  |  |  |  |
|  |  |  |  |  |  |  |
|  |  |  |  |  |  |  |
|  |  |  |  |  |  |  |
|  |  |  |  |  |  |  |
|  |  |  |  |  |  |  |

# Computer Vision Syndrome Patient Questionnaire

**Patient name:** _____

**Doctor name:** _____

### General Visual Information

For the doctor to accurately assess your vision needs and possibly prescribe appropriate eyewear for computer use, **complete the following information**.

Number of hours per day spent at the computer: _____

Work is performed while:

❑ Sitting

❑ Other (please describe): _____

Describe the lighting in your work area: _____

Are you experiencing any of the following symptoms while at your computer (check appropriate boxes)?

❑ Headaches

❑ Blurred near vision

❑ Blurred distance vision

❑ Slowness in focusing

❑ Double vision

❑ Sore or tired eyes (strain)

❑ Glare (light) sensitivity

❑ Dry or watery eyes

❑ Burning, itching, or red eyes

❑ Neck and shoulder pain

❑ Back pain

Do you wear glasses while working at the computer?

❑ No

❑ Yes *If yes, please wear them to the eye exam.*

Do you wear contact lenses while working at the computer?

❑ No

❑ Yes *If yes, please bring them with you to the eye exam.*

Do you view reference materials while working at the computer?

❑ No

❑ Yes

If yes, what percentage of the time? _____

In inches, what is the viewing distance from your eye to the computer screen? _____

In inches, what is the viewing distance from your eye to the keyboard? _____

In inches, what is the viewing distance from your eye to reference material? _____

*Please check where appropriate.*

❑ The center of the screen is above eye level.

❑ The center of the screen is equal to eye level.

❑ The center of the screen is below eye level.

If above or below, by how many inches? _____

❑ Reference material is above eye level.

❑ Reference material is equal to eye level.

❑ Reference material is below eye level.

If above or below, by how many inches? _____

# Consultation Letter

Dear _____:

I recently saw our mutual patient, _____, whom you are currently treating for diabetes.
The eye health examination revealed no presence of retinal disease. Tonometry was _____ OD and _____
OS, within normal limits. Best corrected visual acuity is _____ right eye and _____ left eye, far and near. External slit
lamp examination and internal ophthalmoscopy were both normal.
Enclosed are copies of fundus photographs for your records. As you can see, there are no signs of diabetic retinal change. I also
performed a complete dilated peripheral retinal examination to rule out any other abnormalities.
If there is any additional information you would like, or if there are any other aspects of this patient's care you feel I should know
about, please call.
I plan to see _____ again in 6 months and I will urge him/her to follow your recommendations and continue to
see you on a regular basis.

Sincerely,

   Dr. _____

Enclosure

# CONTACT LENS RECORD

Name: _____  DOB: _____  Exam Date: _____

| | SOLUTIONS | |
|---|---|---|

Lenses Dispensed: _____

OD: _____

OS: _____

Service Agreement Effective thru: _____

SOLUTIONS

SOFT
Optifree _____
Renu _____
Complete _____
AOSept _____
Other _____
_____

RGP
Boston _____
Optimum _____
Claris _____
Other _____
_____

K's
OD_____/_____@_____
OS_____/_____@_____

#7
OD_____
OS_____

Recommended Wearing Schedule: DW_____ EW_____ Flex_____ Replace every_____ Gave written instructions ☐

**CL APPOINTMENT TYPE:   CLD-____ ☐   CLRF-____ ☐   CL CHECK ☐**   If new lenses, lens type_____ Tech Initials_____

**Date:**_____ AWT_____ WTT_____ Replace lenses every_____ Age of lenses_____

**Subjective Symptoms:** Vision: _____
Comfort: _____
Handling: _____

| DIST VA | NEAR VA | AUTOREFRACTION | | SOR | | SCOR | |
|---|---|---|---|---|---|---|---|
| OD 20/ | 20/ | OD | | OD | 20/ | OD | 20/ |
| OS 20/ | 20/ | OS | | OS | 20/ | OS | 20/ |
| OU 20/ | 20/ | | | | | | |

BIOMICROSCOPY
OD          OS

LENS POSITION
Center   OD          OS
Lag      OD          OS
Orient/  OD          OS
Fl.ptn

LENS INSPECTION
OD          OS

Assessment: _____  Plan: _____

Dr.'s Signature: _____  RTC: _____ Dr.____

**CL APPOINTMENT TYPE:   CLD-____ ☐   CLRF-____ ☐   CL CHECK ☐**   If new lenses, lens type_____ Tech Initials_____

**Date:**_____ AWT_____ WTT_____ Replace lenses every_____ Age of lenses_____

**Subjective Symptoms:** Vision: _____
Comfort: _____
Handling: _____

| DIST VA | NEAR VA | AUTOREFRACTION | | SOR | | SCOR | |
|---|---|---|---|---|---|---|---|
| OD 20/ | 20/ | OD | | OD | 20/ | OD | 20/ |
| OS 20/ | 20/ | OS | | OS | 20/ | OS | 20/ |
| OU 20/ | 20/ | | | | | | |

BIOMICROSCOPY
OD          OS

LENS POSITION
Center   OD          OS
Lag      OD          OS
Orient/  OD          OS
Fl.ptn

LENS INSPECTION
OD          OS

Assessment: _____  Plan: _____

Dr.'s Signature: _____  RTC: _____ Dr.____

**CL APPOINTMENT TYPE:   CLD-____ ☐   CLRF-____ ☐   CL CHECK ☐**   If new lenses, lens type_____ Tech Initials_____

**Date:**_____ AWT_____ WTT_____ Replace lenses every_____ Age of lenses_____

**Subjective Symptoms:** Vision: _____
Comfort: _____
Handling: _____

| DIST VA | NEAR VA | AUTOREFRACTION | | SOR | | SCOR | |
|---|---|---|---|---|---|---|---|
| OD 20/ | 20/ | OD | | OD | 20/ | OD | 20/ |
| OS 20/ | 20/ | OS | | OS | 20/ | OS | 20/ |
| OU 20/ | 20/ | | | | | | |

BIOMICROSCOPY
OD          OS

LENS POSITION
Center   OD          OS
Lag      OD          OS
Orient/  OD          OS
Fl.ptn

LENS INSPECTION
OD          OS

Assessment: _____  Plan: _____

Dr.'s Signature: _____  RTC: _____ Dr.____

## CONTACT LENS RECORD—cont'd

**CL APPOINTMENT TYPE: CLD-____ ☐   CLRF-____ ☐   CL CHECK ☐**   If new lenses, lens type_____ Tech Initials_____

**Date:_____ AWT_____ WTT_____ Replace lenses every_____ Age of lenses_____**

**Subjective Symptoms: Vision:** _____

Comfort: _____

Handling: _____

| DIST VA | NEAR VA | AUTOREFRACTION | | SOR | | SCOR | |
|---------|---------|----------------|----|-----|-----|------|-----|
| OD 20/ | 20/ | OD | | OD | 20/ | OD | 20/ |
| OS 20/ | 20/ | OS | | OS | 20/ | OS | 20/ |
| OU 20/ | 20/ | | | | | | |

**BIOMICROSCOPY**     **LENS POSITION**     **LENS INSPECTION**

OD    OS      Center OD    OS      OD    OS

Lag OD    OS

Orient/ OD    OS

Fl.ptn

Assessment: _____    Plan: _____

Dr.'s Signature: _____    RTC:    Dr.____

---

**CL APPOINTMENT TYPE: CLD-____ ☐   CLRF-____ ☐   CL CHECK ☐**   If new lenses, lens type_____ Tech Initials_____

**Date:_____ AWT_____ WTT_____ Replace lenses every_____ Age of lenses_____**

**Subjective Symptoms: Vision:** _____

Comfort: _____

Handling: _____

| DIST VA | NEAR VA | AUTOREFRACTION | | SOR | | SCOR | |
|---------|---------|----------------|----|-----|-----|------|-----|
| OD 20/ | 20/ | OD | | OD | 20/ | OD | 20/ |
| OS 20/ | 20/ | OS | | OS | 20/ | OS | 20/ |
| OU 20/ | 20/ | | | | | | |

**BIOMICROSCOPY**     **LENS POSITION**     **LENS INSPECTION**

OD    OS      Center OD    OS      OD    OS

Lag OD    OS

Orient/ OD    OS

Fl.ptn

Assessment: _____    Plan: _____

Dr.'s Signature: _____    RTC:    Dr.____

---

**CL APPOINTMENT TYPE: CLD-____ ☐   CLRF-____ ☐   CL CHECK ☐**   If new lenses, lens type_____ Tech Initials_____

**Date:_____ AWT_____ WTT_____ Replace lenses every_____ Age of lenses_____**

**Subjective Symptoms: Vision:** _____

Comfort: _____

Handling: _____

| DIST VA | NEAR VA | AUTOREFRACTION | | SOR | | SCOR | |
|---------|---------|----------------|----|-----|-----|------|-----|
| OD 20/ | 20/ | OD | | OD | 20/ | OD | 20/ |
| OS 20/ | 20/ | OS | | OS | 20/ | OS | 20/ |
| OU 20/ | 20/ | | | | | | |

**BIOMICROSCOPY**     **LENS POSITION**     **LENS INSPECTION**

OD    OS      Center OD    OS      OD    OS

Lag OD    OS

Orient/ OD    OS

Fl.ptn

Assessment: _____    Plan: _____

Dr.'s Signature: _____    RTC:    Dr.____

| ORDERED | DISPENSED | OD | OS | LENS BRAND/TYPE | RETURNED DATE |
|---------|-----------|----|----|-----------------|---------------|
| | | | | | |
| | | | | | |
| | | | | | |
| | | | | | |
| | | | | | |
| | | | | | |
| | | | | | |
| | | | | | |
| | | | | | |

# Contact Lens Policies

### Basic Fees During Fitting and Evaluation Period

Our fees for contact lenses include all examinations, progress visits, and materials during the fitting period. There will be no additional charges for changes in lens type or power during this period unless you have a special request not covered by this policy. The fitting period includes all examinations and progress visits until the doctor is satisfied you have a proper fit. Thereafter you will need either annual or semiannual examinations that are not included in the fitting fee.

### Your Responsibility

It is important to periodically evaluate your contact lenses after they have been worn. Depending on the type of lens, this evaluation may be several days, weeks, or months from the initial fitting. Failure to return for a progress examination may jeopardize the health of your eyes as well as cause unnecessary discomfort. If you cannot keep an appointment, please advise our office as soon as possible in advance of the appointment so that we may schedule another patient at your time. It is your responsibility to reschedule any progress examinations that have been cancelled.

### Fees

The total fee for your contact lenses is not due until they are dispensed. If you or the doctor later decide that contact lenses prove to be unsatisfactory for you and a decision is made to terminate the fitting procedure, you will pay only for the professional time spent in examinations and fittings up to that time. A refund will be issued for the balance.

### Loss and Insurance

Contact lens insurance for specialty lenses is available through our office. It is optional and the cost of the insurance is not included in the fitting fee. The replacement cost of a nondisposable contact lens will include one progress visit to evaluate the fit of a replacement lens. If a new or replacement lens performs in a defective manner, please return it to our office as soon as possible. The manufacturer warrants all contact lenses for a limited time period.

If you have any questions concerning either finances or the fitting of your contact lenses, please ask.

Thank you,

Dr. _____ and Staff

# Contact Lens Selection Questionnaire

Please circle the appropriate response for each question. The purpose of this form is to help determine what type of lens will be best for you and how easily you will adapt to contact lenses.

1. Environment you live in
   a. Clean air (rural)
   b. Mildly polluted (suburban)
   c. Polluted (urban)
   d. Highly polluted (industrial)

2. Allergies
   a. None
   b. Mild
   c. Moderate
   d. Severe

3. Skin type
   a. Normal
   b. Dry or oily
   c. Sensitive

4. Medications
   Antihistamines
   a. Never use
   b. Use occasionally for cold
   c. Use more than once a month
   Diuretics
   a. Never use
   b. Use less than once a week
   c. Use frequently
   Birth control pills
   a. No
   b. Yes

5. Tearing
   a. Normal
   b. Mild
   c. Excessive
   d. Dry (gritty feel)

6. Light sensitivity
   a. None
   b. Mild
   c. Moderate
   d. Severe

7. Eye itching
   a. None
   b. Mild
   c. Moderate
   d. Severe

8. Eye infection
   a. Never
   b. Rare (less than one per year)
   c. Frequent (more than one per year)
   d. Continual

9. Sensitivity to smoke and chemicals
   a. None
   b. Mild
   c. Moderate
   d. Severe

10. Anticipated contact lens wearing time
    a. Casual wear (few hours social wear on occasion)
    b. Less than 8 hours
    c. Over 8 hours
    d. Extended wear (more than 24 hours)

# Contact Lens Wearing Schedule

| Day | Date | Hours Worn | Max. Hours Recommended | Comments |
|-----|------|-----------|------------------------|----------|
| 1 | | | | |
| 2 | | | | |
| 3 | | | | |
| 4 | | | | |
| 5 | | | | |
| 6 | | | | |
| 7 | | | | |
| 8 | | | | |
| 9 | | | | |
| 10 | | | | |
| 11 | | | | |
| 12 | | | | |
| 13 | | | | |
| 14 | | | | |

Next appointment:

# Contact Lens "Dos and Don'ts"

To have comfortable and optimal use of your contact lenses, it is important that you follow these basic instructions on the care and cleaning of your lenses. An instructional session will be scheduled with you to teach proper lens insertion and removal as well as proper cleaning and care procedures.

Please review the following list of "dos and don'ts" and ask our staff any questions you may have.

## Dos

1. Before handling lenses, wash your hands with a mild soap.
2. Clean your lenses well.
3. Follow your wearing schedule.
4. Soak your lenses in the recommended soaking/storage solution when not wearing them.
5. Remove your lenses if discomfort or blurring occurs.
6. Use proper eye protection or sunwear when needed.
7. Keep appointment for follow-up care and remember to wear your lenses at least two hours before scheduled evaluations in our office.
8. Contact our office immediately if problems arise.
9. Keep an updated pair of eyeglasses for emergency and know where they are.
10. Use eye makeup designed for contact lens wearers.
11. Have a complete visual examination once a year.
12. Bring your glasses and contact lens case with you each time you come to the office.

## Don'ts

1. Overwear your lenses beyond the maximum recommended wearing schedule.
2. Sleep with your lenses unless specifically advised to do so by your doctor.
3. Shower, sauna, or swim with your lenses (unless you use a mask or goggles for swimming).
4. Wear your lenses near aerosol sprays or noxious fumes.
5. Use any products other than those recommended by your doctor.
6. Take the advice of other contact lens wearers without consulting our office.

# Contact Lens Service Agreement

Date _____

Patient _____

Address _____

City _____ State _____ Zip _____

Fee for one year $ _____ Effective date _____ Expiration _____

Type of contact lens covered: R: _____ L: _____

Type of lens: Soft ___        Toric ___        Bifocal ___        Opaque ___        Gas permeable ___

While this agreement is in effect, we agree to:

Unlimited replacement of the covered contact lenses at the reduced cost of $_____ regardless of loss or damage.

Provide contact lens progress evaluation every _____ months.

Supply contact lens solutions at a discount of _____ %.

Polishing of gas permeable lenses, if required, at a discount of _____%.

All other eyewear (sunglasses, reading glasses, driving glasses, etc.) at a discount of _____%.

Other professional services and materials not specifically listed above will be at our usual and customary fees.

This agreement is only valid for use by the patient named above and at the office where issued.

# Six Contact Lens Comfort Lens Plans

Your eyecare professional will recommend the type of contact lenses and plan that best suits your vision correction needs and lifestyle.

With the Comfort Lens Plan, you know exactly how much you will spend on complete contact lens care for the year, including all the necessary solutions and cleaners.

1. $_____Daily wear/flex-wear
   Lens replacement – quarterly
   4 pairs per year

2. $_____Daily wear/flex-wear
   Lens replacement – biweekly
   26 pairs per year

3. $_____Daily wear/flex-wear
   Tinted lenses
   Lens replacements – quarterly
   4 pairs per year

4. $_____1-Day contact lenses
   Lens replacement – daily
   360 pairs per year

5. $_____Daily wear bifocal lenses
   Lens replacement – quarterly
   4 pairs per year

6. $_____Daily wear/flex-wear
   Tinted lenses
   Lens replacement – biweekly
   26 pairs per year

For as little as one dollar a day, the annual Comfort Lens Plan provides you with the following at no additional charge:

- Annual comprehensive eye examination
- Glaucoma test
- Contact lens check-ups for 1 year
- All solutions for 1 year
- Care and handling instructions
- 20% off prescription glasses for 1 year
- Multiple pairs of contact lenses

# Fresh Lens Planned Replacement Program

## Why Fresh Lens Is Important

The goal of the Fresh Lens Program is to provide you with a convenient, carefree, and safe contact lens regimen.

When your scheduled quarterly contact lens wear period is over, simply throw away the used lenses and replace them with fresh, sterile ones.

By replacing your lenses on a regular schedule, you:

- Minimize lens deposits, a major source of contact lens discomfort and potential eye health complications
- Enjoy cleaner, safer, more comfortable and convenient contact lens wear
- Always have a spare pair

## What's Included

The Fresh Lens Program provides professional eyecare services, planned replacement of your contact lenses, and solutions and cleaning agents for a full year.

## Quarterly Fresh Lens Program

- Yearly comprehensive eye examination
- Care and treatment
- Contact lens check-up for 1 year
- Lenses (four pairs of contact lenses)
- Handling and care instructions
- Solutions

Cost: $ _____

# Contact Lens Maximum Wearing Schedule

Congratulations! The fitting procedures were successful and you are taking your contact lenses home. It is important to adhere to the prescribed *maximum* contact lens wearing schedule. Regular follow-up care is also extremely important.

### Maximum Wearing Schedule

| | |
|---|---|
| Day 1 | 4 hours |
| Day 2 | 5 hours |
| Day 3 | 6 hours |
| Day 4 | 7 hours |
| Day 5 | 8 hours |
| Day 6 | 9 hours |
| Day 7 | 10 hours |

If you are unable to see us 7 days after the dispensing of your lenses, maintain a maximum of 10 hours of wear until you are able to be seen in our office.

Please wear your contact lenses for the next appointment. If your lenses are comfortable and your eyes are not red, wear the lenses for at least 2 hours before the visit.

## Patient Recommendations

1. If at any time you experience any redness, irritation, discomfort, discharge, or blurring of your vision while wearing your lenses, please remove the lens, clean it, and reapply it. If the problem persists, remove the lens and contact us immediately.
2. Your lenses should NOT be worn while sleeping unless your doctor instructs you that it is appropriate.
3. Your lenses should NOT be worn while in the presence of noxious or irritating vapors.
4. Do NOT swim with your lenses in place.
5. Remove your lenses during a cold, influenza, or hospitalization. Clean and place the lenses in your disinfection system as soon as possible.

# Dilation of Your Pupils

We recommend that your pupils be dilated so that we may more thoroughly evaluate the health of the inside of your eyes under the best conditions. Dilating the pupils is necessary for the best evaluation of many eye conditions, such as cataracts, glaucoma, macular degeneration, retinal detachment, and other potentially sight-threatening conditions. It is necessary for the earliest detection of these serious conditions. Without dilation, it is often not possible to detect these conditions.

Drops will be placed in your eyes to enlarge your pupils. When the pupils are enlarged, you will likely find:

- Increased sensitivity to light. Please bring your sunglasses to wear home. We may also provide dilation sunglasses for your comfort.
- Blurred vision, especially close up. You may have difficulty reading or doing desk work.
- Difficulty driving because of increased glare, sensitivity to light, and blurred vision. It is best to have someone drive you.
- The effects of dilation will usually last from 2 to 6 hours.

Please ask us any questions you may have. We provide dilation for the best care of your eyes and your vision. If you experience any problems after dilation, please feel free to call us. We have a doctor on call at all times for our patient's needs.

Your appointment for dilation is:    _____

## EXAMINATION FORM

| Examination Form | Date: | |
|---|---|---|
| Name:<br>Address:<br>City/state:<br>Home: (   )          DOB:<br>Work: (   ) | Present Rx    From_____ Type_____<br>OD_____<br>OS_____<br>Add | **Technician Initials**<br>_____ |

CC: (Location/quality/severity/duration/context/assoc. signs/symptoms)

| | | (D)        (N) | |
|---|---|---|---|
| **AR OD**_____<br>　　**OS** _____<br>**AK OD**_____<br>　　**OS** _____ | **Vsc  OD**<br>　　**OS**<br>　　**OU** | 20/_____ 20/_____<br>20/_____ 20/_____<br>20/_____ 20/_____ | **CT**　　(D)_____ (N)_____<br>**EOMs** ☐ SAFE OU_____<br>**NPC** ☐ TTN _____<br>**Pupils** ☐ ERRL(A)-APD OU_____<br>**CF** ☐ FTFC OU_____ |
| **Color:**　/6OD　　/6OS<br>**Stereo:**　"Circles　PD_____<br>**Phoria: (H)**　　　**(V)** | **Vcc  OD**<br>　　**OS**<br>　　**OU** | 20/_____ 20/_____<br>20/_____ 20/_____<br>20/_____ 20/_____ | **BP**　　/　　@<br>**Pulse**　　bpm |

| | OD | |
|---|---|---|
| | OS | |
| | OD | |
| **MR** | OS | |
| | | |
| | | |
| | | |
| **PRA (−)** | | |
| **NRA (+)** | | |
| **OD** | | **OS** |

**DPAs** | F ☐ Prop. ☐ T0.5% ☐ T1.0% ☐ P2.5% ☐ C1.0% ☐ OD  OS  OU
@

| **SLEx** | **OD** | **OS** |
|---|---|---|
| **L/L** | ☐ Cl | ☐ Cl |
| **Conj.** | ☐ Cl | ☐ Cl |
| **Tears** | ☐ Cl | ☐ Cl |
| **Cornea** | ☐ Cl | ☐ Cl |
| **Iris** | ☐ Flat/Intact | ☐ Flat/Intact |
| **A/C** | ☐ D/Q | ☐ D/Q |
| **Ta** | OD        mm Hg | OD        mm Hg @ |

| **Internal** | **OD** | **OS** |
|---|---|---|
| **Lens**<br>**Media** | ☐ Cl<br>☐ Cl | ☐ Cl<br>☐ Cl |
| **Disc** | C/D | C/D |
| **Vessels** | ☐ 2/3 AV, 1/5 ALR | ☐ 2/3 AV, 1/5 ALR |
| **Macula** | ☐ +FR/Cl | ☐ +FR/Cl |
| **Retina** | ☐ WNLs OD | ☐ WNLs OD |

**Assessment**

|  | HS | EX | DM |
|---|---|---|---|
| | P | P | S |
| | E | E | L |
| | D | D | M |
| | C | C | H |

**Plan**

Patient educated on conditions and recommended treatments.
RTC    3mo    6mo    1yr    2yr_____ for
DR'S. SIGNATURE                              , O.D.

Date    /  /    For: Constant Wear ☐  D ☐  N ☐

| | Sphere | Cylinder | Axis | Prism | Base |
|---|---|---|---|---|---|
| O.D. | | | | | |
| O.S. | | | | | |
| Add | | Seg Ht. | Dist PD | Near PD | |
| O.D. | | | | | |
| O.S. | | | | | |
| Type | | | Tint | | |
| Frame | | | Coating | | |
| Eyesize | | DBL | Color | | |
| Temples | | Inv# | | Lab | |

Date    /  /    For:

| | Sphere | Cylinder | Axis | Prism | Base |
|---|---|---|---|---|---|
| O.D. | | | | | |
| O.S. | | | | | |
| Add | | Seg Ht. | Dist PD | Near PD | |
| O.D. | | | | | |
| O.S. | | | | | |
| Type | | | Tint | | |
| Frame | | | Coating | | |
| Eyesize | | DBL | Color | | |
| Temples | | Inv# | | Lab | |

# Excusal from School (Proof of Appointment Slip)

Date: _____

Patient: _____

To whom it may concern:

The above patient was seen at this office on this day of _____ at _____.

Sincerely,

Receptionist for the office of Dr. _____

## General Eye Exam: Diabetes Study

Patient: _____     Date: _____
           Last Name        First Name

**1. Brief History (including stability of vision):**

**2. Acuity:**    OD:_____/20    OS:_____/20

            OD/ph:_____/20   OS/ph:_____/20

**3. Anterior Segment:**    **OD**           **OS**

                             L/L

                             C/S

                             K

                             AC

                             I

                             L

**4. IOP:**    OD:_____mm Hg    OS:_____mm Hg    Time: _____

**5. Disc Appearence (circle):**    OD normal    OD abnormal [comment:_____]

                                 OS normal    OS abnormal [comment:_____]

**6. Fundus Abnormalities (DR and any other):**

**OD:**                       **OS:**

| Check box | Normal | Abnormal |
|---|---|---|
| M: | | |
| BV: | | |
| P: | | |

| Check box | Normal | Abnormal |
|---|---|---|
| M: | | |
| BV: | | |
| P: | | |

# Care Instructions for Frames and Lenses

Eyeglass frames will get out of adjustment for many reasons. The proper alignment and fit of your frames is critical to ensuring your best vision. For that reason, feel free to return to our office for periodic adjustment. There is no charge for this service.

CARE OF LENSES: Lenses need to be cleaned with care to avoid scratching. Rinse lenses thoroughly under tap water to remove dirt and debris. Use a lens cleaner or mild liquid dishwashing soap and rinse in cool tap water. Dry with a soft cotton cloth. DO NOT use tissues or paper towels. Remember to use a properly maintained case when not wearing your glasses and protect the lens surfaces.

CARE OF FRAMES: Always use two hands when placing frames on or off your face so as not to bend or stress the frames. If frames become too loose, bring them to our office for an adjustment. DO NOT try to bend them yourself.

In case of loss or breakage we always recommend a second pair of eyeglasses as a back-up. If your prior pair will not adequately serve this need, let us know. Our laboratories offer a _____% discount on second pairs when ordered at the same time.

Remember that taking care of your eyewear will prolong its satisfactory use and is important to good vision and comfort!

Dr. _____ and Staff

# Frame Breakage Release

I am aware that by using old or used frames there is a possibility of breakage. I will not hold Dr. _____,
the office staff, or the laboratory responsible if these frames should break during lens insertion or adjustment.

Date _____

Signature _____

# Patient Prescription Laboratory and Frame Inventory Record

| Patient name | Exam date | Order date | Lab | Tray | Name of frame, size, color | Rx received | Frame received | Date received | Date called | Date dispensed | Follow-up or comments |
|---|---|---|---|---|---|---|---|---|---|---|---|
| | | | | | | | | | | | |
| | | | | | | | | | | | |
| | | | | | | | | | | | |
| | | | | | | | | | | | |
| | | | | | | | | | | | |
| | | | | | | | | | | | |
| | | | | | | | | | | | |
| | | | | | | | | | | | |
| | | | | | | | | | | | |
| | | | | | | | | | | | |
| | | | | | | | | | | | |
| | | | | | | | | | | | |
| | | | | | | | | | | | |
| | | | | | | | | | | | |

# Informed Consent or Refusal for Dilated Fundus Exam

Dilation involves instilling eye drops for the purpose of enlarging the pupils of the eyes to better check the health of the inside of the eyes.

The pupils are simply an entry way/opening to the inside of the eye. Looking through an *undilated* pupil is similar to looking into a room through a keyhole in the door; the doctor may see only about 20% to 50% of what is inside. However, looking through a *dilated* pupil is like looking into a room through an open door; the doctor gets a complete view of the inside of the eye.

A dilated fundus exam is recommended routinely at the time of your initial exam for baseline recording and usually every other full eye exam thereafter (about every 2 to 3 years). It should be done annually if you have any of the conditions listed under **Benefits** below.

## Benefits

Dilation allows the doctor a better view of the peripheral retina for disease. It is highly recommended if you or your family has a history of high blood pressure, diabetes, past retinal problems (i.e., retinal detachment/tears), or extreme nearsightedness. It is also recommended if you have experienced sudden cloudiness of vision, especially in one eye, "curtain or veil-like" obstruction of vision, a sudden onset of many "floaters," or flashing lights off to the side of your vision.

## Risks

- Some blurring of vision and glare because of enlarged pupils for about 2 (but up to 6) hours. You should not operate heavy equipment or drive an automobile unless you are comfortable with your vision.
- Difficulty with near reading for 1 to 2 hours. The focusing ability is impaired and may cause a slight headache if you try to read.
- Induced ocular hypertension. Rare cases have been reported in which redness and sharp pain are experienced because of increased eye pressure. If this happens, contact the doctor immediately.

Check one:

❑ I understand the above and consent to have dilation done.

❑ I understand the above and decline dilation at this time. I understand that potential for partial or total loss of vision may exist and, without dilation, may go undetected.

**I have read and understand the above.**

Signature: _____ Date: _____

## GLAUCOMA FLOWSHEET

| PATIENT NAME: | | | | | | | DIAGNOSIS: | | | |

| DATE OF VISIT | DIAGNOSIS VAs | | C/D | | IOP | | | VF/TYPE | PHOTOS | TREATMENT |
|---|---|---|---|---|---|---|---|---|---|---|
| | OD | OS | OD | OS | OD | OS | TIME | | | |
| | | | | | | | | | | |
| | | | | | | | | | | |
| | | | | | | | | | | |
| | | | | | | | | | | |
| | | | | | | | | | | |
| | | | | | | | | | | |
| | | | | | | | | | | |
| | | | | | | | | | | |
| | | | | | | | | | | |
| | | | | | | | | | | |
| | | | | | | | | | | |
| | | | | | | | | | | |
| | | | | | | | | | | |
| | | | | | | | | | | |
| | | | | | | | | | | |
| | | | | | | | | | | |
| | | | | | | | | | | |
| | | | | | | | | | | |
| | | | | | | | | | | |
| | | | | | | | | | | |
| | | | | | | | | | | |
| | | | | | | | | | | |
| | | | | | | | | | | |
| | | | | | | | | | | |
| | | | | | | | | | | |
| | | | | | | | | | | |
| | | | | | | | | | | |
| | | | | | | | | | | |
| | | | | | | | | | | |
| | | | | | | | | | | |
| | | | | | | | | | | |
| | | | | | | | | | | |
| | | | | | | | | | | |

# Health Insurance Portability and Accountability Act (HIPAA) of 1996

## What is HIPAA?

The Health Insurance Portability and Accountability Act (HIPAA) of 1996 was signed into law by former President Bill Clinton on August 21, 1996. Conclusive regulations were issued on August 17, 2000, to be instated by October 16, 2002. HIPAA requires that the transactions of all patient healthcare information be formatted in a standardized electronic style. In addition to protecting the privacy and security of patient information, HIPAA includes legislation on the formation of medical savings accounts, the authorization of a fraud and abuse control program, the easy transport of health insurance coverage, and the simplification of administrative terms and conditions.

## What does HIPAA cover?

HIPAA encompasses three primary areas, and its privacy requirements can be broken down into three types: privacy standards, patients' rights, and administrative requirements.

**1. Privacy Standards.** A central concern of HIPAA is the careful use and disclosure of protected health information (PHI), which generally is electronically controlled health information that is able to be distinguished individually. PHI also refers to verbal communication, although the HIPAA Privacy Rule is not intended to hinder necessary verbal communication. The U.S. Department of Health and Human Services (USDHHS) does not require restructuring, such as soundproofing, architectural changes, and so forth, but some caution is necessary when exchanging health information by conversation.

An Acknowledgment of Receipt Notice of Privacy Practices, which allows patient information to be used or divulged for treatment, payment, or healthcare operations (TPO), should be procured from each patient. A detailed and time-sensitive authorization can also be issued, which allows the optometrist to release information in special circumstances other than TPOs. A *written consent* is also an option. Optometrists can disclose PHI *without* acknowledgment, consent, or authorization in very special situations, for example, perceived child abuse, public health supervision, fraud investigation, or law enforcement with valid permission (i.e., a warrant). When divulging PHI, an optometrist must try to disclose only the *minimum necessary* information, to help safeguard the patient's information as much as possible.

It is important that eye care professionals adhere to HIPAA standards because healthcare providers (as well as healthcare clearinghouses and healthcare plans) who convey *electronically* formatted health information via an outside billing service or merchant are considered *covered entities*. Covered entities may be dealt serious civil and criminal penalties for violation of HIPAA legislation. Failure to comply with HIPAA privacy requirements may result in civil penalties of up to $100 per offense with an annual maximum of $25,000 for repeated failure to comply with the same requirement. Criminal penalties resulting from the illegal mishandling of private health information can range from $50,000 and/or 1 year in prison to $250,000 and/or 10 years in prison.

**2. Patients' Rights.** HIPAA allows patients, authorized representatives, and parents of minors, as well as minors, to become more aware of the health information privacy to which they are entitled. These rights include, but are not limited to, the right to view and copy their health information, the right to dispute alleged breaches of policies and regulations, and the right to request alternative forms of communicating with their optometrist. If any health information is released for any reason other than TPO, the patient is entitled to an account of the transaction. Therefore, it is important for optometrists to keep accurate records of such information and to provide them when necessary.

The HIPAA Privacy Rule determines that the parents of a minor have access to their child's health information. This privilege may be overruled, for example, in cases where there is suspected child abuse or the parent consents to a term of confidentiality between the optometrist and the minor. The parents' rights to access their child's PHI also may be restricted in situations when a legal entity, such as a court, intervenes and when a law does not require a parent's consent. For a full list of patient rights provided by HIPAA, be sure to acquire a copy of the law and to understand it well.

**3. Administrative Requirements.** Complying with HIPAA legislation may seem like a chore, but it does not need to be so. It is recommended that you become appropriately familiar with the law, organize the requirements into simpler tasks, begin compliance early, and document your progress in compliance. An important first step is to evaluate the current information and practices of your office.

Optometrists will need to write a *privacy policy* for their office, a document for their patients detailing the office's practices concerning PHI. It is useful to try to understand the role of healthcare information for your patients and the ways in which they deal with the information while they are visiting your office. Train your staff; make sure they are familiar with the terms of HIPAA and your office's privacy policy and related forms. HIPAA requires that you designate a *privacy officer*, a person in your office who will be responsible for applying the new policies in your office, fielding complaints, and making choices involving the minimum necessary requirements. Another person with the role of *contact person* will process complaints.

A *Notice of Privacy Practices*—a document detailing the patient's rights and the eye care office's obligations concerning PHI—also must be drawn up. Further, any role of a third party with access to PHI must be clearly documented. This third party is known as a *business associate* (BA) and is defined as any entity who, on behalf of the optometrist, takes part in any activity that involves exposure of PHI.

*Continued*

## Health Insurance Portability and Accountability Act (HIPAA) of 1996—cont'd

### For More Information on HIPAA

Web sites that may contain useful information about HIPAA are:

- USDHHS Office of Civil Rights: www.hhs.gov/ocr/hipaa
- Work Group on Electronic Data Interchange: www.wedi.org/SNIP
- Phoenix Health: www.hipaadvisory.com
- USDHHS Office of the Assistant Secretary for Planning and Evaluation: http://aspe.os.dhhs.gov/admnsimp/

# How the Health Insurance Portability and Accountability Act (HIPAA) Will Affect Your Eye Care Visit

The U.S. Department of Health and Human Services has issued national health information privacy standards. The Health Insurance Portability and Accountability Act, a federally mandated law known as HIPAA, is designed to:
- provide protection for the privacy of certain identifiable health data (called *protected health information [PHI]*),
- ensure health insurance coverage when changing employers, and
- provide standards for facilitating electronic transfers of health care–related information.

While the privacy of your personal PHI will remain confidential, certain aspects of this law will permit disclosures of PHI to facilitate public health activities. The following charts review the types of health data disclosure allowed under HIPAA.

---

### PHI can be disclosed with your authorization in the following categories.

You may request a limitation or restriction on the disclosure of this information. You have the right to:
- request a restriction or limit of any of the above disclosures used for treatment, payment, or office operations.
- inspect and copy information that may be used to make decisions about your care.
- request an amendment of this information if you feel it is incorrect or incomplete.
- an accounting of disclosures we have made that were not related to treatment, payment, or operations of this office.

These requests must be submitted in writing to the office manager and you will be informed of the specifics that are required for this request.

*Treatment*—PHI will be used to provide appropriate treatment either by this office or other healthcare providers, diagnostic or fabrication laboratories.

*Payment*—PHI will be used to facilitate payment for treatment rendered. Your health plan requires this information in order to bill, collect payments, or obtain approval prior to treatment.

*Healthcare Operations*—In order to ensure all patients receive timely and quality care, PHI will be used to facilitate the daily operations of our practice. These include, but are not limited to:
- clinical/research studies to improve our practice
- appointment reminders by phone calls or mailings
- sign-in sheets used to notify us of your arrival
- posted appointment schedules
- information regarding your treatment options or related benefits and services
- communications with family or friends that are involved in your care or payment for your care

### PHI can be disclosed without your authorization in the following categories.

| As Required by Law | Judicial and Administrative Proceedings | Oversight |
|---|---|---|
| | | PHI can be disclosed to a health oversight agency as authorized by law for audits, investigations, inspections, and licensure. |
| **Public Health** | **Lawsuits and Disputes** | **Workers' Compensation**<br>PHI may be released to workers' compensation or similar programs that provide benefits for work-related injuries or illness. |
| **Public Health Risks** | **Law Enforcement** | **Military and Veterans** |
| **Health Research**<br>PHI disclosures are permitted when required by federal, state, tribal, or local laws. | **Coroners and Medical Examiners**<br>Release of PHI to officials will occur: in response to a court order, subpoena, discovery request or summons; to identify a suspected fugitive, witness, or missing person; about a victim of crime if unable to obtain permission from the person; to identify a deceased person, determine cause of death, about a death that is believed to be the result of criminal conduct; criminal conduct occurring at the practice; in emergency situations. | **National Security and Intelligence Activities** |
| **Abuse, Neglect, or Domestic Violence**<br>PHI can be disclosed to prevent a threat to your health and safety or the health and safety of others. | **Cadaver Organ, Eye, or Tissue Donations**<br>PHI disclosure can be made to organ banks as necessary to facilitate organ or tissue donation and transplantation. | **Protective Services for the President and Others**<br>PHI may be released as authorized by law when requested by military command authorities, federal officials for national security, and protection of the president and other heads of state. |

# Inactive Notice

Dear _____:

It has been _____ years since we last had the opportunity of seeing you and taking care of your visual needs. We have enjoyed having you as a patient and would like the chance to continue to provide you with the quality eye care service and care that you deserve.

If you have chosen another office to care for your needs, please let us know so we may remove your records from the active file. Our office will always be available to you in the future if the need arises.

Sincerely,

Dr. _____ and Staff

# Informed Consent for In-Office Procedures

Permission is hereby granted for any therapeutic treatment, injections, anesthesia, operations, removal of tissue, and disposal of tissue as may be deemed advisable or necessary by the attending doctors on staff. Risks, complications, and treatment options have been discussed with me by the treating doctor and I understand these.

Date_____

Procedure to be performed_____

Patient Name_____     Signature_____

Witness_____     Signature_____

Physician Name_____ OD Signature_____

# Insurance Information

Name of Employer _____

Name of Insurance Company _____

Insurance Billing Address    _____

_____

Policy # _____ Group # _____

| | |
|---|---|
| Patient name | |
| Patient DOB | |
| Insured's name | |
| Insured DOB | |
| Insured's ID / SS# | |

## Benefits

| | How Often | # Allowed | Insurance to Pay | Patient to Pay |
|---|---|---|---|---|
| Exam | | | | |
| Frame | | | | |
| SV | | | | |
| BF | | | | |
| TF | | | | |
| Prog | | | | |
| Contacts | | | | |

## Eligibility

| | Now Eligible | Not Until |
|---|---|---|
| Exam | yes    no | |
| Frame | yes    no | |
| Lenses | yes    no | |
| Contacts | yes    no | |
| Deductible | | |
| Co-pay | | |
| Auth. % | | |
| | | |
| | | |

# called _____

Date called _____

Person contacted _____

# Vision Insurance Coverage

### Responsibility for Payment

Your employer, management, or union has purchased vision insurance coverage from a selection of plans offered by an insurance company or broker. Each insurance company offers many different plans. The type of vision benefits that are covered relate to the dollar amount spent on the benefit package. Generally, the more money spent on a plan, the more services are covered. Most vision insurance covers only 50% to 80% of the cost of treatment. Laboratory services (frames, lenses and contact lenses) are usually only covered at a 50% rate.

The fees charged for vision treatment reflect the many different parts of a particular procedure or procedures. Treatment for your particular needs may or may not fall within the limits set by your particular vision plan. Many vision procedures may not even be listed in your insurance's procedure/payment schedule. If your vision procedure falls into this category, you may not receive any insurance reimbursement for that procedure. **You are ultimately responsible for paying the entire fee for an accepted vision treatment, regardless of your insurance coverage**.

### Choosing Treatment Options

Our goal through your examination, diagnosis, and treatment phases is to provide you with the best possible vision health. We do not allow the insurance company to tell us how to treat you. We recommend to you those treatments that we believe you need and we will discuss alternative plans with you. Whether or not the recommended treatment is a covered vision benefit is between you and your employer and the insurance carrier.

### Submitting the Claim

We are happy to help you receive the maximum benefits you are allowed from your vision coverage. In order for us to submit your insurance claim, we will need an insurance form with your portion completed and signed. We deal with vision insurance companies on a daily basis; therefore, we have a great deal of experience submitting these claims to insurance carriers. We take great care in submitting claims properly the first time. There are three things we **cannot** do: 1) Alter the date of treatment; 2) Submit a claim for more than the actual fee; 3) Submit a claim for procedures that have not been performed. Because it is not at all uncommon for the insurance carriers to make a mistake, we would prefer to submit the claims ourselves, and then verify proper payment. Insurance carriers may respond to requests for payment of preauthorized treatment in as little as a week or as long as 45 days. Please be patient; we have no control over the post office or the speed with which the insurance carrier processes your claim.

Our office cannot negotiate with your insurance company for reimbursement of eye care expenses. Only the purchaser of the plan (your employer) can negotiate better coverage. If you would like better or more coverage, you will need to talk with your plan purchaser about the features you want in your vision plan.

**If you have any questions about your vision insurance coverage, please feel free to ask us.**

# Vision Insurance: Points to Consider

The following is a plain-language synopsis of most vision insurance contracts. Please read it carefully, and perhaps keep it for future reference.

✓ Vision insurance benefits do not work in the same way as medical insurance. There is ***almost always a co-payment*** due from the patient for ***almost every*** procedure.

✓ There are "deductibles" in all plans.

✓ Insurance companies do not typically provide seminars or instruction books on the best method to obtain the highest financial reimbursement benefits for the patient.

✓ Irrespective of any vision insurance benefits that might exist, the patient is always legally responsible for the entire cost of vision treatment.

✓ The extent of vision coverage is solely dependent on the vision insurance plan purchased by the employer. The higher the premium the employer pays, the greater the vision insurance benefits.

✓ Even if there is a written predetermination of benefits returned from the insurance carrier, it is possible that after treatment is provided, there are no insurance benefits payable.

✓ We (your optometrist's office) have absolutely no power or leverage to deal with the insurance carrier. Only the employee or the contract purchaser has power. Any complaints about benefits, payment, or coverage should be directed to Human Resources or the company owner.

✓ The letters *UCR* on insurance vouchers stand for *Usual, Customary, and Reasonable* fee. The dollar amount you see as UCR has no basis in reality. It is an arbitrary amount determined solely by the plan selected and insurance premium paid by the employee. There is no relationship to the actual office fee. The better the plan (i.e., the more premium paid), the higher the UCR will be.

✓ A single insurance carrier may have a dozen different UCR fees for the same procedure, same office, and same optometrist.

✓ There is no universal coverage and payment schedule established. Just because an insurance code describing a eye care service exists, it does not guarantee that it will be a paid benefit under your policy. There are many eye care procedures that are necessary, and many of them are preventive or cosmetic, but are not covered benefits.

✓ Financial benefits cannot be saved and carried over into the next year.

Your vision benefits almost always have a yearly maximum contribution level. This amount is the MOST your insurance carrier is contractually obligated to pay during a defined year (calendar or otherwise). When this amount is reached, there will be no further vision benefits payable until the next benefit year. If you have already begun some additional vision treatment prior to the maximum being reached, the insurance carrier has no payment obligation beyond that of the annual maximum.

# Determination of Insurance Benefits

(Date)

Dear (patient name),

We have received the completed predetermination of benefits from your insurance carrier. You may also have received a copy of this predetermination of benefits form.

When you are ready to begin treatment, please call our office to review the treatment plan details and make the appropriate financial arrangements. Please note that your plan may have a limitation that requires treatment to begin within a set time period. When treatment does not begin within the set time period, the predetermination status may be canceled by your insurance carrier.

Sincerely,

# Information Request

Date:

Dear (Patient):

In order to properly process and submit your vision insurance claim form for treatment provided on (date), we will need the following information (see below). For your convenience, a self-addressed stamped return envelope has been enclosed.

❑ Please fill out the entire enclosed form.

❑ Please fill out the entire patient portion of the enclosed form.

❑ Please sign the enclosed form in all places marked with an X.

❑ Please contact us concerning your claim form.

Thank you in advance for your prompt attention to this matter.

Sincerely,

# Preauthorization of Payment

I, (name of payer), authorize (name of eye care office) to keep my signature on file and to charge my
      ❑ VISA        ❑ MasterCard      ❑ Other _____
the balance of charges not paid by vision insurance immediately on receipt of vision insurance co-payment or the balance of charges not paid within 30 days of completion of eye care treatment and not to exceed $_____ for ❑ this appointment only ❑ all appointments this year.
     Recurring charges for ongoing treatment or completed treatment of $_____ every
❑ week    ❑ month from (date) to (date). I assign my vision insurance benefits to the above-named provider. I understand that this form is valid for 1 year from the date noted below unless I cancel authorization of the provider in writing.


    Patient Name:
    Cardholder Name:
    Cardholder Address:
    City, State, and Zip Code:
    Credit Card Account #:          Expiration Date:


    _____     _____

    Cardholder Signature     Date

# Lifestyle Questionnaire

**Name** _____ **Date** _____

To better meet your visual needs, the doctor would like to know which activities you participate in. Please circle all that apply.

Bowling
Golf
Tennis
Fishing
Flying
Driving
Hunting
Exercise
Playing piano/other instruments
Sewing/arts and crafts
Bookkeeping
Computer
Reading
Boating
Playing cards
Biking

| | | |
|---|---|---|
| Are you satisfied with your distance and reading vision? | Yes | No |
| Are you satisfied with your present frames and types of lenses? | Yes | No |
| Do you wear sunglasses? | Yes | No |
| Does the glare from headlights bother your eyes? | Yes | No |
| Are you interested in information on LASIK refractive surgery? | Yes | No |

How many hours a day do you operate a computer? _____

# Patient Information Form

Name_____ DOB_____

Address_____ Telephone_____

City_____ State_____ Zip_____

Occupational or School _____

Relative or Friend:     Name_____

Address_____

City_____ State_____ Zip_____

Telephone_____ Relationship_____

Last eye examination: Approximate date_____ Doctor_____

Are you currently under treatment by an eye doctor? _____ If so, who? _____

Has your vision changed in the past 6 months? _____

Do you have eyeglasses? _____ Magnifiers?_____ Special vision aids? _____

Check which tasks listed below are difficult because of your vision problems:

Reading news headlines                 _____

Reading newsprint                      _____

Walking outdoors                       _____

Driving                                _____

Cooking                                _____

Shopping                               _____

Hobbies                                _____

Work or school activities              _____

Feel free to comment on any of the previous tasks that are difficult for you: _____

*Continued*

# Patient Information Form—cont'd

What visual tasks would you like us to help you with? _____

_____

_____

_____

List any problems with your general health: _____

_____

_____

_____

List any medications that you take regularly: _____

_____

Do you have health insurance such as Medicare or private insurance?

Specify insurance _____ Member number _____

Are you a United States veteran? _____

Who may we thank for referring you to our office? _____

# REFERRAL INFORMATION FORM

Dear Doctor:

This patient is making an appointment in our low vision center. We would greatly appreciate
your assistance in supplying the information requested below.

Patient's Name: _____

Date of Birth: _____

Address: _____

_____

Telephone: _____

**I request that the following information
be released to** _____

_____

_____
**(Patient's signature)**

\*　\*　\*　\*　\*　\*

Date of Last Examination: _____

Diagnosis: _____

_____

_____

Visual Acuity: _____

_____

Other: _____

_____

**Doctor's Signature:** _____

**Doctor's Name (Print):** _____

**Address:** _____

_____

**City/State/Zip:** _____

**Telephone:** _____

**UPIN #:** _____

# LOW VISION BILLING FORM

**Patient's Name:** _____   **Date:** _____

☐ Medicare              ☐ Private              ☐ Other:
_____

## PRESCRIBED DEVICES/AIDS

| CPT Code (V) | Catalog ID# (MI) | Item | Autorization Amount ($) | Status/Date | | | |
|---|---|---|---|---|---|---|---|
| | | | | O | A | H | D |
| | | | | | | | |
| | | | | | | | |
| | | | | | | | |
| | | | | | | | |
| | | | | | | | |
| | | | | | | | |
| | | | | | | | |

**Status Codes:** O = To be ordered; A = Awaiting approval; H = Held; D = Dispensed
**Codes:**
**V2600 =** hh low vision aids/tints/misc.
**V2610 =** sinigle lens - spectacle mounted (hi-add/optivisor/loops)
**V2615 =** telescopic/compound lens system

## PRESCRIBED GLASSES

| CPT Code (V) | Item | Autorization Amount ($) | Status/Date | | | |
|---|---|---|---|---|---|---|
| | | | O | A | H | D |
| | | | | | | |
| | | | | | | |
| | | | | | | |
| | | | | | | |
| | | | | | | |
| | | | | | | |
| | | | | | | |

| | | |
|---|---|---|
| **V2020 =** Frames | **V2799 =** Polycarb or misc. | **V2780** = Oversize lens |
| **V____** = SV, BF, etc. | **V2700 =** Balance lens | **V____** = Lenticular |
| | | **V____** = Tint |

# LOW VISION PRECERTIFICATION REQUEST FORM

IMPORTANT: Please type or print clearly. Incomplete requests will be returned or denied.

Date: _____          Member ID #: _____

Doctor Name: _____          Patient Name: _____

Address: _____          Patient Date of Birth: _____

_____          Authorization #: _____

Phone: _____          Member Name: _____

Fax: _____          Address: _____

_____

This request is for:  ☐ Low Vision Evaluation          ☐ Low Vision Aids

Attachments:          ☐ Invoice(s) and/or Catalog Sheet(s)          ☐ Other Attachments
(Required for each low vision aid requested)

Patient's Diagnoses
Indicate the patient's low vision diagnosis first, followed by any related medical or refractive diagnoses.

ICD-9:          1. _____          2. _____          3. _____          4. _____

Vision Loss Is:          ☐ Permanent ☐ Reversible  Describe: _____

Trial Frame Subjective:                              Add:          Best Corrected Visual Acuity:

Right:  Sphere _____  Cyl_____ x _____   _____   Distance ____/____ Near ____/____

Left:   Sphere _____  Cyl_____ x _____   _____   Distance ____/____ Near ____/____

Visual Field Width (in degrees):                     Sector Defect:

Right:  Horizontal _____ Vertical _____   ☐ None  ☐ Hemianopia  ☐ Other

Left:   Horizontal _____ Vertical _____   ☐ None  ☐ Hemianopia  ☐ Other

Additional documentation of medical necessity and/or benefit(s) to patient: _____

### Complete this section for Low Vision Evaluation

Level of low vision evaluation proposed:          ☐ Comprehensive          ☐ Limited

Your total usual and customary fee for the proposed evaluation procedures: $ _____

Proposed evaluation procedures:          ☐ Tint/Flash/Illumination          ☐ Trial Frame Refraction
(check all that apply)                   ☐ Field Expansion                   ☐ Magnifiers/Microscopics
☐ Telescopic Evaluation             ☐ Other (Describe) _____

### Complete this section for Low Vision Aids

| Description of Aid* | Model # | CPT or HCPCS | MON/ BIN | Rx Inc. | Visual Acuity | Patient Use/ Activity | Wholesale Cost | Total Fee |
|---|---|---|---|---|---|---|---|---|
| | | | M B | Yes No | | | $ | $ |
| | | | M B | Yes No | | | $ | $ |
| | | | M B | Yes No | | | $ | $ |

*A copy of the invoice or catalog sheet is required for each low vision aid requested.

# New Resident Letter

Dear Neighbor,

One of the most difficult "just moved" decisions you will make is finding a new family eye doctor you can trust.
Don't wait for an emergency to select your optometrist.
We hope you will not just pick an eye doctor from the Yellow pages or from a sign on the side of a building.
You'll benefit in our office from our high-quality, unrushed vision care, friendly and knowledgeable staff, and state-of-the-art equipment.
For your convenience, we offer morning, afternoon, and evening hours to accommodate most working schedules, and free parking is not a problem. You'll be happy to know we accept most insurance carriers, including Medicare, and will help you with your insurance paperwork.
Because your eyes are sensitive and precious, we welcome open discussions and consultations concerning visual problems, headaches, contact lenses, eye health treatment, and sports vision.
As a way of welcoming you to our community, we are offering a comprehensive eye examination for adults and children for
$ _____. The usual cost is $ _____.
My staff and I are anxious to provide quality eye care for you and your family.
Feel free to call our office to schedule an appointment.

Sincerely,

Dr. _____

# No-Show Policy

Office hours are by appointment and we do value your time. This office is a private practice office and not a "clinic." Appointment time is reserved for you alone. Where appropriate, we prefer to schedule longer appointments so we can complete as much needed treatment as possible during one appointment. We feel this type of scheduling will cause minimal disruption to your daily schedule and will provide efficiency in completing your care. When you make an appointment, please be sure that you will be able to keep it. Morning appointments are best for more complicated procedures.

Emergencies and unforeseen patient treatment problems may arise, causing schedule changes. Emergencies are unexpected and seem to come at the most inconvenient times. If you have an emergency that needs immediate attention, we will always offer to see you at once. We expect that other patients who might be slightly inconvenienced by this will be understanding of the emergency situation. At some point, they may need the same courtesy.

Unlike many offices, this office does not call to confirm your appointment. Please make a note of any appointments we have scheduled in a place where you will be easily reminded. If you cannot make an appointment as scheduled, please notify the office. There will be a charge of $_____ per 30 minutes of scheduled time for a broken appointment or cancellation with less than 24 hours notice for appointments before 4 p.m., weekdays. For appointments broken or canceled without 24 hours notice after 4 p.m., weekdays or Saturdays, the charge is $_____ per 30 minutes of scheduled time.

If our staff is successful in filling your appointment time with another patient, there will be no broken appointment charge.

**If you have any questions about our appointment, cancellation and no-show policy, please feel free to ask us.**

# Ocular Emergency Report Form

Patient name: _____

Current phone: _____    Previous patient? Y N

Call handled by: _____    Date: _____ Time: _____

Chief complaint: _____
_____
_____

Did the patient describe any of the following situations? If so, tell Dr. IMMEDIATELY:
flashing lights    loss of vision    curtain/veil blocking vision
many floaters    extreme pain    chemical in eye
different-sized pupils    sudden double vision    foreign object lodged in eye
Which eye is affected?        Right    Left    Both
When did it start? _____
Have you had any injury to your head? _____
Is it getting better or worse? _____
Has it ever happened before? _____
Are you wearing contact lenses now?    N    Y    If yes, remove ASAP.
Have you slept with your contacts in?    N    Y    If yes, how long?
Type of contacts:    soft    daily wear    extended wear    gas perm    hard

**Are You Experiencing:**        **If Yes, Describe:**

Redness?  N or Y    _____
If yes, where is it on eye?        _____
Decreased vision?    N or Y        _____
If yes, sudden or gradual?        _____
Blurry, distorted, or missing?        _____
Pain?    N or Y    _____
If yes, describe the pain.
Sensitivity to light?    N or Y        _____
Double vision?    N or Y        _____
Pupils same size?    N or Y        _____
Burning?  N or Y    _____
Itching?   N or Y    _____
Tearing?  N or Y    _____
Discharge, mucus in eye?        N or Y    _____
If yes, what color is it?        _____
The sensation that something is in your eye?    N or Y    _____
Swollen eyelids?    N or Y    _____
What have you (patient) done (eye drops, eyewash, emergency department)?
_____
_____

What action has been taken by staff? _____
_____

Follow-up call placed to patient:
By _____ Time _____ Date _____

# Patient History

Patient name: _____

Date: _____

Referring physician: _____

List any medications you currently take, **including** eye drops: _____

_____

Do you have allergies to any medications?   ❑ Yes   ❑ No

If yes, list drug allergies: _____

## Personal History

Have you ever had the following diseases?

| YES | NO | | YES | NO | |
|---|---|---|---|---|---|
| ❑ | ❑ | Glaucoma (eye - right, left) | ❑ | ❑ | Have you ever used IV drugs? |
| ❑ | ❑ | Cataract (eye - right, left) | ❑ | ❑ | Are you pregnant? |
| ❑ | ❑ | Retinal detachment (eye - right, left) | ❑ | ❑ | Emphysema |
| ❑ | ❑ | Eye injury (eye - right, left) | ❑ | ❑ | Asthma |
| ❑ | ❑ | Eye infection (eye - right, left) | ❑ | ❑ | Pneumonia |
| ❑ | ❑ | Diabetes | ❑ | ❑ | Hepatitis |
| ❑ | ❑ | High blood pressure | ❑ | ❑ | Arthritis |
| ❑ | ❑ | Stroke | ❑ | ❑ | Thyroid problems |
| ❑ | ❑ | Heart attack | ❑ | ❑ | Multiple sclerosis |
| ❑ | ❑ | Coronary artery disease | ❑ | ❑ | Epilepsy |
| ❑ | ❑ | Congestive heart failure | ❑ | ❑ | Tuberculosis (TB) |
| ❑ | ❑ | Cancer | ❑ | ❑ | Migraine headaches |
| ❑ | ❑ | Anemia | ❑ | ❑ | Stomach ulcers |
| ❑ | ❑ | Venereal disease (STD) | ❑ | ❑ | Herpes |
| | | | ❑ | ❑ | Shingles |
| | | | ❑ | ❑ | Lupus |
| | | | ❑ | ❑ | Have you been exposed to the AIDS virus (HIV)? |

List all major illnesses, injuries, or surgery not described above:

_____

_____

## Social History

Current occupation: _____

Do you smoke?   ❑ Yes   ❑ No

If yes, how many packs a day? _____

Do you drive?   ❑ Yes   ❑ No

Do you have visual difficulty when driving?   ❑ Yes   ❑ No

Have you ever had a blood transfusion?   ❑ Yes   ❑ No

Do you drink alcohol? ❑ Yes   ❑ No

If yes, how often? _____

Do you currently wear glasses?   ❑ Yes   ❑ No

Have you ever lived outside the United States?   ❑ Yes   ❑ No

When: _____   Where: _____

## Family History

Has anyone in your family had:

❑ Diabetes

❑ Migraine headache

❑ Heart disease

❑ Cancer

❑ Stroke

❑ Tuberculosis

❑ Glaucoma

❑ Blindness

❑ High blood pressure

*Continued*

# Patient History—cont'd

Patient Name:
Account #:
Date:
Referring Physician:

## Review of Systems

Do you currently have any problems in the following areas?
Constitutional Symptoms

| YES | NO | |
|-----|-----|-----|
| ❏ | ❏ | Fever |
| ❏ | ❏ | Weight loss/poor appetite |
| ❏ | ❏ | Fatigue/tire easily |

Eyes

| YES | NO | |
|-----|-----|-----|
| ❏ | ❏ | Loss of vision |
| ❏ | ❏ | Distorted vision |
| ❏ | ❏ | Double vision |
| ❏ | ❏ | Floating objects in vision |
| ❏ | ❏ | Flashing lights |
| ❏ | ❏ | Dryness of eyes |
| ❏ | ❏ | Redness |
| ❏ | ❏ | Itching |
| ❏ | ❏ | Burning |
| ❏ | ❏ | Excess tearing |
| ❏ | ❏ | Glare/light sensitivity |
| ❏ | ❏ | Eye pain or soreness |
| ❏ | ❏ | Crossed eyes |
| ❏ | ❏ | Lazy eye (amblyopia) |
| ❏ | ❏ | Past eye surgery |
| | | Type of surgery _____ |

Ears, Nose, Mouth, Throat

| YES | NO | |
|-----|-----|-----|
| ❏ | ❏ | Recent viral infection |
| ❏ | ❏ | Sore throat |
| ❏ | ❏ | Loss of hearing or deafness |
| ❏ | ❏ | Dryness of mouth |

Endocrine

| YES | NO | |
|-----|-----|-----|
| ❏ | ❏ | Thyroid problems |

Allergic/Immunologic

| YES | NO | |
|-----|-----|-----|
| ❏ | ❏ | Hay fever symptoms |
| ❏ | ❏ | Skin or respiratory |

Skin

| YES | NO | |
|-----|-----|-----|
| ❏ | ❏ | Easy bruising |
| ❏ | ❏ | Rashes/facial acne |

Neurological

| YES | NO | |
|-----|-----|-----|
| ❏ | ❏ | Severe headache |
| ❏ | ❏ | Numbness or tingling of extremities |
| ❏ | ❏ | Seizures |
| ❏ | ❏ | Depression/psychiatric conditions |

Cardiovascular (heart/blood vessels)

| YES | NO | |
|-----|-----|-----|
| ❏ | ❏ | Chest pain |
| ❏ | ❏ | Irregular heart beat |

Respiratory

| YES | NO | |
|-----|-----|-----|
| ❏ | ❏ | Chronic bronchitis/emphysema |
| ❏ | ❏ | Chronic cough |
| ❏ | ❏ | Shortness of breath |

Gastrointestinal

| YES | NO | |
|-----|-----|-----|
| ❏ | ❏ | Stomach pain |
| ❏ | ❏ | Diarrhea |

Genitourinary (genitals/kidney/bladder)

| YES | NO | |
|-----|-----|-----|
| ❏ | ❏ | Burning with urination |
| ❏ | ❏ | Genital sores |
| ❏ | ❏ | Kidney infection or bleeding |

Musculoskeletal

| YES | NO | |
|-----|-----|-----|
| ❏ | ❏ | Muscle or neck pains |
| ❏ | ❏ | Back pain or stiffness |
| ❏ | ❏ | Joint pains or stiffness |

Doctor's Signature _____ Date _____

**Confidential Medical History**                                    **Date:**

Name:_____ Date of birth:_____ ☐ Male ☐ Female
Address:_____ Phone:_____
City/zip:_____ Social Security #:_____
Name of medical doctor:_____ Dr.'s phone #:_____

List any allergies to medicines:_____

List any medications you take (including birth control pills, aspirin, over-the-counter medications, and home remedies)

_____
_____

List all major injuries, surgeries, and hospitalization you have had:_____

_____

Last physical exam:_____ Are you pregnant or nursing?  ☐ Yes  ☐ No

Do you wear glasses?      ☐ Yes  ☐ No  If yes, how old are your lenses?_____

Do you wear contact lenses? ☐ Yes  ☐ No  If yes, how old are your current pair?_____

What type of contact lenses: ☐ Disposable soft lenses  ☐ Standard soft lenses  ☐ Rigid

If you use disposable lenses, how often do you throw them away?_____

What solutions do you use?_____ Do you ever sleep with your lenses on?  ☐ Yes  ☐ No

Have you ever had refractive surgery?  ☐ Yes  ☐ No    If yes, specify type:  ☐ RK  ☐ PRK  ☐ LASIK
Are you interested in refractive surgery?  ☐ Yes  ☐ No

**Personal/Family History**
Please answer the question below regarding you or your immediate family (parents. grandparents, siblings, children)
for the following:

| | **You** | | **Family** | | | |
|---|---|---|---|---|---|---|
| | Yes | No | Yes | No | ? | **Relationship** |
| Blindness/loss of vision | ☐ | ☐ | ☐ | ☐ | ☐ | _____ |
| Crossed eyes | ☐ | ☐ | ☐ | ☐ | ☐ | _____ |
| Glaucoma | ☐ | ☐ | ☐ | ☐ | ☐ | _____ |
| Macular degeneration | ☐ | ☐ | ☐ | ☐ | ☐ | _____ |
| Retinal detachment | ☐ | ☐ | ☐ | ☐ | ☐ | _____ |
| Retinal disease | ☐ | ☐ | ☐ | ☐ | ☐ | _____ |
| Cancer | ☐ | ☐ | ☐ | ☐ | ☐ | _____ |
| Diabetes | ☐ | ☐ | ☐ | ☐ | ☐ | _____ |
| Heart disease | ☐ | ☐ | ☐ | ☐ | ☐ | _____ |
| High blood pressure | ☐ | ☐ | ☐ | ☐ | ☐ | _____ |
| Lupus | ☐ | ☐ | ☐ | ☐ | ☐ | _____ |
| Thyroid disease | ☐ | ☐ | ☐ | ☐ | ☐ | _____ |
| Other_____ | ☐ | ☐ | ☐ | ☐ | ☐ | _____ |

*Continued*

## Confidential Medical History—cont'd

<u>Social History</u> **(If you do not want to give a written response, please discuss the information with your clinician.)**

Do you drive? ☐ Yes ☐ No If yes, do you have difficulty with vision while driving? ☐ Yes ☐ No

Do you use tobacco products? ☐ Yes ☐ No If yes, type/amount/howlong: _____

Do you drink alcohol? ☐ Yes ☐ No If yes, type/amount/howlong: _____

### <u>Review of Systems</u>

Do you currently have or ever had any problems in the following areas:

| | Yes | No | ? | | Yes | No | ? |
|---|---|---|---|---|---|---|---|
| *Constitutional* | | | | *Ears/Nose, Mouth, Throat* | | | |
| Fever/weight changes | ☐ | ☐ | ☐ | Allergies/hay fever | ☐ | ☐ | ☐ |
| *Integumentary (Skin)* | ☐ | ☐ | ☐ | Sinus congestion | ☐ | ☐ | ☐ |
| Rosacea | ☐ | ☐ | ☐ | Dry throat, mouth | ☐ | ☐ | ☐ |
| *Neurological* | | | | *Respiratory* | ☐ | ☐ | ☐ |
| Headaches | ☐ | ☐ | ☐ | Asthma | ☐ | ☐ | ☐ |
| Migraines | ☐ | ☐ | ☐ | Emphysema | ☐ | ☐ | ☐ |
| Seizures | ☐ | ☐ | ☐ | Chronic bronchitis | ☐ | ☐ | ☐ |
| *Eyes* | | | | *Vascular/Cardiovascular* | | | |
| Blurred vision | ☐ | ☐ | ☐ | Diabetes | ☐ | ☐ | ☐ |
| Distorted vision/halos | ☐ | ☐ | ☐ | Vascular disease | ☐ | ☐ | ☐ |
| Loss of side vision | ☐ | ☐ | ☐ | High cholesterol | ☐ | ☐ | ☐ |
| Double vision | ☐ | ☐ | ☐ | High blood pressure | ☐ | ☐ | ☐ |
| Dryness | ☐ | ☐ | ☐ | *Gastrointestinal* | | | |
| Mucous discharge | ☐ | ☐ | ☐ | Chronic diarrhea | ☐ | ☐ | ☐ |
| Redness | ☐ | ☐ | ☐ | *Genitourinary* | | | |
| Sandy or gritty feeling | ☐ | ☐ | ☐ | Kidney/bladder | ☐ | ☐ | ☐ |
| Itching | ☐ | ☐ | ☐ | *Bones/Joints/Muscles* | | | |
| Burning | ☐ | ☐ | ☐ | Rheumatoid arthritis | ☐ | ☐ | ☐ |
| Foreign body sensation | ☐ | ☐ | ☐ | *Lymphatic/Hematologic* | | | |
| Glare/light sensitivity | ☐ | ☐ | ☐ | Anemia | ☐ | ☐ | ☐ |
| Eye pain or soreness | ☐ | ☐ | ☐ | Bleeding problems | ☐ | ☐ | ☐ |
| Eye trauma injury | ☐ | ☐ | ☐ | *Endocrine* | | | |
| Flashes | ☐ | ☐ | ☐ | Thyroid | ☐ | ☐ | ☐ |
| Floaters in vision | ☐ | ☐ | ☐ | *Psychiatric/Depression* | ☐ | ☐ | ☐ |
| Tired eyes | ☐ | ☐ | ☐ | *Other* | ☐ | ☐ | ☐ |

I understand that information contained in this form and collected during my examination may be used for teaching purposes or statistical analysis. My identity will remain confidential.

Patient Signature:_____ Date:_____

**Reviewed at annual exam:**

Clinician:_____ Date:_____

Clinician:_____ Date:_____

Clinician:_____ Date:_____

## PATIENT INFORMATION

Name _____     Date of Birth _____

Address _____     Home Phone _____

City _____  State _____  Zip _____

Employer _____  Position _____  Phone (     ) _____

Spouse's Employer _____  Position _____  Phone (     ) _____

Date of last visual examination: _____/_____/_____
Whom may we thank for referring you to this office?  Name _____
Family members living at home:

    Spouse _____  Age _____

    Name _____  Age _____

    Name _____  Age _____

_Please answer the following questions to help us give you a complete and comprehensive examination. Thank you for your cooperation._

1. Any difficulty seeing clearly at a distance?  Approx. how long? _____
   Night Vision _____ Driving _____ T.V. _____ Movies _____ Other _____

2. Any problem focusing clearly at close range?  Approx. how long? _____
   Reading _____ Sewing _____ Phone Book _____ Work _____ Other _____

3. Do your eyes: Burn _____ Ache _____ Tire _____ Itch _____ Water _____

4. Sensitive to light?  Yes _____ No _____
   Fluorescent Lights _____ Glare _____ Snow _____ Sun _____

5. Do you wear glasses? Sunglasses _____ Sport _____ Work ____ Dress _____ Other _____

6. Hobbies _____ Sports _____

7. Do you work with a computer? Yes _____ No ____

8. Have you ever worm contact lenses? _____ Soft _____ Other _____
   Currently wearing contact lenses? _____ Soft _____ Other _____
   Interested in learning more about the benefits of contacts? Yes ____ No____

9. Family history of the following:
   Allergies _____     Sinus Problems _____     Diabetes _____
   High Blood Pressure _____     Cataracts _____     Glaucoma _____

10. Headaches? _____ How often? _____ Spots or Floaters? _____ Double Vision? _____

11. Family physician _____ Dentist _____

12. Medications currently taking _____

Payment method: Cash _____  Check _____  Credit Card ____  Insurance _____

_____          _____
Signature of Party Responsible for Payment          Relationship

# Questionnaire for Children

Child's name _____

Age _____     Date _____

1. Do the words in your book blur or run together when you read for a little while?
    YES      NO           SOMETIMES
2. Do you ever see two words or numbers on your page when you know there is really only one?
    YES      NO
3. Do you feel you have to close or cover one eye to help you get your reading or homework finished?
    YES      NO           SOMETIMES
4. Do your eyes ever sting or burn after you have been reading for a while?
    YES      NO           S0METIMES
5. Do you ever want to rub your eyes after you have been reading or writing?
    YES      NO           SOMETIMES
6. Do you ever have to wait for your eyes to get clear when you look up from reading and try to see what the teacher has written on the chalkboard?
    YES      NO           SOMETIMES
7. Does reading or writing ever make your eyes "cry" or "water" or get "teary"?
    YES      NO           SOMETIMES
8. Do you have trouble seeing what the teacher has written on the chalkboard?
    YES      NO           SOMETIMES
9. Do you ever have to move closer to see what the teacher has written on the chalkboard?
    YES      NO           SOMETIMES
10. Do you make too many mistakes in copying words and numbers even when you know how to do the work?
    YES      NO           SOMETIMES
11. How often do you have headaches? DAILY   WEEKLY   MONTHLY   RARELY   NEVER
12. If you get headaches, do they usually come after you have been reading or writing?
    YES      NO           SOMETIMES
13. Do you lose your place often when reading?
    YES      NO           SOMETIMES
14. Do bright lights bother your eyes?
    YES      NO           SOMETIMES
    What type of lights?      SUNLIGHT    INDOOR    LIGHTING
15. Is there anything else that you feel would be important for us to know about your eyes?

_____

_____

_____

# Questionnaire for Parent

To the parents of _____

Address _____

Gathering this information before your appointment will ensure the best use of your visit. It also helps tell us what examination routines will best apply to your child's problem.

Parent's name _____ Occupation _____

Child's full name _____ Phone no. _____

Name of school _____ Grade _____

School address _____ Teacher's name _____

In what areas does your child seem to have visual difficulty?

_____
_____
_____

How does your child complain about his or her vision?

_____
_____
_____

Does your child report any of the following? If so, when?

Headaches:       Yes    No      When _____

Blurred vision:      Yes    No      When _____

Blurred vision at distance:      Yes    No

Blurred vision at near (reading): Yes    No

Double vision:      Yes    No      When _____

Eyes "hurt" or are "tired":      Yes    No      When _____

Have you or anyone else ever noted the following (check as indicated):

| | Yes | No | If Yes, When? |
|---|---|---|---|
| 1. Holding reading close | | | |
| 2. Closing one eye | | | |
| 3. Covering one eye | | | |
| 4. Eyes frequently bloodshot | | | |
| 5. Frequent styes | | | |
| 6. Excessive eye rubbing | | | |
| 7. Excessive blinking | | | |
| 8. Getting lost in book (not aware of surroundings) | | | |
| 9. Tilting head when reading | | | |
| 10. Reading in bed | | | |
| 11. Inability to see distant objects | | | |
| 12. Bumping into objects | | | |
| 13. Poor general coordination | | | |
| 14. Large pupils in normal light | | | |
| 15. Bothered by light | | | |

## School

1. Age at time of entrance? _____ Kindergarten _____ First grade _____
2. Does child like school? Yes _____ No _____ Teacher? Yes _____ No _____
3. Has a grade been repeated? Yes _____ No _____ Which? _____

*Continued*

## Questionnaire for Parent—cont'd

4. Have there been any school difficulties? Yes _____ No _____
5. Is school work average _____ better than average _____ below average _____
6. Is there any subject or subjects that seem particularly easy for the child?

_____

7. Is there any subject or subjects that seem particularly difficult for the child?

_____

### Developmental History

1. Full term pregnancy? _____ Normal birth? _____ Any complications before, during, or immediately after delivery?

_____
2. Did your child crawl? _____ All fours? Age _____
3. At what age did child walk? _____
4. Speech: First words? _____ Sentences? _____ Was speech clear to others? _____
5. Was child active? _____
6. When fatigued, child does which of following? Sags _____ Becomes irritable _____ Becomes excited _____
7. When under tension, is there any pattern of behavior, such as thumb sucking, nail biting, etc.?

_____

8. List illnesses:              Age                  Mild                    Severe

_____
_____
_____

### Visual History

1.      How long has difficulty been noticed? _____
2.      Previous visual examinations:
        Name    Doctor's name    Results

_____
_____
_____

3.      Members of family who have had visual attention and why:
        Name                     Age      Visual situation




4.      Give a brief description of your child's personality.

_____
_____
_____

As you complete this history questionnaire you will recognize the thoroughness with which your child's problem will be considered. The office examination will take up enough time to permit a complete optometric investigation of the problem. It is desirable to have one or both parents present during the examination. Your child's future deserves the fullest consideration that you as parents and our office can provide.
Thank you.

Date _____

Doctor _____

# Recommendations for Additional Care

Patient's name: _____ Date of exam: _____

❏ Annual vision examination
❏ Anti-reflective coating
❏ Bifocal lenses
❏ Blood pressure
❏ Computer Rx
❏ Contact lens evaluation
❏ Contact lenses
❏ Dilation exam
❏ Glaucoma test
❏ Glaucoma work-up
❏ High-index lenses
❏ Indoor Rx
❏ LASIK evaluation
❏ Outdoor Rx
❏ Photochromic lenses
❏ Polarized lenses
❏ Polycarbonate lenses
❏ Progressive lenses
❏ Retinal photos
❏ Second pair of glasses
❏ Semiannual contact lens exam
❏ Solutions for contact lenses
❏ Sports goggles
❏ Sunwear
❏ Tint
❏ Trifocal lenses
❏ UV protection
❏ Visual fields
Remarks:

_____

_____

Office use only:    Carrier # _____    Acct. type _____    Acct. # _____

# Patient Registration Form

Responsible party _____
First name        Initial        Last name

Address _____
_____

City _____ State _____ Zip_____

Phone: (home) _____ (work) _____

Employer _____

Address _____

Name and address of nearest relative not living with you
_____

Phone _____

Referring physician _____

## Family Member Information

First name   Last name   Sex   Relationship (I-S-C-O*)   Birthday

Pt #

(1) _____

(2) _____

(3) _____

(4) _____

Please list additional members on next page.

* I = Insured, S = Spouse, C = Child, O = Other dependent

## Medical Insurance Information

Subscriber name _____ SS # _____ Pt. # _____

Carrier name and address _____
_____

Group name _____

Group number _____

Does this plan cover all family members? _____ Yes _____ No

If no, specify those NOT covered. _____

| Assignment of Benefits | Release of Information |
|---|---|
| I authorize payment of medical benefits to myself or the named provider for professional services rendered.<br>Signed _____ Date _____<br>(Subscriber) | I authorize the release of any medical information necessary to process this claim.<br>Signed _____ Date _____<br>(Patient, or parent if minor) |

Additional medical coverage: _____ Yes _____ No

If yes, please complete below.

If spouse works, complete Employer section on below.

Additional medical insurance coverage _____

Subscriber name _____

Carrier name and address _____
_____

Employer name and address _____
_____

Group name _____ Group number _____

Does this plan cover all family members? _____ Yes _____ No

If no, please specify members NOT covered by plan.
_____

## Patient Registration Form—cont'd

### Assignment of Benefits

I authorize payment of medical benefits to myself or the named provider for professional services rendered.

Signed _____ Date _____

(Subscriber)

### Release of Information

I authorize the release of any medical information necessary to process this claim.

Signed _____ Date _____

(Patient, or parent if minor)

**Additional Family Members**

(5) _____

(6) _____

(7) _____

(8) _____

(9) _____

# Notice of Privacy Practices

**This notice describes how medical information about you may be used and disclosed and how you can get access to this information. Please review it carefully.**

This notice is effective until _____ or until further notice.

## Right to Notice

As a patient, you have the right to adequate notice of the uses and disclosures of your protected health information. Under the Health Insurance Portability and Accountability Act (HIPAA), this office can use your protected health information for treatment, payment, and health care operations.

1. Treatment: We may use or disclose your health information to a physician or other health care provider providing treatment to you.
2. Payment: We may use and disclose your health information to obtain payment for services we provide you.
3. Health care operations: We may use and disclose your health information in connection with our health care operations. Health care operations include financial or billing audits, internal quality assurance, participation in managed care plans, defense of legal matters, and business planning.

## Your Authorization

Most uses and disclosures that do not fall under treatment, payment, or health care operations will require your written authorization. Upon signing, you may revoke your authorization (in writing) through our practice at any time.

## Uses and Disclosures for Other Reasons Without Permission

In some limited situations, the law allows or requires us to use or disclose your health information without your permission. Such uses or disclosures are:

1. When a state or federal law mandates that certain health information be reported for a specific purpose.
2. For public health purposes, such as contagious disease reporting, investigation, or surveillance and notices to and from the federal Food and Drug Administration regarding drugs or medical devices.
3. Disclosures to governmental authorities about victims of suspected abuse, neglect, or domestic violence.
4. Disclosures for judicial and administrative proceedings, such as in response to subpoenas or orders of courts.
5. Disclosures for law enforcement purposes.
6. Uses or disclosures for health-related research.
7. Uses or disclosures for national security to Armed Forces personnel under certain circumstances.
8. Disclosures relating to worker's compensation programs.
9. Disclosures to "business associates" who perform health care operations for us and who commit to respect the privacy of your health information.
10. Unless you object, we will also share relevant information about your care with your family or friends who are helping you with your eye care.
11. Marketing communications about our own health care products or services.

## Appointment Reminders

Unless you tell us otherwise, we will mail you an appointment reminder on a postcard, and/or leave you a reminder message on your home answering machine or with someone who answers your phone if you are not at home.

## Your Rights as a Patient

You have the right to restrict the disclosure of your protected health information (in writing). The request for restriction may be denied if the information is required for treatment, payment, or health care operations.

1. You have the right to receive confidential communications regarding your protected health care information.
2. You have the right to inspect and copy your protected health care information within 5 business days of asking us (in writing).
3. You have the right to amend your protected health care information if you think it is incorrect or incomplete. If we agree, we will amend the information within 60 days from when you ask us. If we do not agree, you can write a statement of your position, and we will include it with your health information along with any rebuttal statement that we may write.
4. You have a right to receive an account of disclosures of your protected health information.
5. You have the right to a paper copy of this notice of privacy practices.

## Legal Requirements

This office is required by law to maintain the privacy of your protected health information. We are required by law to abide by the terms of this notice as it is currently stated and reserve the right to change this notice. If we change our Notice of Privacy Practices, we will post the new notice in our office, have copies available in our office, and post it on our Web site.

## Notice of Privacy Practices—cont'd

### Complaints

If you have complaints about the way your protected health information was handled, you may submit a complaint in writing to our office or to the U.S. Department of Health and Human Services, Office for Civil Rights.

### Contact Information

If you want more information about our privacy practices, please contact _____,
Privacy Officer, in this office.

### Acknowledgment of Receipt

I acknowledge that I received a copy of this Notice of Privacy Practices.

Patient Name _____

Signature _____ Date _____

# Reschedule of Missed Appointment

Dear _____ :




We missed you! Sorry that you missed your appointment. We hope everything is all right. Your
_____ exam was scheduled for _____ at _____.
Your vision is very important and precious. Remember, many diseases or changes in your eyesight can only be detected by having a complete examination. Your complete eye health involves much more than merely having your eyes examined when you notice that your glasses or contact lenses need replacement. We should check regularly for signs of glaucoma, cataracts, macular degeneration, and complications caused by high blood pressure or diabetes. These vision problems may show no symptoms until they are in their later stages.

We will call you in the next few days to reschedule your eye health examination. See you soon!

Sincerely,

Dr. _____ and Staff

# Teen's or Child's Vision Examination Recall

Dear Parents of _____:

Your child's last vision evaluation was on _____. It is time to schedule another eye health exam.

Your child's eyes mature rapidly while visual demands at school steadily increase. Reading demands increase and print size decreases as your child gets older.

Because of the potential for rapid change during these formative years, we feel that a vision examination is advisable every 12 months. Please call our office to make an appointment.

Sincerely,

Dr._____ and Staff

## LASER VISION CORRECTION SCREENING FORM

Name:_____ Date:_____ Age:_____

Address:_____ State:_____ Zip:_____

Phone:  home (_____)_____  work (_____) _____

How did you hear about vision correction surgery? *(please check one)*

[ ] Optometrist     [ ] Mailer     [ ] Newspaper     [ ] Yellow Pages     [ ] Radio     [ ] Friend

I am interested in knowing if I am a suitable candidate for excimer laser correction surgery. I understand that this is only a screening evaluation that will establish whether  I can have excimer laser surgery and that there is no charge for this screening evaluation.

**Signature:**_____    **Date:**_____

**Current Visual Information:**

I currently wear:     [ ] Glasses     [ ] Contacts     [ ] RGP     [ ] Soft     [ ] EW     [ ] Daily Wear

Last eye exam:_____     Dr._____

Ocular and general health: *(please circle any that apply)*
        Diabetes  Arthritis  High blood pressure  Glaucoma  Cataracts   Retinal disease  Pregnant

Other:_____

Medications:_____

---

### FOR OFFICE USE ONLY

ADD

Rx:     OD _____ - _____ x _____ _____     VA:  20/

Rx:     OS _____ - _____ x _____ _____     VA:  20/

**Surgery Candidate:**     YES     NO

| PRE | | PRE |
|---|---|---|

## LASER VISION CORRECTION **PRE** OPERATIVE EXAM FORM
### LASIK:[ ] OD [ ] OS [ ] OU   PRK:[ ] OD [ ] OS [ ] OU ENHANCEMENT:[ ] OD [ ] OS [ ] OU

Name:_____ DOB:_____ Age:_____ Date:_____

Phone (H): (   )_____ - _____    Phone (W): (   )_____ - _____    [ ]Male   [ ]Female   Occupation:_____
                                                            Referring doctor: _____

Address:_____ City: _____ Zip: _____ Surgeon: _____

**Uncorrected VA:** OD: 20/_____    **Dominant Eye:** [ ] OD     **Pupils:**        OD:____mm
                   OS: 20/_____                [ ] OS    *(dim illumination)*   OS:____mm

**Subjective OD:** _____ - _____ x_____ 20/____   **Vertex Distance:** _____**mm** Stereo:
**Refraction: OS:** _____ - _____ x_____ 20/____   **Vertex Distance:** _____**mm** _____ sec of arc

**Cycloplegic OD:** _____ - _____ x_____ 20/___   **K OD:**_____@_____ ;_____@ _____

**Refraction: OS:** _____ - _____ x_____ 20/___   **K OD:**_____@_____ ;_____@ _____
            Use same cylinder as subjective refraction.            [ ] Keratometer [ ] Autokeratometer [ ] Topographer

**Stable Refraction?** [ ] yes [ ] no   **Previous CL wearer?** [ ] yes [ ] no   **Type:** _____   **Time out of CLs:** _____

| **History:** | **Examination:** | **Informed Consent:** [ ] Sent [ ] Needed |
|---|---|---|
| Check Applicable | Media opacities: Y   N | **Topography:** [ ] Sent [ ] Needed |
| [ ] Prior ocular herpes | Cornea disease: Y   N | |
| [ ] Keloid formation | Lid disease:    Y   N | *Discussed with patient:* [ ] Infection |
| [ ] Diabetes | Dry eye:      Y   N | [ ] VA fluctuation, halo / glare, pain |
| [ ] Vascular disease |    If yes degree of dry eyes: | [ ] Undercorrection / overcorrection |
| [ ] **None of the above** |    mild/ moderate / severe   TBUT: _____ | [ ] Possible need for enhancement |
| | **IOP:** _____   _____ | [ ] Presbyopia: eventual / imminent |

**Medication Allergies:** _____

**Systemic Medications:** _____

**Comments:** _____

       **Recommended amount of laser treatment**    **OD:** _____ - _____ x_____
           **at spectacle plane (not corneal):**    **OS:** _____ - _____ x_____

**Monovision:** [ ] yes [ ] no    **Target Rx (Goal) for RIGHT eye:** _____    **LEFT eye:** _____

If enhancement: [ ] LASIK   [ ] PRK   Reason:_____    Date of original Tx:_____

**Procedure Date&Time:** ___/___/___ @_____     **1-Day Post-Op:** ___/___/___ @_____
                                                         **Place:** _____

**Instructions:** _____
_____ Patient fee quoted $:_____

**Referring doctor:** _____ (____)____ - _____    (____)____ - _____
                   (Signature)            (Phone)            (After-hours phone)

Exam Date:_____

## LASER VISION CORRECTION **POST** OPERATIVE EXAM FORM

☐ PLEASE CALL        ☐ PLEASE FAX REPLY        ☐ NO REPLY REQUESTED

Patient Name: _____ Time since treatment:____ Days ___ Weeks___ Months

Managing Doctor: _____ Dr. Phone: (   ) _____-_____ Surgeon:_____

Patient Comments: _____

---

**Operative Eye:** [ ]OD [ ]OS [ ]OU  [ ]LASIK [ ]PRK/LASEK [ ]Enhance Date of procedure: ___/___/___

**Medications:**   [ ]Vigamox   [ ]Ciloxan   [ ]Flarex   [ ]Flur-op   [ ]Lubrication   [ ]Other_____

Frequency:        ____        ____        ____        ____        ____        ____

---

|  | (Distance) | (Monovisiom Tx?) | (Near Vision) | (PH-optional) |
|---|---|---|---|---|
| Uncorrected | OD:20/_____ | For D  N | OD: _____ | OD: 20/_____ |
| Vision | OS:20/_____ | For D  N | OS: _____ | OS: 20/_____ |

Stereo: _____ sec of arc

Subjective Refraction   OD: _____-_____x_____ VA: 20/_____   IOP OD _____ mm Hg

*(Not required on 1 day post-op visit)*   OS: _____-_____x_____ VA: 20/_____   OS_____mg Hg

(IOP no earlier than 8 weeks)

---

Slit Lamp Exam

**LASIK**
OD OS

Epithelium: [ ] [ ] Intact
[ ] [ ] Defect
_____ mm

Flap:   [ ] [ ] Smooth
[ ] [ ] Microstria
[ ] [ ] Folds

Interface:
[ ] [ ] Clear
[ ] [ ] Debris / cells
[ ] [ ] Inflammation
[ ] [ ] Epithelial ingrowth

Hinge:
[ ] [ ] Superior
[ ] [ ] Nasal

OD

OS

**PRK**
OD OS

Epithelium: [ ] [ ] Healed
[ ] [ ] Defect
_____ mm

Stroma:   [ ] [ ] Clear
(haze)   [ ] [ ] Trace
[ ] [ ] 1+
[ ] [ ] 2+
[ ] [ ] 3+

OD   CORNEA  OS

---

Impression/Plan:_____     Meds: _____

_____     _____

_____     _____

Dr.'s Signature                                        Next Visit

# LASER VISION CORRECTION
## Preoperative Patient Questionnaire

Today's Date: _____

Patient Name: _____

City:_____ State:_____ Zip: _____

Telephone: home (____)_____ work (____)_____

1. What is your primary reason for considering a refractive surgery procedure?
   [ ] Want to be free from glasses
   [ ] Contact lens intolerance
   [ ] Occupational requirements
   [ ] Function problems with glasses/contacts
   [ ] Cosmetic reasons

2. How long have you been considering having this surgery?
   [ ] 1 - 6 months
   [ ] 6 months - 1 year
   [ ] 1 - 2 years
   [ ] 2 years or longer

3. Do you know anyone who has had refractive surgery?
   [ ] Yes
   [ ] No

4. What type of refractive problem do you have? Check all that apply.
   [ ] Astigmatism
   [ ] Nearsighted
   [ ] Farsighted

5. Do you currently wear any type of visual correction?
   [ ] Yes
   [ ] No
   If yes, which?
   [ ] Contact lenses      [ ] Distance
   [ ] Glasses             [ ] Reading

6. If you wear contacts, are you having difficulties?
   [ ] Yes
   [ ] No

7. Are you experiencing any problems related to dry eyes?
   [ ] Yes
   [ ] No

8. Do you think that after undergoing refractive surgery you will have to wear contact lenses or glasses again?
   [ ] Yes
   [ ] No

9. Are you experiencing any glare/light sensitivity?
   [ ] Yes
   [ ] No
   If yes, when?
   [ ] Day
   [ ] Night
   [ ] Indoor
   [ ] Outdoor
   [ ] With bright lights

10. When do you feel your vision is best?
   [ ] Day
   [ ] Night
   [ ] Both

*Continued*

## LASER VISION CORRECTION
### Preoperative Patient Questionnaire—cont'd

11. Do you notice fluctuation in your vision?
    [ ] Day to day
    [ ] During the day

12. Can you drive without glasses?
    [ ] Yes
    [ ] No

13. Are you experiencing problems with excessive tearing?
    [ ] Yes
    [ ] No

14. Are you experiencing any double vision?
    [ ] Yes
    [ ] No
    If yes, when?
    [ ] Day
    [ ] Night
    [ ] Indoor
    [ ] Outdoor
    [ ] With bright lights

15. Do you ever have difficulty seeing at night?
    [ ] Yes
    [ ] No

16. Are you experiencing any color vision problems?
    [ ] Yes
    [ ] No

17. Has your refraction (vision with glasses and/or contacts) been stable over the past year?
    [ ] Yes
    [ ] No

18. Have you ever had any prior eye surgery?
    [ ] Yes
    [ ] No
    If yes, specify:
    [ ] Radial keratotomy
    [ ] Astigmatic keratotomy
    [ ] PRK
    [ ] LTK
    [ ] Lamellar keratoplasty
    [ ] Hexagonal keratotomy
    [ ] Cataract
    [ ] Glaucoma
    [ ] Retina
    [ ] Other

19. Does anyone in your family have any eye disorders besides wearing glasses?
    [ ] Yes
    [ ] No
    If yes, specify _____

20. Do you participate in any contact sports?
    [ ] Yes
    [ ] No
    If yes, specify _____

21. How would you rate the quality of your vision without correction?
    [ ] Excellent
    [ ] Good
    [ ] Fair
    [ ] Poor

22. How would you rate the quality of your vision with correction?
    [ ] Excellent
    [ ] Good
    [ ] Fair
    [ ] Poor

# LASER VISION CORRECTION
## Postoperative Patient Questionnaire

Patient Name: _____       Today's Date: _____/_____/_____
Patient Address: _____       Telephone: _____
City: _____ State: _____ Zip: _____

**Operative Eye:  [ ] Right   [ ] Left**

1. How satisfied are you with the results
   of your surgery?
   [ ] Very satisfied
   [ ] Satisfied
   [ ] Unsatisfied
   [ ] Very unsatisfied

2. How highly would you recommend this
   to a friend or family member?
   [ ] Very highly
   [ ] Highly
   [ ] Somewhat highly
   [ ] Don't know
   [ ] Not at all

3. Are you experiencing any glare/
   light sensitivity?
   [ ] Yes
   [ ] No
   If yes, when?
   [ ] Day          [ ] Outdoor
   [ ] Night        [ ] With bright lights
   [ ] Indoor

4. Are you experiencing any double vision?
   [ ] Yes
   [ ] No
   If yes, when?
   [ ] Day          [ ] Outdoor
   [ ] Night        [ ] With bright lights
   [ ] Indoor

5. Do you currently wear any type of visual
   corrections?
   [ ] Yes
   [ ] No
   If yes, what?       If yes, for:
   [ ] Contact lenses  [ ] Distance
   [ ] Glasses         [ ] Reading
                       [ ] Both

6. Can you drive without glasses?
   [ ] Yes
   [ ] No

7. Are you experiencing any problems
   related to dry eyes?
   [ ] Yes
   [ ] No

8. Are you experiencing any problems
   with excessive tearing?
   [ ] Yes
   [ ] No

9. Are you experiencing any color vision
   problems?
   [ ] Yes
   [ ] No

10. How would you rate the quality of your
    vision without correction?
    [ ] Excellent
    [ ] Good
    [ ] Fair
    [ ] Poor

11. How would you rate the quality of your
    vision with correction?
    [ ] Excellent
    [ ] Good
    [ ] Fair
    [ ] Poor

12. Do you notice fluctuation in your vision?
    [ ] No
    [ ] Day to day
    [ ] During the day

13. Do you ever have difficulty seeing at night?
    [ ] Yes
    [ ] No

## Professional Request for Patient Information

| Date/Time | Date/Time | Referring Optometrist Physician | Optometrist, Physician Phone # | Subject |
|---|---|---|---|---|
| | | | | |
| | | | | |
| | | | | |
| | | | | |
| | | | | |
| | | | | |
| | | | | |

■ When patients, other optometrists or physicians call in relation to a patient's treatment, please record the patient's name and information called for in this log.

■ Be sure to note the call details in the patient's chart as well. Initial both this log and the patient's chart.

■ If the message is long, the appropriate portion of this log may be duplicated for the patient's chart.

■ The treating optometrist will review this log daily.

## Authorization for Release of Health Information

**Patient Name:** _____ **Date of Birth:** _____

The office is authorized to: (check one below)

_____ release health information to **OR** _____ receive health information from

_____

**Name of person or facility to receive or give health information**

_____

**Street Address, City, State, Zip Code**

( _____ ) _____     ( _____ ) _____

**Phone Number**                          **Fax Number**

_____

**Health information to be released**

**The purpose of this release is for (check one or more):**

_____ At the request of the patient/patient representative

_____ Other (state reason) _____

### NOTICE

Health organizations are required by law to keep your health information confidential. If you have authorized the disclosure of your health information to someone who is not legally required to keep it confidential, it may no longer be protected by state or federal confidentiality laws.

### YOUR RIGHTS

- This authorization to release health information is voluntary. Treatment, payment, and eligibility for benefits may not be conditioned on signing this authorization except in the following cases: (1) to conduct research-related treatment, (2) to obtain information in connection with eligibility or enrollment in a health plan, (3) to determine an entity's obligation to pay a claim, or (4) to create health information to provide to a third party.
- This authorization may be revoked at any time. The revocation must be in writing, signed by you or your patient representative, and delivered to the clinic Privacy Officer. The revocation will take effect when the office receives it, except to the extent that we or others have already relied on it.
- You are entitled to receive a copy of this authorization.

### EXPIRATION OF AUTHORIZATION

Unless otherwise revoked, this authorization expires _____ (insert applicable date or event).

**I have read and understand this form. I am signing it voluntarily. I authorize the disclosure of my health information as described above.**

_____       _____

Print Name                              Signature (Patient, Parent, Guardian)

_____       _____

Date                                  Relationship to Patient (Parent, Guardian, Conservator, Patient Representative)

**For Internal Use:** Information released: _____ / _____

                                       Initials            Date

Copy of authorization to patient: _____       Authorization revoked: _____

                                 Initials                              Date

# Reminder of Scheduled Exam

Dear _____:

You have an eye health examination scheduled on _____ at _____.

If you cannot keep this appointment because of an emergency, please call our office to reschedule and give another patient an opportunity to use your time.

We look forward to seeing you.

Sincerely,

Dr. _____ and Staff

# Report to Physician for Routine Eye Examination

_____

(date)

_____, MD

_____

_____

Re: _____, age _____

Dear Dr. _____:

_____ was seen for a routine eye examination today. There is a history of

_____ and _____ in the patient's family.

The patient is a _____ with best-corrected acuity of 20/ _____ in the right eye and 20/

_____ in the left eye.

Intraocular pressures were normal at _____ mm Hg in the right eye and _____ mm Hg in the left eye. The patient's retinas appeared healthy, with no signs of hypertensive or diabetic retinopathy. Nor were there signs of macular degeneration. Lenticular changes are normal for the patient's age.

We have taken/recommended baseline visual field tests and retinal photos, which we can forward to you upon request.

Please do not hesitate to contact us should you wish additional information.

Sincerely,

_____ , OD

# Missed Contact Lens Appointment

Dear _____ :

Contact lens wear requires routine follow-up visits to ensure good ocular health and proper fit of your lenses.

When you received your contact lenses, we agreed on a specific schedule for follow-up visits. Our records indicate you missed a follow-up visit on _____ .

We want to help to ensure both comfortable vision and good ocular health, thus the reason for this important reminder.

Please call our office to reschedule this appointment as soon as possible.

Sincerely,

Dr. _____ and Staff

# Confirming Appointment for New Patient

Dear _____:

Thank you for choosing our office and entrusting us with your vision!

Enclosed you will find an appointment card confirming your appointment as well as a copy of our office brochure.

We make every effort to give you the finest vision care. Our office is equipped with the latest technology and our experienced staff is extremely well trained.

Please bring your most recent pair of glasses and sunglasses to your appointment. If applicable, try to wear your contact lenses for two hours before your exam and bring a storage case for after they are checked and removed.

We look forward to seeing you.

Sincerely,

Dr. _____ and Staff

## SUPER BILL

Date of Service: _____

Dr. Seymour Clearly,
125 Main Street
Anytown
USA-999

Patient _____

Insurance Coverage _____ Vision Plan _____

Department Code _____

____ FPS ____ CCLS ____ OD ____ MES ____ TIRR
____ Pediatrics & Binocular Vision ____ Development
____ Diplopia ____ Center for Sight Enhancement

Faculty _____ Student Clinician _____

Acct #: _____

**A Doctor's signature is not required. This form is authentication in itself**
**Notice to Insurance:** This form has been adopted in an effort to keep our costs and paperwork down. If for any reason you require your own form or itemized bill, we will be happy to complete the same upon receipt of: **$20.00**

FILE #: _____

### OFFICE VISITS:

| OFFICE VISITS: | CODE | REF | FEE |
|---|---|---|---|
| **New Patient** | | | |
| Level 1 | 99201 | | |
| Level 2 | 99202 | | |
| Level 3 | 99203 | | |
| Level 4 | 99204 | | |
| Level 5 | 99205 | | |
| **Established Patient** | | | |
| Level 1 | 99211 | | |
| Level 2 | 99212 | | |
| Level 3 | 99213 | | |
| Level 4 | 99214 | | |
| Level 5 | 99215 | | |
| **Other** | | | |
| Postoperative management | 99024 | | |
| Work related examination | 99456 | | |
| **Medicare** | | | |
| Glaucoma Screening | G0117 | | |

| OFFICE VISITS: | CODE | REF | FEE |
|---|---|---|---|
| **Complete Eye Exam (Routine)** | | | |
| complete Eye Exam (New Patient) | S0620 | | |
| complete Eye Exam (Estab. Patient) | S0621 | | |
| **Ophthalmological New Patient** | | | |
| Intermediate Ophthalmological | 92002 | | |
| Comprehensive Ophthalmological | 92004 | | |
| **Ophthalmological Established** | | | |
| Intermediate Ophthalmological | 92012 | | |
| Comprehensive Ophthalmological | 92014 | | |
| **Consultation New or Established** | | | |
| Level 1 Consultation | 99241 | | |
| Level 2 Consultation | 99242 | | |
| Level 3 Consultation | 99243 | | |
| Level 4 Consultation | 99244 | | |
| Level 5 Consultation | 99245 | | |
| **Hospital Inpatient Services** | | | |
| Hospital Care, Initial | 9925 | | |
| Hospital Subsequent Care | 9923 | | |

| OFFICE VISITS: | CODE | REF | FEE |
|---|---|---|---|
| **After Hours in Addition to State Services** | | | |
| Services after posted office hours | 99271 | | |
| Services between 10PM and 8AM | 99272 | | |
| Services on Sundays and Holidays | 99273 | | |
| **Modifiers** | | | |
| Greater than usual procedural service | 22 | | |
| Medicare waiver signed | GA | | |
| Postoperative management only | 55 | | |
| Preoperative management only | 56 | | |
| Prolonged E&M | 21 | | |
| Reduced services | 52 | | |
| Separate E & M, same day as minor proc. | 25 | | |
| Left Upper Eyelid | E1 | | |
| Left Lower Eyelid | E2 | | |
| Right Upper Eyelid | E3 | | |
| Right Lower Eyelip | E4 | | |

### PROCEDURES:

| PROCEDURES: | QTY | CODE | REF | FEE |
|---|---|---|---|---|
| ALP (Hole, Tear) .......... OD, OS, OU | | 67145 | | |
| ALP (Focal) ................. OD, OS, OU | | 67210 | | |
| ALP (PRP) ................... OD, OS, OU | | 67228 | | |
| Angiography Fluorescein | | 92235 | | |
| Ant Stromal Puncture | | 65600 | | |
| Collagen Punctal Closure | | 68731 | | |
| Color Vision, Extended .. OD, OS, OU | | 92283 | | |
| Color Vision, Screening .. OD, OS, OU | | 99172 | | |
| Contrast Sensitivity ...... OD, OS, OU | | 92499A | | |
| Corneal Debridement .... OD, OS, OU | | 65435 | | |
| Corneal Topography | | S0820 | | |
| Electroretinography ........ OD, OS, OU | | 92275 | | |
| Endothelial Microscopy ..... OD, OS, OU | | 92286 | | |
| Epilation, Forceps | | 67820 | | |
| Excision, Chalazion (Single) | | 67800 | | |
| Excision, Chalazion (Multiple) | | 67801 | | |
| Excision Eye Lid Lesion | | 67850 | | |
| FB Removal, Superl. Conj. | | 65205 | | |
| FB Removal, Embedded Conj. | | 65210 | | |
| FB Removal, Cornea | | 65222 | | |
| GDX Screening | | 92135B | | |
| Gonloscopy ................... OD, OS, OU | | 92020 | | |
| Incision, Conj. Cyst | | 68020 | | |
| Iridoplasty ................... OD, OS, OU | | 66762 | | |
| Iridotomy ..................... OD, OS, OU | | 66761 | | |
| Laser Coherence Tomography ................. OD, OS, OU | | 92135 | | |
| Laser Interferometry ........ OD, OS, OU | | 92499C | | |
| Mf-ERG | | 92275A | | |
| Ophthalmoscopy, Extended .. OD, OS, OU | | 92225 | | |
| OPTOS Imaging ............. OD, OS, OU | | 92250A | | |
| Pachymetry ................... OD, OS, OU | | 76514 | | |
| Photography, External ... OD, OS, OU | | 92285 | | |
| Photography, Fundus ...... OD, OS, OU | | 92250 | | |
| Puncturn dilation / Imgation . OD, OS, OU | | 68801 | | |
| Refraction | | 92015 | | |
| Scraping Cornea (Smear or CX) | | 65430 | | |
| S L O ........................... OD, OS, OU | | 92135A | | |
| Serial Tonometry | | 92100 | | |
| Silicone Punctal Closure | | 68761 | | |
| Steroid Injection (External) | | 68200 | | |
| Trabeculoplasty ............. OD, OS, OU | | 65855 | | |
| Ultrasound, A-Scan ........ OD, OS, OU | | 76516 | | |
| Ultrasound, B-Scan ......... OD, OS, OU | | 76512 | | |
| Ultrasound, B-Scan (LS) .. OD, OS, OU | | 76512-52 | | |
| Visual Field Tangent ....... OD, OS, OU | | 92081 | | |
| Visual Field, Screen ...... OD, OS, OU | | 92082 | | |
| Visual Field, Comp Thresh .. OD, OS, OU | | 92083 | | |
| Visual Evoked Potential ...OD, OS, OU | | 95930 | | |
| YAG Capsulotomy ......... OD, OS, OU | | 66821 | | |
| Silicone Punctal Plug (Material) | | 99070B | | |
| Collagen Punctal Plug (Material) | | 99070C | | |

| PROCEDURES: | QTY | CODE | REF | FEE |
|---|---|---|---|---|
| **Pediatric Binocular Services** | | | | |
| Strabismus / Amblyopia Exam | | 92060 | | |
| Binocular Vision Therapy - Initial | | 92065 | | |
| Binocular Vision Therapy - Follow-up | | 92065A | | |
| Developmental Screening | | 96110 | | |
| Auditory / Language Assmt. | | 96111 | | |
| Visual Spatial Cognitive Assmt. | | 96115 | | |
| Visual Perceptual Therapy | | 97532 | | |
| Nystagmus Test, With Report | | 92451 | | |
| Supply V.T. Materials | | 99070A | | |
| **Low Vision Rehabilitation Services** | | | | |
| *SPECIAL EVALUATIONS* | | | | |
| Neuro Re-education | | 97112 | | |
| Cognitive Skill Training | | 97532 | | |
| Sensory Training | | 97533 | | |
| Adaptive Instruction | | 97535 | | |
| Work Reintegration | | 97537 | | |
| Visual Field Tangent ...... OD, OS, OU | | 92081 | | |
| Mag / Refract - New | | LV1 | | |
| Mag / Refract - Estab | | LV2 | | |
| Low Vision Materials | | | | |
| Shipping & handling | | | | |
| Low Vision Rehabilitation | | G9043 | | |
| **Contracts** | | | | |
| Comprehensive Evaluation | | | | |
| Follow-up evaluation | | | | |
| Low Vision Evaluation - Initial | | TCB01 | | |
| Low Vision Evaluation - Brief | | TCB02 | | |
| Low Vision Evaluation - Intermediate | | TCB03 | | |
| Low Vision Evaluation - Extended | | TCB04 | | |
| Low Vision Dispensing Fee | | TCB05 | | |
| Beecher Fit | | TCB10 | | |
| Fitting Fee | | 92354 | | |
| Fitting Fee, Bioplic | | 92355 | | |
| **Laboratory** | | | | |
| Blood Glucose | | 92948 | | |
| Ancillary Lab Test | | | | |
| Conjunctival Smears | | 87205 | | |
| Culture and Sensitivity.... OD, OS, OU | | 87070 | | |
| Venlpuncture | | G0001 | | |

Form of Payment

____ Credit Card ____ Medicare _____%
____ Cash ____ Medicaid ____ Courtesy
____ Check ____ Opticare
____ Other _____

### PROCEDURES:

| PROCEDURES: | | CODE | REF | FEE |
|---|---|---|---|---|
| **Contact Lens Services** | | | | |
| Routine Fitting (Soft or GP) | | 92310 | | |
| Complex Fitting (Soft or GP) | | 92310-21 | | |
| Therapeutic Fitting (Soft or GP) | | 92070 | | |
| Corneal Reshaping (Includes Lenses) | | 92070-21 | | |
| Aphakia (Fitting-Monoc (Includes Lens) | | 92311 | | |
| Aphakia Fitting-Binoc (Includes Lens) | | 92312 | | |
| CL Inspection / Modification | | 92325 | | |
| CL Office Visit / Follow-up | | | | |
| Adaptive F/U Visit (90 Days) | | | | |
| Lens Polish / Cleaning | | | | |

| Contact Lens Materials | DIV | QTY | Unit Cost | Total Cost |
|---|---|---|---|---|
| *Soft Disposable / Planned Replacement* | | | | |
| Single Vision | | | | |
| Toric | | | | |
| Multifocal | | | | |
| Other | | | | |
| *Soft Conventional Lenses* | | | | |
| Single Vision | | | | |
| Toric | | | | |
| Multifocal | | | | |
| Other | | | | |
| *GP Lenses* | | | | |
| Single Vision | | | | |
| Toric | | | | |
| Multifocal | | | | |
| Other | | | | |
| Add-Ons | | | | |
| Contact Lens Supplies | | | | |

Handling Fee _____

Professional Services $ _____

Professional Adjustment _____

Contact Lens Materials ............... _____

Other Materials ......................... _____

DOS: _____ PREVIOUS BALANCE _____

TOTAL _____

AMT PAID _____

BALANCE DUE $ _____

RETURN: _____ Days _____ Weeks _____ Months

| THIS CONDITION RELATES TO | YES | NO | Date of Injury |
|---|---|---|---|
| Patient's Employment | | | |
| ACCIDENT | | | |
| DX1 | DX3 | | |
| DX2 | DX4 | | |

Vision RX Given to Patient: _____ Yes _____ No

_____
**Doctor's Signature**

**ASSIGNMENT AND RELEASE:** I hereby authorize my insurance benefits to be paid directly to Dr. Seymour Clearly. I understand that I am financially responsible for noncovered services. I also authorize the release of any information acuired during the course of my examination treatment.

Signed: _____

*Continued*

## SUPER BILL—cont'd

*Please indicate the appropriate diagnosis(es) by their numerical order of significance.*

| Code | # | Diagnosis |
|---|---|---|
| | | **COLOR VISION DEFECTS** |
| 368.55 | | Acquired color vision deficiency |
| 368.52 | | Deutan defect |
| 368.51 | | Protan defect |
| 368.53 | | Tritan defect |
| | | **CONJUNCTIVA / SCLERA** |
| 918.2 | | Abrasion, conjunctival |
| 372.20 | | Blepharoconjunctivitis - unspecified |
| 372.54 | | Conjunctival concretions |
| 372.75 | | Conjunctival cysts |
| 372.72 | | Conjunctival hemorrhage |
| 372.02 | | Conjunctivitis - acute follicular |
| 372.05 | | Conjunctivitis - acute, allergic |
| 372.03 | | Conjunctivitis - acute, mucopurulent |
| 372.12 | | Conjunctivitis - chronic follicular |
| 372.14 | | Conjunctivitis - chronic, allergic |
| 372.11 | | Conjunctivitis - simple chronic |
| 372.13 | | Conjunctivitis - Vernal |
| 379.01 | | Episcleritis |
| 372.51 | | Pinguecula |
| 372.43 | | Pterygium, central |
| 372.42 | | Pterygium, peripheral, progressive |
| 372.41 | | Pterygium, peripheral, stationary |
| 379.00 | | Scleritis, unspecified |
| | | **CORNEA** |
| 918.1 | | Abrasion, Corneal |
| 371.03 | | Central opacity of cornea |
| 371.40 | | Corneal degeneration |
| 371.50 | | Corneat dystrophy |
| 371.24 | | Corneal edema due to wearing contact lenses |
| 371.21 | | Idiopathic corneal edema |
| 371.62 | | Keratoconus, acute hydrops |
| 371.61 | | Keratoconus, stable condition |
| 371.48 | | Marginal degeneration |
| 371.01 | | Minor opacity of cornea |
| 371.02 | | Peripheral opacity of cornea |
| 371.13 | | Posterior pigmentations |
| 371.42 | | Recurrent erosion of cornea |
| 371.22 | | Secondary corneal edema |
| 371.41 | | Senile corneal changes |
| 371.12 | | Stromal pigmentations |
| | | **EYELIDS DISORDERS OF** |
| 374.34 | | Blepharochalasis |
| 374.87 | | Dermatochalasis |
| 374.82 | | Edema of eyelid |
| 743.63 | | Epicanthal folds |
| 374.20 | | Lagophthalmos |
| 374.30 | | Ptosis of eyelid |
| 374.05 | | Trichiasis without entropion |
| | | **EYELIDS. INF LAMINATION OF** |
| 373.2 | | Chalazion |
| 373.32 | | Contact and allergic dermatitis of eyelid |
| 133.8 | | Demodicosis |
| 373.11 | | Hordeolum extemum (slaphylococcal blepharitis) |
| 373.12 | | Hordeoium intemum - Meibomianitis |
| 373.13 | | Perseptal cellulitis |
| 706.1 | | Rosacea |
| 373.00 | | Seborrheic blepharitis |
| 373.01 | | Ulcerative blepharitis |
| | | **GLAUCOMA** |
| 365.22 | | Acute angle-closure glaucorna |
| 365.02 | | Anatomical narrow angel (boderline) |
| 365.83 | | Aqueous misdirection |
| 743.20 | | Buphthalmos |
| 365.23 | | Chronic angle-closure glaucoma |
| 365.41 | | Glaucoma assoc. with chamber angle anomalies |
| 365.62 | | Glaucoma associated with ocular inflammations |
| 365.61 | | Glaucoma associated with pupillary block |
| 362.63 | | Glaucoma associated with vascular disorders |
| V80.1 | | Glaucoma screening |
| 365.01 | | Glaucoma suspect |
| 365.14 | | Glaucoma, infantite / juvenite |
| 364.22 | | Glaucomatocyclitic crisis |
| 365.31 | | Glaucomatous state (corticosteroid-induced) |
| 365.21 | | Intermittent angle-closure glaucoma |
| 365.12 | | Low tension glaucoma |
| 365.04 | | Ocular hypertension |
| 365.51 | | Phacolytic glaucoma |
| 365.13 | | Pigmentary glaucoma (open-angle) |
| 365.11 | | Primary open angle glaucoma |
| 365.52 | | Pseudoexfoliation glaucoma |
| 364.77 | | Recession of chamber angle |
| 365.32 | | Residual stage (corticosteroid-induced) |
| 365.24 | | Residual stage of angle-closure glaucoma |
| 365.03 | | Steroid responders |
| | | **INJURY TO THE EYE** |
| 940.3 | | Acid chemical bum of cornea and conjunctival sac |
| 940.2 | | Alkaline chemical burn of cornea and conjuctival sac |
| 921.0 | | Black eye not other wise specified |
| 940.0 | | Chemical burn of eyelids and periocular area |
| 921.3 | | Contusion of eyeball |
| 921.1 | | Contusion of eyelids and periocular area |
| 921.2 | | Contusion of orbital tissue |
| 930.0 | | Corneal foreign body |
| 930.1 | | Foreign body in conjunctival sac |
| 918.0 | | Superficial injury of eyelids and periocular area |
| | | **IRIS & CILLARY BODY** |
| 743.45 | | Aniridia |
| 364.72 | | Anterior synechiae |
| 743.46 | | Coloboma of iris |
| 364.54 | | Degeneration of pupilary margin |
| 364.41 | | Hyphema |
| 364.05 | | Hypopyon |
| 364.53 | | Pigmentary iris degeneration |
| 364.71 | | Posterior synechiae |
| 364.01 | | Primary iridocyclitis |
| 364.02 | | Recurrent Iridocyclitis |
| 364.03 | | Secondary Iridocyclitis, Infection |
| 364.04 | | Secondary Iridocyclitis, noninfectious |
| | | **V-CODES** |
| V72.0 | | Examination of eye and vision |
| V65.5 | | Feared condition not demonstrated |
| V80.1 | | Glaucoma screening |
| | | |

| Code | # | Diagnosis |
|---|---|---|
| | | **KERATITIS** |
| 370.03 | | Central corneal ulcer |
| 370.55 | | Corneal abscess |
| 370.62 | | Deep vascularization of cornea |
| 370.52 | | Diffuse interstitial keratitis |
| 370.34 | | Exposure keratoconjunctivitis |
| 370.23 | | Filamentary keratitis |
| 370.64 | | Ghost vessels (corneal) |
| 054.42 | | HSV dendritic keratitis |
| 054.43 | | HSV keratitis (disciform, interstitial) |
| 370.04 | | Hypopyon ulcer |
| 370.33 | | Keratoconjunctivitis sicca |
| 370.61 | | Localized vascularization of cornea |
| 370.22 | | Macular keratitis |
| 370.01 | | Marginal corneal ulcer |
| 370.07 | | Mooren's ulcer |
| 370.05 | | Mycotic corneal ulcer |
| 370.62 | | Pannus (corneal) |
| 370.06 | | Perforated corneal ulcer |
| 370.31 | | Phlyctenular keratoconjunctivitis |
| 370.21 | | Punctate keratitis |
| 370.02 | | Ring corneal ulcer |
| | | **LACRIMAL SYSTEM** |
| 375.32 | | Acute dacryocystitis |
| 375.42 | | Chronic dacryocystitis |
| 375.20 | | Excessive tearing |
| 375.15 | | Dry eye |
| 375.21 | | Epiphora due to excess lacrimation |
| 375.22 | | Epiphora due to insufficient drainage |
| | | **LENS** |
| 366.53 | | After-cataract, obscuring vision |
| 366.13 | | Anterior subcapsular cataract |
| 379.31 | | Aphakia (acquired) |
| 366.19 | | Combined forms-senile |
| 366.15 | | Cortical senile cataract |
| 366.18 | | Hypermature cataract |
| 366.12 | | Incipient cataract |
| 366.16 | | Nuclear scterosis |
| 366.14 | | Posterior subcapsular cataract |
| 366.11 | | Pseudoexfoliation of lens capsule |
| V43.1 | | Pseudophakia |
| 379.32 | | Subluxation of lens |
| 366.17 | | Total or mature cataract |
| | | **NEOPLASMS BENIGN** |
| 224.6 | | Choroid |
| 224.3 | | Conjunctiva |
| 224.4 | | Cornea |
| 216.1 | | Eyelid, including skin |
| 224.7 | | Lacrimal Duct |
| 224.2 | | Lacrimal gland |
| 224.1 | | Orbit |
| 224.5 | | Retina |
| | | **OPTIC NERVE** |
| 377.21 | | Drusen of optic disc |
| 377.14 | | Glaucomatous atrophy (cupping) of optic disc |
| 377.41 | | Ischemic optic neuropathy |
| 377.10 | | Optic atrophy |
| 377.00 | | Optic disc edema |
| 374.10 | | Optic hypoplasia |
| 377.32 | | Optic papillitis |
| 377.24 | | Pseudopapilledema |
| | | **ORBIT** |
| 376.00 | | Acute inflammation of orbit, unspecified |
| 376.10 | | Chronic inflammation of orbit, unspecified |
| 376.31 | | Constant exophthaimos |
| 376.50 | | Enophthalmos |
| 376.22 | | Exophthalmic ophthalmoplegia |
| 376.30 | | Exophthalmos, unspecified |
| 376.36 | | Lateral displacement of globe |
| 376.01 | | Orbital cellulitis |
| 376.11 | | Orbital granuloma |
| 376.32 | | Orbital herriorrhage |
| 376.12 | | Orbital myositis |
| 376.21 | | Thyrotoxic exophthalmos |
| | | **OTHER** |
| 270.2 | | Albinism |
| 315.02 | | Developmental dyslexia |
| 250.51 | | Diabetes, type 1 with ophthalmic manifestations |
| 250.01 | | Diabetes, type 1 without mention of complications |
| 250.50 | | Diabetes, type 2 with ophthalmic manifestations |
| 250.00 | | Diabetes, type 2 without mention of complications |
| 796.2 | | Elevated blood pressure reading w/o dx of HTN |
| 228.00 | | Hemangioma |
| 315.2 | | Other specified learning difficulties |
| 315.2 | | Perceptual disorders |
| 710.0 | | Systemic lupus erythematosus |
| | | **REFRACTION & ACCOMMODATION** |
| 367.32 | | Aniseikonia |
| 367.31 | | Anisometropia |
| 367.20 | | Astigmatism |
| 367.0 | | Hyperopia |
| 367.1 | | Myopia |
| 367.51 | | Paresis of accommodation |
| 367.4 | | Presbyopia |
| 367.53 | | Spasm of accommodation |
| 367.52 | | Total or complete internal ophthalmoplegia |
| 367.81 | | Transient refraction change |
| | | **PUPILS** |
| 379.46 | | Adie's pupil |
| 376.41 | | Anisocoria |
| 337.9 | | Homer's syndrome |
| 379.42 | | Miosis, not due to miotics |
| 379.43 | | Mydriasis, not due to mydriatics |
| | | **VISUAL IMPAIRMENT** |

| | BETTER EYE | | | | |
|---|---|---|---|---|---|
| WORSE EYE | NLP | VA<20/1000 VF <5° | VA 20/500-1000 VF <10° | VA 20/200-400 VF <20° | VA 20/70-160 |
| NLP | 369.01 | 369.03 | 369.06 | 369.12 | 369.16 |
| VA<20/1000 VF <5° | | 369.04 | 369.07 | 369.13 | 369.17 |
| VA 20/500-1000 VF <10° | | | 369.08 | 369.14 | 369.18 |
| VA 20/200-400 VF <20° | | | | 369.22 | 369.24 |
| VA 20/70-160 | | | | | 369.25 |

| Code | # | Diagnosis |
|---|---|---|
| | | **RETINA & CHOROID** |
| 362.32 | | Arterial branch occlusion |
| 362.31 | | Central retinal artery occlusion |
| 362.35 | | Central retinal vein occlusion |
| 363.20 | | Choroiditis |
| 743.56 | | Coloboma of retina |
| 921.3 | | Commotio retinae |
| 362.75 | | Cone (-rod) dystrophy |
| 362.63 | | Degeneration - lattice |
| 362.62 | | Degeneration - microcystoid |
| 362.61 | | Degeneration - pavingstone |
| 362.64 | | Degeneration - senile reticular |
| 362.60 | | Degeneration - retinal (peripheral) |
| 362.07 | | Diabetic macular edema |
| 362.04 | | Diabetic retinopathy - mild nonproliferative |
| 362.05 | | Diabetic retinopathy - moderate nonproliferative |
| 362.02 | | Diabetic retinopahty - proliferative |
| 362.06 | | Diabetic retinopathy - servere nonproliferative |
| 361.32 | | Horseshoe tear without detachment |
| 362.57 | | Macular - Drusen (degenerative) |
| 362.75 | | Macular - Stargardt's disease |
| 362.54 | | Macular - cyst, hole, or pseudohole |
| 362.53 | | Macular degeneration - cystoid |
| 362.52 | | Macular degeneration - exudative senile |
| 362.51 | | Macular degeneration - nonexudative senile |
| 362.56 | | Macular puckering |
| 363.32 | | Macular scars |
| 363.21 | | Pars planitis |
| 362.33 | | Partial arterial occlusion |
| 363.34 | | Peripheral scars |
| 362.83 | | Retinal edema |
| 362.81 | | Retinal hernorrhage |
| 362.16 | | Retinal neovascularization |
| 362.85 | | Retinal nerve fiber bundle defects |
| 362.74 | | Retinitis plgmentosa |
| 363.20 | | Retinochoroiditis |
| 362.13 | | Retinopathy - atherosclerotic / arteriosclerotic |
| 362.41 | | Retinopathy - central serous |
| 362.11 | | Retinopathy - hypertensive |
| 362.21 | | Retinopathy of prematurity |
| 361.31 | | Round hole of retina without detachment |
| 362.42 | | Serous detachment of retinal pigment epithelium |
| 362.55 | | Toxic maculopathy |
| 362.37 | | Venous engorgement |
| 362.36 | | Venous tributary (branch) occlusion |
| | | **RETINAL DETACHMENT** |
| 361.12 | | Bullous retinoschisis |
| 361.2 | | Exudative detachment |
| 361.11 | | Flat retinoschisis |
| 361.13 | | Primary retinat cysts |
| 361.00 | | Rhegmatogenous detachment |
| 361.14 | | Secondary retinat cysts |
| 361.30 | | Serous detachment |
| 361.81 | | Traction detachment of retina |
| | | **SIGNS & SYMPTOMS PAIN GENERAL** |
| 436 | | Acute, ill defined, cerebrovascular disease |
| 368.8 | | Blurring vision |
| 346.00 | | Classical migraine / migraine with aura |
| 346.10 | | Common migraine' |
| 692.9 | | Dermatitis, contact, unspecified |
| 693.0 | | Dermatitis, due to drugs/medications |
| 379.91 | | Eye pain (ocular irritation) |
| 784.0 | | Headache (excel. migraine & tension) |
| 346.90 | | Migraine, unspecified |
| 346.80 | | Ophthalmic migraine |
| | | **STRABISMUS & BINOCULAR EYE MOVEMENT** |
| 368.34 | | Abnormal retinal correspondence |
| 368.02 | | Amblyopia, deprivation |
| 368.03 | | Amblyopia, refractive |
| 368.01 | | Amblyopia, strabismic |
| 378.85 | | Anomalies of divergence |
| 378.84 | | Convergence excess or spasm |
| 378.83 | | Convergence insufficiency or palsy |
| 378.51 | | Cranial nerve III palsy, partial |
| 378.52 | | Cranial nerve III palsy, total |
| 378.53 | | Cranial nerve IV palsy |
| 378.54 | | Cranial nerve VI palsy |
| 378.41 | | Esophoria |
| 378.05 | | Esotropia, alternating |
| 378.01 | | Esotropia, monocular |
| 378.42 | | Exophoria |
| 378.15 | | Exotropia, alternating |
| 378.11 | | Exotropia, monocular |
| 378.55 | | External ophthalmoplegia |
| 368.33 | | Fusion with defective stereopsis |
| 378.31 | | Hypertropia |
| 378.32 | | Hypotropia |
| 378.34 | | Microtropia (monofixation syndrome) |
| 379.50 | | Nystagmus, acquired |
| 379.51 | | Nystagmus, congenital |
| 379.52 | | Nystagmus, latent |
| 368.32 | | Simultaneous visual perception without fusion |
| 368.31 | | Suppression of binocular vision |
| 378.56 | | Total ophthalmopiegia |
| 378.43 | | Vertical neterophoria |
| | | **VISUAL DISTURBANCES / FIELD DEFECTS** |
| 377.75 | | Cortical visual impairment |
| 368.2 | | Diplopia |
| 368.45 | | Generalized contraction or constriction of VF |
| 368.47 | | Heteronymous bilateral field defects |
| 368.46 | | Homonymous bilateral field defects |
| 368.44 | | Other localized visual defect |
| 368.41 | | Scotoma involving central area |
| 368.42 | | Scotoma of blind spot area |
| 368.43 | | Sector or arcuate defects |
| 368.11 | | Sudden visual loss |
| 368.12 | | Transient visual loss |
| 368.10 | | Vision disturbance, subjective |
| 368.13 | | Visual discomfort / asthenopia |
| | | **VITREOUS** |
| 362.21 | | Fibrovascular proliferation |
| 379.21 | | PVD, liquefaction |
| 379.24 | | Vitreous floaters |
| 379.23 | | Vitreous hemorrhage |
| 379.26 | | Vitreous prolapse |

## SUPPLEMENTAL SERVICES
### RECORD OF VISIT

Name _____    DOB _____    Phone _____

| DATE | DOCTOR | OBSERVATIONS, SYMPTOMS, INSTRUCTIONS |
|------|--------|-------------------------------------|
|  |  |  |
|  |  |  |
|  |  |  |
|  |  |  |
|  |  |  |
|  |  |  |
|  |  |  |
|  |  |  |
|  |  |  |
|  |  |  |
|  |  |  |
|  |  |  |
|  |  |  |
|  |  |  |
|  |  |  |
|  |  |  |
|  |  |  |
|  |  |  |
|  |  |  |
|  |  |  |
|  |  |  |
|  |  |  |
|  |  |  |
|  |  |  |
|  |  |  |
|  |  |  |
|  |  |  |
|  |  |  |
|  |  |  |
|  |  |  |
|  |  |  |
|  |  |  |
|  |  |  |
|  |  |  |
|  |  |  |
|  |  |  |
|  |  |  |
|  |  |  |
|  |  |  |
|  |  |  |
|  |  |  |
|  |  |  |
|  |  |  |
|  |  |  |

# Patient Survey

Dear _____:

Our practice continues to grow because of referrals from satisfied and enthusiastic patients. Would you kindly take a moment to answer the following questions so that we may use this information to improve our services?

1. When you made your appointment, were you treated politely on the telephone? Yes _____ No _____
2. When you made your appointment, was the telephone answered promptly? Yes _____ No _____
3. Are you pleased with your new glasses and/or contact lenses? Yes _____ No _____
4. Is there a staff member who stands out as giving exceptionally friendly or courteous service? Yes _____ No _____
   Name _____
5. Is there a staff member who stands out as being unfriendly or discourteous?
Yes _____ No _____ Name _____
6. Did Dr. _____ give you a full explanation of your visual condition and recommendation for correction?
Yes _____ No _____

Comments:
_____
_____

Was there any confusion between the doctor, our staff, and you about the doctor's recommendations?
Yes _____ No _____

Comments:
_____
_____

8. How would you rate the overall quality of care received in our office (circle one)?
Fair     Average     Above average     Outstanding
9. How would you rate the overall appearance of our staff and office (circle one)?
Fair     Average     Above average     Outstanding
10. Would you recommend Dr. _____ and our office to your friends?
Yes _____ No _____
11. How can we improve our service?
Comments: _____
Please feel free to add any other comments you may wish to make.
_____
_____

Please return anonymously in the envelope provided.

Thank you,

Dr. _____ and Staff

# Telephone Inquiry

Name: _____ Phone: _____ Date: _____

Address: _____ City: _____ State: _____ Zip: _____

Inquiry Regarding: _____Eye exam _____Contact lens exam _____LASIK _____ Office hours
_____ Experience of doctors

Calling for self or someone else? _____ Age _____

Currently wearing contact lenses? Yes _____ No _____

Type: Soft_____ Extended wear_____ Gas permeable_____

Were fees quoted? Yes _____ No _____ If yes, amount and for what? _____

Years since last exam: _____

Appointment made: Yes _____ Date/Time: _____

No _____ Reason: _____

How did the caller find us? _____ Yellow Pages ____ Internet ____ Friend/relative ____ Other

Information Requested: Yes ____ No____ Information sent: Yes ____ no_____

Comments: _____

When to call again: _____

Follow-up comments: _____

# Thank You to Current Patient

Dear _____ ,

We want to let you know how much we appreciate you continuing to rely on our office for your vision care needs. We are very aware of the trust and the responsibility placed on us and we intend to live up to your expectations.

If there is any aspect of our care we can improve, please let us know. We hope to continue our relationship with you, and we value your comments. Your vision is precious and our goal is to help you protect it.

Thanks again for the trust you've shown in selecting our office. We look forward to seeing you again in the near future.

Sincerely,

Dr._____ and Staff

# Thank You to New Patient

Dear _____:

I would like to take this opportunity to welcome you to our office and to thank you for becoming a patient. We are delighted you chose our office for your vision care. We pride ourselves in making our patients feel welcomed and cared for.

Your support is appreciated and we would be grateful for any opportunity to provide vision care to other members of your family and your friends. You can be assured when referring them that we will give them the same careful attention and quality of care you receive.

If you have any questions or if we can be of assistance to you before your next scheduled visit, please call.

Again, welcome and thank you for choosing us!

Sincerely,

Dr. _____ and Staff

# Thank You for Your Referral

Dear _____:

Thank you for referring _____ to our office.

It is a pleasure to receive referrals from our patients because that indicates you are satisfied with our services and care. We appreciate the opportunity to demonstrate that the confidence you express by sending a family member or friend is not misplaced. I assure you that any relatives or friends you recommend will receive our thorough attention and the same quality of care you have experienced.

Thanks again. We value your loyalty.

Sincerely,

Dr. _____ and Staff

# Transfer of Spectacle Information

To: _____ Re: _____

Address: _____

Dear Doctor:

[ ] I am referring the above patient to you for continued vision care and submitting the following information.
[ ] The patient named above has come to me for continued vision care. Please supply the indicated information listed below.
Thank you.

Pertinent refractive, ocular, and general health information (use reverse side if necessary):

_____

Date of last examination: _____

Chief complaint at last examination: _____

Unaided VA at last exam:      Far    Near
             OD 20/ _____      20/ _____
             OS 20/ _____      20/ _____
Best corrected VA at last exam:      Far Near
             OD 20/ _____      20/ _____
             OS 20/ _____      20/ _____

Were new glasses prescribed? Yes _____      No _____
Ks OD _____ OS _____

Last Rx dispensed:

| Sph | Cyl | Axis | Prism | Base | Add | Type | PD |
|-----|-----|------|-------|------|-----|------|-----|
|     |     |      |       |      |     |      |     |
|     |     |      |       |      |     |      |     |

Tint _____ Glass _____ Hard resin _____
Prescribed to wear: Far only _____ Near only _____ Constantly _____
Comments: _____
_____

I hereby grant permission for the above-named doctor to exchange information from my patient records.

[ ] Parent or [ ] Guardian Signature: _____ Date:_____

# Triage Sheet

Date/time _____ Patient name _____

Patient telephone (home) _____ (work) _____

Staff member _____

Which eye? Right / Left / Both  When symptoms began: _____

Has there been any sudden changes in vision?    Yes / No

If yes, was it: Suddenly blurry / **Suddenly dim or black** / Suddenly double

Is there any pain or discomfort?     Yes / No

If yes, is it:    Throbbing pain / Dull pain / Sharp pain / Itch

Did you get anything in your eye? Yes / No / Don't know

If yes, was it:    A **chemical** / other _____

If a chemical, instruct patient to irrigate immediately with water for 20 minutes and call back.

Is there any discharge?      Yes / No _____

Has there been any trauma to the eye or head? Yes / No _____

Is the eye red?     Yes / No _____

Do you see flashes of light?     Yes / No      _____

Do you have a sudden increase in floaters or spots? Yes / No _____

Do you wear contact lenses?     Yes / No _____

If yes, instruct to remove if any redness, pain, or discharge is present.

_____ Emergency – Any Bold answer – Schedule immediately or refer to ER

_____ Urgent – If any YES is circled (except for contact lenses) – Schedule within 24 hours

_____ Routine – Any call with no YES responses – Schedule at patient's convenience

Appointment (day and time) _____

---

Optometrist review:

_____ Appointment approved

_____ Reschedule for immediate appointment

_____ Reschedule for urgent appointment

# Visual Field Examination

A highly sophisticated computerized visual field testing instrument allows us to provide a more thorough medical analysis of your eyes. This instrument electronically measures retinal and optic nerve function and sensitivity to light in both the central (straight-ahead) and peripheral (side-view) areas. This measurement can assist us in early detection of many disorders, including brain tumors, glaucoma, diabetic retinopathy, and retinal disorders.

We strongly recommend that all our patients receive the screening version of this exam. It is especially important for people who:

- Have Headaches
- See spots or flashes of light
- Have A history of diabetes
- Have A history of high blood pressure
- Have Circulatory problems
- Have A strong eyeglass prescription

There is an additional charge of $_____ for this screening exam. Many major medical insurance plans will reimburse you for this medical procedure.

Please check the appropriate line below and sign the bottom.

_____ I do want a visual field exam.

_____ I do not want a visual field exam.

Patient's name (print) _____

Patient's signature _____ Date _____

# Welcome to Our Office

Patient name _____

Who pays the bills at your house? _____

How did you hear of our practice?

❏ Patient referral: Whom may we thank for referring you? _____

❏ Yellow Pages

❏ Insurance plan

❏ Doctor referral

❏ Location

❏ Other _____

Patient birth date _____ ❏ M  ❏ F  E-mail address _____

Mailing address _____  Apt# _____

City _____ State _____ Zip _____

Phone: Home (   ) _____ Work (   ) _____

Vision insurance company _____

Patient ID# (if none, use SS#) _____

Whose insurance is this? _____

Subscriber ID# or SS# _____

How is patient related (circle one)?     Self      Spouse      Child

Secondary or medical insurance company _____

Whose insurance is this? _____

Subscriber ID# or SS# _____

How is patient related (circle one)?     Self      Spouse      Child

Occupation? _____

Employer/School _____

I authorize my insurance company to pay for the above services. I understand that I am responsible for any charges denied by my insurance company.

Signature _____

## Health Form

Patient name _____

Have you or your relatives been diagnosed with any of the following?

| You | Your family | You | Your family |
|---|---|---|---|
| ❏ | ❏ Glaucoma | ❏ | ❏ Cancer |
| ❏ | ❏ Cataracts | ❏ | ❏ Stroke |
| ❏ | ❏ Turned or crossed eye | ❏ | ❏ Heart disease |
| ❏ | ❏ Diabetes | ❏ | ❏ Neurological disorders |
| ❏ | ❏ High blood pressure | ❏ | ❏ Kidney/thyroid disease |

Who is your primary care physician? _____

Please list all medications you are currently taking:

(include vitamins and over-the-counter medications; check here if none ❏)

Are you allergic to any medications? _____

Are you a smoker (circle one)?          Yes        No

Please describe any eye injuries or surgeries you have had. _____

When was your last eye examination? _____

Do you wear contact lenses (circle one)?          Yes        No

Would you be interested in learning more about contact lenses (circle one)?      Yes        No

If you do wear contact lenses, are you having any problems? _____

Do you have seasonal (hay fever) allergies? _____

## Patients Who Need to Be Rescheduled

| Patient | Phone # (home, work, etc.) | Treatment | With Whom | Desired Time | Call Result | Date | Initials |
|---------|----------------------------|-----------|-----------|--------------|-------------|------|----------|
|         |                            |           |           |              |             |      |          |
|         |                            |           |           |              |             |      |          |
|         |                            |           |           |              |             |      |          |
|         |                            |           |           |              |             |      |          |
|         |                            |           |           |              |             |      |          |
|         |                            |           |           |              |             |      |          |
|         |                            |           |           |              |             |      |          |
|         |                            |           |           |              |             |      |          |
|         |                            |           |           |              |             |      |          |
|         |                            |           |           |              |             |      |          |

- Keep this form near the phone.
- Place patient name and information on list, one patient per row.
- Contact when the desired opening occurs in the schedule.
- Record results of contact (coming in, etc.), call date, and intials of person placing the call.
- Bring list to doctor's attention weekly for reveiw.
- After three attempts to contact and if no appointment is scheduled, bring to attention of doctor.

## Priority Rescheduling

| Patient | Treatment | Phone # (home, work, etc.) | Desired Time | Result | Date | Initials |
|---------|-----------|----------------------------|--------------|--------|------|----------|
|  |  |  |  |  |  |  |
|  |  |  |  |  |  |  |
|  |  |  |  |  |  |  |
|  |  |  |  |  |  |  |
|  |  |  |  |  |  |  |
|  |  |  |  |  |  |  |
|  |  |  |  |  |  |  |
|  |  |  |  |  |  |  |
|  |  |  |  |  |  |  |
|  |  |  |  |  |  |  |
|  |  |  |  |  |  |  |

■ Keep this form near the phone.

■ Place patient name and information on list, one patient per row.

■ Contact when the desired opening occurs in the schedule.

■ Record results of contact (coming in, etc.), call date, and initials of person placing the call.

■ Bring list to doctor's attention weekly for reveiw.

■ After three attempts to contact and if no appointment is scheduled, bring to attention of doctor.

# Part 3

# Practice Administration and Sample Contracts

# Introduction to Using These Samples (Disclaimer and Recommendation for Legal Consult)

The following pages contain documents that are intended for use as examples only. Please use these examples to simplify discussions with attorneys and accountants and make those discussions more efficient. Do not assume that you can use these agreements or forms in your state without the advice of an attorney and/or accountant. Laws vary from state to state. For example, in some states it is permissible to have a covenant not-to-compete in employment agreements, but in other states such restrictions are not enforceable without a transfer of equity (i.e., between partners or upon a sale). The publishers are not responsible for the legal consequences you incur as a result of using these documents. Again, it is strongly recommended that you seek the advice of a lawyer for information about the validity and consequences of using the documents contained in this section.

# Application for Employment

So that your application may be properly evaluated, please answer all questions on this application carefully and completely.

You will be considered for employment without regard to your race, color, creed, sex, religion, marital status, national origin, status with regard to public assistance, disability, or age.

## Please Print

Name in full _____

Present address _____

Phone number _____ How long have you lived here? _____

Permanent address _____
         (if different from above)

Position desired _____ Salary desired _____ Are you now employed? ____

Where? _____ May we contact your present employer? _____

Are you acquainted with or related to any person employed here? _____

Who? _____ Relationship _____

Date available for work _____ Are you willing to be bonded? _____

Physical disabilities or chronic illnesses _____

Days absent from work last year due to sickness _____ Can you work overtime? _____

Any professional license _____ Current license # _____ State issued _____

*Secretarial, clerical, and office applicants only*

Can you type?        Yes        No        Speed (wpm) _____

Operate computer equipment?    Yes        No

Run 10-key adding machine?     Yes        No

Do you know ophthalmic terminology?    Yes        No

List other secretarial, clerical, and accounting skills _____

## Education

High school _____

College or university _____

## Employment Record

Company name _____

Address _____

City, state, zip _____

Phone number _____

Immediate supervisor _____

Dates of employment _____

Salary/hourly wage _____

Duties _____

Reason for leaving _____

## Personal References (Do Not List Relatives)

| Name | Address | Phone | Business |
|------|---------|-------|----------|
|      |         |       |          |
|      |         |       |          |
|      |         |       |          |
|      |         |       |          |

## Read Carefully Before Signing (We Bond All Employees)

1. All statements made by me on this application are true to the best of my knowledge and belief. If I have submitted any false information, it is cause for my immediate discharge.

2. Should I desire to leave your employ, I agree to give my written resignation 2 weeks before my termination date.

3. At no time, whether I am an employee or not, will I reveal any information regarding patients to anyone unless I have been specifically instructed to do so.

Date _____ Signature _____

## To Be Completed on the Date Employment Begins

Date of birth _____ Height _____ Weight _____ SS# _____

Number of dependents _____ Marital status: Single    Married    Divorced    Widowed

Are you covered by a spouse's health insurance?  Yes    No

# Telephone Reference Check

Applicant's name _____

Reference source _____

Relationship to applicant _____

1. State your identity and the purpose of your call. Give the reference source some basic information about the job the applicant is being considered for.

2. Confirm: Previous position _____

Starting date _____ Salary _____

Ending date _____ Salary _____

Reason for leaving _____

_____

Tardiness or absenteeism? _____

3. What can you tell me about this employee? _____

_____

_____

4. Strengths _____

_____

5. Weaknesses _____

_____

6. Would you rehire? _____ Reason _____

_____

7. Additional comments _____

_____

References checked by _____ Date _____

# Offer of Employment

Dear _____ :

We are pleased to confirm our offer for you to join _____ as an optometric assistant. We are confident your acceptance will make a positive addition to our practice. The basic terms of the offer are as follows:

1. Your starting pay will be $____ per hour. After a 3-month probationary period, your salary will be $_____ per month. Your starting schedule will be Monday from 8:30 AM to 12:30 PM; Tuesday, Thursday, and Friday from 8:30 AM to 5:30 PM with a 1-hour lunch; Wednesday from 9:30 AM to 6:30 PM with a 1-hour lunch, and Saturdays as needed (Saturday hours are typically 9 AM to 2 PM). Not including any Saturday hours, this is 36 hours per week.

2. The first 3 months of employment are considered probationary, or at will. This is our opportunity to assess how well you integrate into our office work structure and your opportunity to assess us as well. During this time you may resign or we may discontinue your employment without notice. After 3 months, a 30-day notice is requested.

3. After 3 months, at your election you will be eligible for full-time benefits, including _____ medical coverage, 5 days paid vacation, 10 paid holidays, and 5 days sick leave annually. (Sick leave is not to be used as additional vacation but only for medical necessity.) Salaried employees are also eligible for "comp time," that is, replacing a holiday not taken because of the employee's work schedule, or for extra hours worked with the approval of the office manager. Comp time must be taken within the current calendar year. Vacation is accrued and prorated on a yearly basis. Our policy is to offer _____ medical coverage for our salaried employees, for which you will be eligible after the 3-month probationary period. Deductions can be made to add dependents on a before-tax basis. You will also be eligible to participate in the employee retirement and pension plan after your first full year of employment. Cost of living, merit, and benefit increases are normally considered in January of each year.

We look forward to working with you!

Sincerely,

_____ , OD

# Employee Evaluation Report

Name: _____     Date: _____

E = Excellent
S = Satisfactory
P = Progressing
N = Needs improvement

## Personal Qualities

A. Individuality
    1. Personal appearance
        a. Neatness, cleanliness, appropriateness
    2. Behavior/disposition
    3. Communication skills
        a. Thoughtful
        b. Impulsive
        c. Attitude, morale, work ethic
B. Dependability and initiative
    1. Punctuality/keeping to scheduled work hours
    2. Recording hours worked as well as sick/vacation days
    3. Responsiveness
        a. Completion and focus on tasks assigned without interfering with other staff members' assigned tasks
        b. Initiative toward tasks unassigned but necessary
        c. To needs of doctors
        d. Carries out procedures/attention to detail
C. Productivity
    1. Quantity of work accomplished
    2. Quality of work accomplished
D. Cooperation
    1. Willingness to help
    2. Willingness to learn and be trained
    3. Willingness to accept responsibility for work not up to par
E. Patient relations
    1. Listens carefully to the needs of the patient and acts on those needs
    2. Friendly and courteous
    3. Tactful with the patients as well as staff in front of patients
F. Adaptability
    1. Offers new ideas
    2. Accepts new changes that are not necessarily his or her own
    3. Implements new methods and is willing to maintain them

## Front Office Skills

A. Telephone etiquette
B. Bookkeeping procedures
    1. Accuracy in figuring patients' balances
C. Appointment scheduling
D. Filing procedures
E. Insurance claims
F. Typing accuracy
G. Keeping patient flow smooth

## Dispensing/Lab/Optical Skills

A. PDs
B. Seg heights for bifocals, trifocals, and PALS
C. Appropriate frame selection
    1. For Rx
    2. For patient's physical needs
    3. For patient's lifestyle
    4. For patient's personal aesthetics

*Continued*

## Employee Evaluation Report—cont'd

D. Appropriate lens selection
E. Frame adjustment
F. Frame repairs
G. Lensometer
   1. Accuracy in neutralization
   2. Corroboration of orders (e.g., correct frame, PDs, lens material, segs, tints)
H. Contact lenses
   1. Accuracy in neutralization
   2. Corroboration of orders (e.g., lens material, diameter, OZD, tints)
   3. Insertion and removal
   4. Care
I. Autoperimeter
   1. Use of instrument
   2. Accuracy in determining lenses to aid patient

### Office Administration

A. Office management
   1. Puts effort toward success of daily operations
   2. Supports executive structure
   3. Maintains priorities in accordance with office policy
   4. Willingness to maintain the physical appearance, cleanliness, and order of the office
   5. Tracks inventory of solutions, office supplies, and maintenance of equipment
   6. Anticipates challenges
   7. Offers solutions
   8. Adheres to policies on safety
   9. Practice promotions
B. Statistics
   1. Proficiency in calculation and analysis
C. Reconciliation
   1. Statements/invoices
D. Returns
   1. Accuracy and timeliness in return of frames and contact lenses for credit
E. Recall cards

### Employee Feedback

A. Assessment of employee, management, and office policy performance

### Employee Goals

A. Short- and long-term goals
B. Suggestions for improving office procedures, work conditions, and assistance needed in achieving goals

# Employee Self-Evaluation

## Job Performance Self-Evaluation

E = Excellent          G = Good          RI = Room for improvement

Staff member _____ Date _____

|  | E | G | RI |
|---|---|---|---|

### I. Personal: Are you bringing the best you can to each patient?

| | E | G | RI |
|---|---|---|---|
| A. How do you rate your clothing/uniform appearance? (style, cleanliness) | —— | —— | —— |
| B. How do you rate your personal appearance? (hair, nails, makeup, hands, neatness, etc.) | —— | —— | —— |
| C. How do you rate your enthusiasm? | —— | —— | —— |

### II. General: Is this office better because of you?

| | E | G | RI |
|---|---|---|---|
| A. How do you rate your punctuality? | —— | —— | —— |
| B. How do you rate your willingness to work? | —— | —— | —— |
| C. How do you work at saving expenses? | —— | —— | —— |
| D. How do you rate your ability to act professionally? | —— | —— | —— |
| E. How do you rate your ability to keep office information confidential? | —— | —— | —— |

### III. Duties: Do you earn your wages?

| | E | G | RI |
|---|---|---|---|
| A. How do you rate your ability to find work during slack time? | —— | —— | —— |
| B. How do you rate the efficiency of your work? | —— | —— | —— |
| C. How do you rate your striving for self-improvement? | —— | —— | —— |
| D. How do you rate your growth in job abilities? | —— | —— | —— |
| E. How do you rate your ability to conserve supplies and stock? | —— | —— | —— |
| F. How do you rate your positive mental attitude? | —— | —— | —— |
| G. How do you rate your ability to leave your home problems at home? | —— | —— | —— |
| H. How do you rate your ability to take responsibility? (Carrying out jobs, finding solutions, etc.) | —— | —— | —— |

### IV. Patient relations

| | E | G | RI |
|---|---|---|---|
| A. How do you rate your ability to make each patient feel special? | —— | —— | —— |
| B. How do you rate your ability to treat everyone alike? | —— | —— | —— |
| C. How do you rate your ability to visit with patients? | —— | —— | —— |
| D. How do you rate your striving to sell "optometry"? | —— | —— | —— |
| E. How do you rate your ability to handle difficult patients? | —— | —— | —— |
| F. How do you rate your ability to alert the doctor to something special in a patient's life? | —— | —— | —— |

### V. Staff relations: Are you good to work with?

| | E | G | RI |
|---|---|---|---|
| A. How do you rate your ability to pitch in and help out? | —— | —— | —— |
| B. How do you rate your ability to be friendly with other members of the staff? | —— | —— | —— |
| C. How do you rate your "member of the team" attitude? | —— | —— | —— |

### VI. Employer relations

| | E | G | RI |
|---|---|---|---|
| A. How do you rate your willingness to learn? | —— | —— | —— |
| B. How do you rate your ability to accept constructive help and direction? | —— | —— | —— |

### VII. Comments: _____

_____

_____

_____

_____

_____

_____

_____

_____

_____

*Continued*

## Employee Self-Evaluation—cont'd

### VIII. Staff members' comments

A. How could this office be a better place to work? _____

B. What would you like to see changed? _____

C. Are you happy with your job? _____

D. Do you feel your salary and fringe benefits are fair? _____

E. What do you feel is your strongest attribute? _____

F. What do you feel is your weakest attribute? _____

G. What are your goals for the next 12 months? _____


_____          _____

Date                                              Signature of employee

# Personnel Performance Evaluation

## Instructions

Evaluate each component of performance on the following scale:

5 = Performance in all aspects materially exceeds the requirements and is outstanding and deserving of special commendation.

4 = Performance is in the upper limit of acceptability, being substantially above average but not meriting special commendation: needs very little improvement.

3 = Performance is in the middle limit of acceptability; average.

2 = Performance is satisfactory but is in the lower limit of acceptability.

1 = Performance is considered to be unacceptable, being deficient to such a degree as to require major improvement.

## Attitude

Influence on others

    Cheerful and considerate toward patients         _____

    Cheerful and considerate toward staff         _____

    Sympathetic and confidential with patient problems         _____

    Helps and teaches others willingly         _____

    Contributes ideas         _____

    Shows enthusiasm in discharge of duties         _____

    Is loyal to employer         _____

Mental flexibility

    Is cooperative         _____

    Is receptive to suggestions and ideas         _____

    Accepts constructive criticism         _____

Initiative

    Is willing to undertake and learn new responsibilities         _____

    Seeks self-improvement         _____

    Keeps busy finding duties when defined work is done         _____

Manners and disposition

    Looks people in the eye when speaking to them         _____

    Honest in discharge of duties         _____

    Keeps personal finances and affairs unknown to office         _____

Appearance

    Exhibits good posture         _____

    Exhibits good personal hygiene         _____

    Shows pride in personal appearance and grooming         _____

## Availability

Punctuality

Arrives at work on time         _____

Is ready to work on time         _____

## Attendance

    Exhibits good attendance on the job         _____

    ___ days office open for business

    ___ days absent, illness

    ___ days absent, vacation

    ___ days absent, other

    Remarks _____

    Is considerate in notifying others of absences         _____

## Ability

Quality of work

    Writes legibly and with correct grammar         _____

    Speaks clearly and with correct grammar         _____

    Is proficient in required skills of duties assigned         _____

Comprehension and judgment

    Able to understand assignments clearly and perform them at once         _____

    Shows mental alertness         _____

    Able to reason and reach a logical conclusion         _____

    Responsive to directions and instructions         _____

Staff member _____

Evaluated by _____ Date _____

# Employee Performance Review

This form is to be used to appraise the performance of all employees at time of formal review and upon separation from the company for reasons other than retirement or death. If any items are deemed not applicable, mark "NA."

| Name | | Title | | | | Division | | |
|---|---|---|---|---|---|---|---|---|
| Date of Employment | Date of Present Assignment | Current Salary | **Last Increase** | | **Appraisal Period** | | Type of Review | |
| | | | Amount | Date | From | To | | |

## Rating Categories

O = Outstanding

This level of performance over a sustained period approaches the best we can possibly expect of an employee in a given position. An outstanding employee should have mastered the essential elements of the assigned position and should be performing at a level well beyond that normally expected of the vast majority of incumbents with similar duties.

V = Very good; exceeds position requirements

A very good employee should be meeting all of the position requirements in a manner indicating full understanding of all the required functions. The results achieved are consistently better than would be expected of most incumbents.

G = Good; meets position requirements

A good employee should be meeting the requirements of the position in a fully acceptable manner. The results achieved are those one would expect of employee at this level.

I = Improvement needed to meet position requirements

A rating level for inexperienced employees or others whose performance is below the acceptance level. Some elements of the position may still require considerable supervision and/or learning before performance is satisfactory.

U = Unacceptable

Employee is considered on probation and not eligible for a salary increase. A specific period of time should be established for the employee to improve his or her performance. If improvement is not made, termination of the employee should result.

## Employee Process Factors

A. Administrative skills      O      V      G      I      U
                              ❑      ❑      ❑      ❑      ❑

Sets priorities and organizes work; uses available resources; controls and follows through on all work activities; completes tasks and delegates responsibility; communicates clearly and accurately in written and oral form with all levels of the organization. Describe performance citing examples, then rate.

Strengths:

Areas for improvement:

B. Personal work characteristics      O      V      G      I      U
                                       ❑      ❑      ❑      ❑      ❑

Initiates action; works well under pressure and for sustained periods; is self-disciplined; completes routine work objectives with minimal supervision; responds to work with a sense of urgency; accepts responsibility for his or her personal growth and development. Describe performance citing examples, then rate.

Strengths:

Areas for improvement:

## Accomplishment

A. Statistics

Attach the appropriate statistical or budget performance summary and rate.

O      V      G      I      U
❑      ❑      ❑      ❑      ❑

# Employee Performance Review—cont'd

B. Objectives
Attach a copy of objectives assigned and agreed upon for this rating period.

| O | V | G | I | U |
|---|---|---|---|---|
| ❑ | ❑ | ❑ | ❑ | ❑ |

C. Describe this employee's chief statistical and nonstatistical accomplishments for this rating period, citing examples when possible. Explain why employee achieved or failed to achieve desired accomplishments.

Evaluation of total accomplishment for this period

| O | V | G | I | U |
|---|---|---|---|---|
| ❑ | ❑ | ❑ | ❑ | ❑ |

Rate this employee's total accomplishment. This rating is based on the process by which the accomplishment were achieved and the actual accomplishments.

Summary of the employee's performance

| O | V | G | I | U |
|---|---|---|---|---|
| ❑ | ❑ | ❑ | ❑ | ❑ |

Describe this employee as an asset to the company. Summarize major strengths and areas for improvement. Then rate this employee, giving consideration to circumstances that may have affected the employee's performance favorably or adversely. Include this employee's potential for continued growth and contribution to the company.

## Action to Be Taken

| No Change in Salary | Current Salary | New Salary | Other |
|---|---|---|---|
| | Increase Salary by | Effective Date | |

| Appraisal by: |
|---|
| Name (print) |
| Signature/date |

| Appraisal by: |
|---|
| Name (print) |
| Signature/date |

## Post Interview Action

A. Employee being reviewed
I have read and discussed my evaluation with my supervisor.
Reviewed employee signature _____ Date _____

B. Employee's comments (*if any*) _____
_____
_____

C. Reviewing executive
Did the employee understand and agree with this evaluation? If not, what was the area of disagreement?
How was it resolved? _____
_____
Reviewing executive name (print) _____
Reviewing executive signature _____ Date _____

*Continued*

# Employee Performance Review—cont'd

| Employee | Pay Scale | | | | Performance | | | | | Current Wage per Hour | Current Wage per Month | Raise per Hour | Raise per Month |
|---|---|---|---|---|---|---|---|---|---|---|---|---|---|
| | Lowest Quartile | Below Avg. Quartile | Above Avg. Quartile | Highest Quartile | Meets Few Expecta-tions | Meets Some Expecta-tions | Meets Expecta-tions | Exceeds Expecta-tions | Far Exceeds Expecta-tions | | | | |
| | | | | | | | | | | | | | |
| | | | | | | | | | | | | | |
| | | | | | | | | | | | | | |
| | | | | | | | | | | | | | |
| | | | | | | | | | | | | | |
| | | | | | | | | | | | | | |
| | | | | | | | | | | | | | |
| | | | | | | | | | | | | | |
| | | | | | | | | | | | | | |
| | | | | | | | | | | | | | |
| | | | | | | | | | | | | | |
| | | | | | | | | | | | | | |
| | | | | | | | | | | | | | |
| | | | | | | | | | | | | | |
| | | | | | | | | | | | | | |

# Progress Evaluation

Employee _____ Date _____

1. Job knowledge
   - Knows technical requirements of job and completes requirements in a timely manner.
   - Follows office policy and procedures.
   - Keeps accurate, complete, and neat records of all forms and transactions.
   - Has thorough knowledge of paperwork flow and distribution.
   - Meets the pace of the office workload.

   Strengths _____

   _____

   _____

   To improve, employee should _____

   _____

   _____

   _____

2. Job-related responsibilities
   - Practices good safety habits by taking precautions that will avoid accidents by reporting dangerous conditions.
   - Is neat, clean, and organized in own work area and takes initiative to keep area and office clean.
   - Is pleasant, courteous, and attentive to patients and other employees, treating them as first priority.
   - Meets promised dates for delivery, adjustment, or repair with follow-up to patient and/or other employees if date cannot be met.
   - Practices good follow-up and completes transactions and paperwork in a timely manner.

   Strengths _____

   _____

   _____

   To improve, employee should _____

   _____

   _____

   _____

3. Work relationships
   - Gets along well with co-workers and supervisor. Works with an attitude of team effort toward the common interest of the office.
   - Accepts and adapts to suggestions for improvement.
   - Can be counted on to complete tasks and assignments in spite of difficulties and works well under pressure.
   - Does not create rumors, untruths, or actions that may create an unpleasant and disruptive work environment

   Strengths _____

   _____

   _____

   To improve, employee should _____

   _____

   _____

   _____

4. Initiative
   - Seeks opportunities to improve job knowledge, professional skill, and growth of the office.
   - Organizes work time efficiently and effectively; recognizes and sets priorities appropriately.
   - Assumes responsibility without being asked or told; requires minimal supervision.
   - Knows when to refer problems to supervisor; exercises sound judgment with patients and co-workers.

   Strengths _____

   _____

   _____

   To improve, employee should _____

   _____

   _____

   _____

5. Attendance
   Absences/tardies _____
6. Overall comments and goals _____

   _____

Supervisor's signature _____ Date _____
Personnel manager's signature _____ Date _____
Employee's signature _____ Date _____

# Employment Agreement

This Employment Agreement ("Agreement") is made effective as of January 1, 20____, by and between Eye Center Optometry ("Employer"), of 123 Main Street, Anytown, USA 99999 and Seymour Clearly, OD ("Employee"), of 456 Home Street, Anytown, USA 99999.

A. Employer is engaged in the business of optometry. The Employee will primarily perform the job duties at the following location: 123 Main Street, Anytown, USA.

B. Employer desires to have the services of the Employee.

C. Employee is willing to be employed by Employer.

Therefore the parties agree as follows:

**1. Employment.** Employer shall employ Employee as a _____ (state) Licensed Doctor of Optometry. Employee shall provide to Employer the following services: optometric patient care, management, community involvement, and marketing of the practice. This Employment Contract does not prohibit Employee from employment outside Eye Center Optometry for the one day each week that is not scheduled at Eye Center Optometry. Additionally, it is agreed that the intent of both parties is to form a partnership in the operation of Eye Center Optometry. To that end, both parties will work toward establishing that agreement during the one year of this Employment Contract. Employee accepts and agrees to such employment, subject to the general supervision, advice, and direction of Employer and the Employer's supervisory personnel. Employee shall also perform (i) such other duties as are customarily performed by an employee in a similar position, and (ii) such other and unrelated services and duties as may be assigned to Employee from time to time by Employer.

**2. Best efforts of employee.** Employee agrees to perform faithfully, industriously, and to the best of Employee's ability, experience, and talents, all the duties that may be required by the express and implicit terms of this Agreement, to the reasonable satisfaction of Employer. Such duties shall be provided at such place(s) as the needs, business, or opportunities of the Employer may require from time to time.

**3. Compensation of employee.** As compensation for the services provided by Employee under this Agreement, Employer will pay Employee an annual salary of $_____ payable every two weeks on Friday. Upon termination of this Agreement, payments under this paragraph shall cease, provided, however, that the Employee shall be entitled to payments for periods or partial periods that occurred before the date of termination and for which the Employee has not yet been paid. Accrued vacation will be paid in accordance with state law and the Employer's customary procedures. This section of the Agreement is included only for accounting and payroll purposes and should not be construed as establishing a minimum or definite term of employment.

**4. Commission payments.** In addition to the payments under the preceding paragraph, Employer will make commission payments to the Employee based on _____% of each comprehensive examination billed by Dr. Clearly. This commission will be paid every two weeks, no later than three days after the payroll period that ended on the preceding Tuesday.

*a. Accounting.* The Employer shall maintain records in sufficient detail for purposes of determining the amount of the commission. The Employer shall provide to Employee a written accounting that sets forth the manner in which the commission payment was calculated.

*b. Right to inspect.* The Employee, or the Employee's agent, shall have the right to inspect Employer's records for the limited purpose of verifying the calculation of the commission payments, subject to such restrictions as Employer may reasonably impose to protect the confidentiality of the records. Such inspections shall be made during reasonable business hours as may be set by Employer.

*c. Death of the Employee.* If Employee dies during the term of this Agreement, Employee shall be entitled to payments or partial commission payments for the period ending with the date of Employee's death.

**5. Reimbursement for expenses in accordance with employer policy.** The Employer will reimburse Employee for the following "out-of-pocket" expenses in accordance with Employer policies in effect from time to time:

a. Community promotional activities including dues and expenses up to $500 attendant to memberships in service organizations

b. Other authorized expenses related to practice promotion

**6. Recommendations for improving operations.** Employee shall provide Employer with all information, suggestions, and recommendations regarding Employer's business, of which Employee has knowledge, that will be of benefit to Employer.

**7. Confidentiality.** Employee recognizes that Employer has and will have information regarding the following:

a. Prices

b. Costs

c. Discounts

d. Future plans

e. Business affairs

f. Trade secrets

g. Technical matters

h. Patient medical/optometric records

i. Patient/customer lists

and other vital information (collectively, "Information") that is valuable, special, and unique assets of Employer. Employee agrees that the Employee will not at any time or in any manner, either directly or indirectly, divulge, disclose, or communicate any Information to any third party without the prior written consent of the Employer. Employee will protect the Information and treat it as strictly confidential. A violation by Employee of this paragraph shall be a material violation of this Agreement and will justify legal and/or equitable relief.

## Employment Agreement—cont'd

**8. Confidentiality after termination of employment.** The confidentiality provisions of this Agreement shall remain in full force and effect for a one-year period after the termination of Employee's employment. During such one-year period, neither party shall make or permit the making of any public announcement or statement of any kind that Employee was formerly employed by or connected with Employer.

**9. Noncompete agreement.** Employee recognizes that the various items of information are special and unique assets of the company and need to be protected from improper disclosure. In consideration of the disclosure of the Information to Employee, Employee agrees and covenants that for a period of one year after the termination of this Agreement, whether such termination is voluntary or involuntary, Employee will not directly or indirectly engage in any business competitive with Employer. This covenant shall apply to the geographical area that includes the City of Anytown, USA. Directly or indirectly engaging in any competitive business includes, but is not limited to, (i) engaging in a business as owner, partner, or agent; (ii) becoming an employee of any third party that is engaged in such business; (iii) becoming interested directly or indirectly in any such business; or (iv) soliciting any customer of Employer for the benefit of a third party that is engaged in such business. Employee agrees that this noncompete provision will not adversely affect the Employee's livelihood.

**10. Employee's inability to contract for employer.** Employee shall not have the right to make any contracts or commitments for or on behalf of Employer without first obtaining the express written consent of Employer.

**11. Vacation.** Employee shall be entitled to _____ hours of paid vacation for each year of employment beginning on the first day of Employee's employment. Such vacation must be taken at a time mutually convenient to Employer and Employee, and must be approved by Employer. Requests for vacation shall be submitted to Employee's immediate supervisor before March 10th of each year.

**12. Sick leave.** Employee shall be entitled to _____ hour(s) paid time for illness each year of employment beginning on the first date of Employee's employment. Unused sick leave benefits as of January 1 of each year may be converted into cash compensation at a rate of $_____ per hour. Sick leave may be accumulated from year to year up to a total of 120 hours.

If Employee is unable to work for more than seven days because of sickness or total disability, and if Employee's unused sick leave is insufficient for such period, a maximum of all of Employee's unused vacation time shall be applied to such absence.

All requests for sick days off shall be made by Employee in accordance with Employer policies in effect from time to time

**13. Holidays.** Employee shall be entitled to nine holidays with pay during each calendar year.

**14. Insurance benefits.** Employee shall be entitled to insurance benefits in accordance with the Employer's applicable insurance contract(s) and policies and applicable state law. These benefits shall include:

    a. Health insurance

    b. Life insurance

**15. Other benefits.** Employee shall be entitled to the following additional benefits:

    a. Profit sharing

    b. Retail warehouse membership

    c. Malpractice insurance for practice at Eye Center Optometry.

as such benefits are provided in accordance with Employer policies in effect from time to time.

**16. Term/termination.** Employee's employment under this Agreement shall be for one year, beginning on January 1, 20___. This Agreement may be terminated by either party upon thirty days written notice. If Employee is in violation of this Agreement, Employer may terminate employment without notice and with compensation to Employee only to the date of such termination. The compensation paid under this Agreement shall be the Employee's exclusive remedy.

**17. Termination for disability.** Employer shall have the option to terminate this Agreement, if Employee becomes permanently disabled and is no longer able to perform the essential functions of the position with reasonable accommodation. Employer shall exercise this option by giving two weeks written notice to Employee.

**18. Compliance with employer's rules.** Employee agrees to comply with all of the rules and regulations of Employer.

**19. Return of property.** Upon termination of this Agreement, the Employee shall deliver all property (including keys, records, notes, data, memoranda, models, and equipment) that is in the Employee's possession or under the Employee's control that is Employer's property or related to Employer's business. Such obligation shall be governed by any separate confidentiality or proprietary rights agreement signed by the Employee.

**20. Notices.** All notices required or permitted under this Agreement shall be in writing and shall be deemed delivered when delivered in person or deposited in the United States mail, postage paid, addressed as follows:

    Employer:

    Eye Center Optometry.

    Joe Eyedoctor, OD

    Owner

    123 Main Street

    Anytown, USA 99999

    Employee:

    Seymour Clearly, OD

    456 Home Street

    Anytown, USA 99999

Such addresses may be changed from time to time by either party by providing written notice in the manner set forth above.

*Continued*

## Employment Agreement—cont'd

**21. Entire agreement.** This Agreement contains the entire agreement of the parties and there are no other promises or conditions in any other agreement whether oral or written. This Agreement supersedes any prior written or oral agreements between the parties.

**22. Amendment.** This Agreement may be modified or amended, if the amendment is made in writing and is signed by both parties.

**23. Severability.** If any provisions of this Agreement shall be held to be invalid or unenforceable for any reason, the remaining provisions shall continue to be valid and enforceable. If a court finds that any provision of this Agreement is invalid or unenforceable, but that by limiting such provision it would become valid or enforceable, then such provision shall be deemed to be written, construed, and enforced as so limited.

**24. Waiver of contractual right.** The failure of either party to enforce any provision of this Agreement shall not be construed as a waiver or limitation of that party's right to subsequently enforce and compel strict compliance with every provision of this Agreement.

**25. Applicable law.** This Agreement shall be governed by the laws of the State of _____.

Employer:

Eye Center Optometry.

By: _____

        Joe Eyedoctor, OD

        Owner

Agreed to and accepted.

Employee:

By: _____

        Seymour Clearly, OD

# Agreement Between Independent Contractor and Client

WHEREAS, DR. JOE EYEDOCTOR ("CLIENT") intends to contract with DR. SEYMOUR CLEARLY (independent contractor, "IC") for the performance of certain tasks; and

WHEREAS, IC's principal place of business is at the following address: 456 Home Street, Anytown, USA 99999; and

WHEREAS, CLIENT's principal place of business is located at the following address: 123 Main Street, Anytown, USA 99999; and

WHEREAS, IC declares that IC is engaged in an independent business and has complied with all federal, state, and local laws regarding business permits and licenses of any kind that may be required to carry out the said business and the tasks to be performed under this agreement; and

WHEREAS, IC declares that IC is engaged in the same or similar activities for other clients and that CLIENT is not IC's sole and only client.

THEREFORE, IN CONSIDERATION OF THE FOREGOING REPRESENTATIONS AND THE FOLLOWING TERMS AND CONDITIONS, THE PARTIES AGREE:

1. SERVICES TO BE PERFORMED. CLIENT engages IC to perform the following tasks or services: optometric examinations, contact lens evaluations, treatment of ocular disease for which IC is properly trained and licensed, and low vision consultations.
2. TERMS OF PAYMENT. CLIENT shall pay IC according to the following terms and conditions: _____ per day and payments to be made on the 16th and 1st of each month for the previous period. IC shall submit invoices to CLIENT for the payments called for in this paragraph.
3. INSTRUMENTALITIES. IC shall supply his own hand held diagnostic equipment and tools to accomplish the designated tasks.
4. GENERAL SUPERVISION. IC retains the sole right to control or direct the manner in which the services described herein are to be performed. Subject to the foregoing, CLIENT retains the right to inspect, stop work, prescribe alterations, and generally supervise the work to ensure its conformity with that specified herein.
5. NO PAYROLL OR EMPLOYMENT TAXES. No payroll or employment taxes of any kind shall be withheld or paid with respect to payments to IC. The payroll or employment taxes that are the subject of this paragraph include but are not limited to FICA, FUTA, federal personal income tax, state personal income tax, state disability insurance tax, and state unemployment insurance tax.
6. NO WORKER'S COMPENSATION. No worker's compensation insurance has been or will be obtained by the CLIENT on account of IC.
7. SCHEDULING OF SERVICES. IC shall provide CLIENT a schedule of availability for services at least 30 days in advance of dates services to be performed.
8. TERMINATION. This agreement shall end on _____ and may not be terminated earlier (except for cause) without 60 days prior written notice from one party to the other.

Agreed to this _____ day of _____, _____ at Anytown, USA.

CLIENT:  INDEPENDENT CONTRACTOR:

By: _____    By: _____

Joe Eyedoctor, OD    Seymour Clearly, OD

# Letter of Intent

The purpose of this document is to provide a guideline for the drafting of a partnership agreement between Dr. Joe Eyedoctor (Seller) and Dr. Seymour Clearly (Buyer) which will insure the orderly transfer of equity and management responsibility for the optometric practice known as "Eye Center Optometry" at 123 Main Street, Anytown, USA 99999.

## Value

Buyer and Seller agree that a conventional practice appraisal is not applicable for the following reasons:

1. The practice has been recently remodeled and new equipment purchased. These expenses distort practice value for the applicable years normally used to establish economic value.
2. The value, as would be based on net income, will be greatly influenced by future factors such as Buyer's efficiency in management, salary, and cost containment.
3. Historical calculations that use a capitalization approach could be distorted based on what assumptions are made regarding the effects of managed care programs and changes in the competitive environment.
4. Future value is based on potential; management, internal and external marketing expenses, and effectiveness will not be solely within the purview of Seller.
5. Value will reflect the time, understanding, and interest invested in patients. Good communication, follow-up, and bonding will establish patient confidence.

Therefore value will be that of the following components:

- Ophthalmic equipment
- Leasehold improvements
- Frame and contact lens inventory
- Office supplies
- Office furniture and equipment
- Prepaid expenses
- Current accounts receivable
- Goodwill/records
- Covenant not to compete

Total value: $_____

No representations of value, income, or expenses are being relied upon other than that stated above.

## Effective Date

The effective date of the partnership will be January 1, 20___.

## Rent

Buyer is aware that Seller owns the building for which a rental agreement has been entered into. The agreement (attached) is comparable on a square-foot basis with similar space. The terms of the current lease are:

Rent:     $_____ per month
Expiration: December 31, 20_____
Options:   Five-year option to renew at a minimum monthly rent of $_____ or a sum computed from the Consumer Price Index as per section _____ of lease, whichever is lesser.

This lease will be assigned to the partnership: Dr. Joe Eyedoctor and Dr. Seymour Clearly, as individuals.

## Personal Property

Personal property of Seller, not a part of this agreement, includes:

- Personal library
- Personal diagnostic equipment and tools
- Antique collection of frames, equipment, etc.
- Artwork
- Projectors, slide trays, and films

## Management Responsibilities

Effective January 1, 20___, Buyer will be responsible for all patient orders, recalls, billings, and accounts receivable.
Effective January 1, 20___, Buyer will be additionally responsible for accounts payable, salaries, employee taxes, and reporting.

## Ownership of Patient Records

All patient files, records, etc. are the property of "Eye Center Optometry" No records, regardless of format, will be removed from the premises without the express permission of each partner.

# Letter of Intent—cont'd

## Compensation

Both Buyer and Seller will be entitled to an equal division of net income. No draws or distributions will be made without the consent of both partners. A final adjustment will be made for each year after December 31 so that the total of all draws will not exceed 90% of net annual earnings, unless both partners agree to make a special distribution.

## Partnership Agreement

The agreement will be prepared by an attorney. This letter of intent and "Draft Agreement" below shall form the basis of that agreement. Attorney fees will be paid equally by Buyer and Seller. The agreement will contain provisions, to the extent allowable by law, for Seller to retain rights for the benefits of depreciation on equipment, furnishings, and leasehold improvements made by and paid by Seller, until such time as all payments required by paragraph 6 of draft agreement have been paid.

## Capitalization of Partnership Checking Account

Each partner will contribute $10,000 to a partnership checking account. It is a goal of this partnership to maintain a balance equal to two months operating expenses.

## Draft Agreement

WHEREAS, the parties hereto desire to engage in the practice of optometry together; and

WHEREAS, the parties desire to practice together under a long-term arrangement for more effective and efficient practice of optometry and on a basis that will progressively reflect the experience and contribution of each party to the practice:

NOW, THEREFORE, this Agreement is executed this day of January 3, 20____, but is effective as of January 1, 20____, by and between Joe Eyedoctor and Seymour Clearly as follows:

1. There is hereby created a partnership between the parties to this Agreement that shall be known as "Eye Center Optometry." The parties to this Agreement shall engage in the practice of optometry solely under the true name of each party as that name is set forth in the license granted to him by the State Board of Optometry and shall not use or practice under the name of any optometry clinic, partnership, trade name, business name, or any entity or association whatsoever.

2. Each of the undersigned represents that he is duly admitted to the practice of optometry under the laws of the State of _____ and agrees that he will conduct his practice according to the standards set by the American Optometric Association. Any failure to act as aforesaid shall be treated as an election to withdraw from the partnership.

3. The principal place of business of the partnership shall be 123 Main Street, Anytown, USA 99999, County of _____, State of _____, and at such other localities within the State of _____ as may be decided upon by both of the partners.

4. The purpose of this partnership shall be for the practice of optometry and such allied and related endeavors as may be agreed upon by the partners. Each partner shall devote the majority of his working time to the practice of optometry and not engage in any other business or hold any office or appointment without the consent of the other. Exceptions include teaching or research appointments. No partner shall be required to devote his full time or attention to the business of the partnership. However, each shall be required to devote as much time to the conduct of the partnership business as is deemed necessary for the reasonable success of the partnership business.

5. The partnership shall commence on the first day of January, 20___, and shall continue until terminated as hereinafter provided.

6. Dr. Eyedoctor hereby agrees to sell and Dr. Clearly hereby agrees to buy an undivided one-half (1/2) interest in Dr. Eyedoctor's existing optometry practice, including but not limited to, the equipment, supplies, accounts receivable, records, and goodwill as of December 31, 20___, for a total purchase price of $_____ as follows:
   a. One-half (1/2) interest in equipment and furniture
   b. One-half (1/2) interest in supplies
   c. One-half (1/2) interest in leasehold improvements
   d. One-half (1/2) interest in prepaid taxes and insurance
   e. One-half (1/2) interest in value of lease and option
   f. One-half (1/2) interest in goodwill
   g. One-half (1/2) interest in current accounts receivable
   Said purchase price shall be payable in annual installments of not less than $_____, including interest at the rate of _____ percent per annum upon the unpaid balance. Payment of purchase installments shall be due on the first day of December of each and every year thereafter until the entire purchase price has been paid.

7. The partnership shall provide the parties with all necessary facilities and equipment and with complete office and technical services, including keeping of files, books, records, preparation of professional and other reports and correspondence, making appointments for patients, handling all arrangements for laboratory work and services and shall hire and pay for all laboratory, secretarial and clerical personnel required and all expenses incurred by the parties in the conduct of their practice, with the exception of licenses, malpractice, and other personal insurance, and professional memberships and dues.

*Continued*

# Letter of Intent—cont'd

8. All withdrawals from partnership bank accounts shall be made by check signed by either partner and shall be supported by appropriate statements, bills, etc.

9. The partnership books of account and records shall be maintained at the office of the partnership and shall be kept on a calendar year basis, January 1 through December 31, and shall be closed and balanced at the end of the year and at such other time or times as may be desirable. An audit by an independent accountant shall be made as of the closing date if requested in writing by either partner to the other partner.

10. The net income and loss-sharing ratios of the partnership, except as otherwise adjusted by the partnership, are as follows:
    Dr. Eyedoctor  50%
    Dr. Clearly     50%
    Net income is understood to be gross income resulting from the practice of optometry, plus gain on the sale of equipment, less losses on sale of equipment, reduced by all normal expenses in the operation of the optometry practice.

11. No partner shall convey any interest in the partnership or its profits to anyone who is not a partner except with the consent of the other partner, and full compliance with provisions contained herein concerning voluntary and involuntary withdrawals.

12a. A partner shall not, without the consent of the other:
    1. Borrow money in the firm name for any purpose or use collateral owned by the partnership as security for such loans.
    2. Assign, transfer, pledge, compromise, or release any of the claims of, or debts due, the partnership except upon payment in full, or arbitration or consent to the arbitration of any of the disputes or controversies of the partnership.
    3. Make, execute, or deliver any assignment for the benefit of creditors or any bond, judgment, chattel, mortgage, deed, guarantee, indemnity bond, surety bond, or contract to sell or contract of sale of any portion of the property of the partnership.

12b. No partner shall, on behalf of the partnership, negotiate any lease, incur any expense in excess of $500.00, engage any personnel, or enter into any contract for special service in excess of $500.00 without the consent of the other partner.

13. Each partner shall personally keep in force adequate and reasonable amounts of malpractice insurance and public liability and property damage automobile insurance as mutually agreed by the partners as reasonable. Professional liability individual limits will be no less than $3,000,000 general aggregate and $1,000,000 each occurrence.

14. The partners agree that the general conduct of the partnership business in respect to relations with patients, employees, and others and the general control of the partnership funds shall be supervised by the managing partner. Dr. Eyedoctor shall be the managing partner until the entire purchase price has been paid as described in paragraph 6. After that time each partner shall have equal rights in the management and conduct of the partnership business.

15a. The total value of the practice after January 1, 20___, shall be the average of no more than the previous 36 months' gross receipts of the partnership, multiplied by twelve.

15b. Effective January 1, 20___, Dr. Eyedoctor's share shall be 50% of the total as per paragraph 15a hereof, plus the unpaid balance of Dr. Clearly's original purchase price as in paragraph 6.

15c. Effective January 1, 20____, Dr. Clearly's share shall be 50% of the total value as per paragraph 15a hereof, less his unpaid balance on the original purchase price as in paragraph 6.

16. If a physician determines that a partner is mentally or physically disabled, that partner shall suffer no reduction in distribution for the first six months. He shall receive three-fourths (3/4) of his normal distribution for the following six months and one-half (1/2) of his normal distribution for the following twelve months. Two years after the disability occurs, the disabled partner may be forced to sell his share of the practice for 90% of the valuation set forth in paragraph 15. After three months, an optometrist shall be hired (to cover the normal work days of the disabled partner) and his or her salary shall be paid by the disabled partner. The employed optometrist's salary shall not exceed one-half (1/2) the disabled partner's distribution.
    If the disabled partner is able to spend at least 50% of his regular office hours performing his full professional duties, he is entitled to receive his full salary for a period of three years from the date of disability. After six months, an optometrist shall be hired part time and his or her salary shall be paid by the partially disabled partner.
    If the disabled partner wished to sell his share of the practice, the price anytime after the disability shall be 90% of the valuation set forth in paragraph 15.

17. Insurance policies to partially cover the purchase of the share of a deceased partner shall be obtained by each partner on the life of the other; the details of which are set forth in the Partnership Insurance Agreement, attached hereto and made a part hereof by reference, entitled "Addendum I."
    In the event of death of either partner, the remaining partner shall purchase the deceased's share as valued in paragraph 16 hereof and pay the heirs the balance not covered by insurance within five years in equal annual installments. No interest shall be charged on this balance.

18. Before the year 20____ Dr. Eyedoctor may elect to gradually retire from the practice of optometry by offering his share of the partnership to any licensed optometrists agreeable to Dr. Clearly at an amount to be decided by Dr. Eyedoctor. Approval of buyers will not be unreasonably withheld. Any such additional owner shall agree to be bound by the terms of this agreement.

# Letter of Intent—cont'd

After the year 20___ Dr. Eyedoctor may elect to gradually retire from the practice of optometry by first offering his share of the partnership to Dr. Clearly for a price not to exceed the valuation of Dr. Eyedoctor's share as per paragraph 15 hereof. Dr. Clearly shall pay Dr. Eyedoctor his amount within ten years, in equal annual installments. No restrictions exist with regard to the transfer of ownership to Dr. Eyedoctor's or Dr. Clearly's children should they also be licensed optometrists.

19. The partnership shall maintain bank accounts in such banks or institutions as the partners from time to time shall elect, and such account or accounts shall be drawn by check signed by the partners in such manner as may be designated by the partners. All monies of the partnership and all instruments for the payment of monies to it shall be deposited in the bank account or accounts of the partnership and all debts and obligations of the partnership shall be paid by check, except petty expense items. Correct books of accounts of the partnership business shall be kept on a cash basis by or under the direction of the partners.

20. Within sixty days after the end of each fiscal year of the partnership, the partnership shall furnish to each partner an annual report. This report shall consist of (a) a copy of the partnership's federal income tax return for that fiscal year, (b) supporting profit and loss statements, and (c) any additional information that the partners may require for the preparation of their individual federal and state income tax returns.

21. This agreement shall remain valid until termination by mutual agreement, death of one of the partners, incapacity of one of the partners, voluntary retirement of one of the partners, voluntary withdrawal of one of the partners, or upon termination of the right of either of the partners to practice as a doctor of optometry.
    For the first two years of this agreement, either partner may, with reasonable cause, give 90 days notice of termination, after which the partnership may be dissolved. Should Seller terminate this agreement, any installments paid by Buyer in accordance with paragraph 6 will be returned to Buyer.

22. It is agreed among the parties hereto that any controversy or claim arising out of or relating to this contract or the breach thereof shall be settled by arbitration in agreement with the rules of the American Arbitration Association and judgment upon the award rendered by the arbitrators may be entered in any court having jurisdiction thereof.

23. Any partner who shall elect to withdraw or retire from the partnership shall not engage in the practice of optometry within a radius of five miles of Anytown, County of _____, State of _____, for a period of two years.

24. This agreement may be amended at any time and from time to time, as long as in writing and signed by each partner.

25. Any written notice required or permitted under this Agreement shall be deemed to have been duly given on the date of service if served personally on the party to whom notice is given, or five days after deposit in the United States mail addressed to the partnership at its principal place of business, by first-class mail, return receipt requested, postage prepaid.

26. This agreement shall be construed pursuant to the laws of the State of _____.

27. This instrument contains the entire agreement of the parties relating to the rights granted and obligations assumed in this instrument. Any oral representations or modifications concerning this instrument shall be of no course or effect unless contained in a subsequent written amendment signed by all partners.

IN WITNESS WHEREOF, the parties have hereunto set their hands and seals this day and date first above written.

Dr. Joe Eyedoctor          Dr. Seymour Clearly

_____    _____

# Agreement of Partnership of Eye Center Optometry

# Dated as of January 1, 20___

**Table of Contents**

Recitals

# Agreement of Partnership of Eye Center Optometry—cont'd

*Continued*

## Agreement of Partnership of
## Eye Center Optometry—cont'd

# Agreement of Partnership of
# Eye Center Optometry—cont'd

THIS AGREEMENT OF PARTNERSHIP is made as of January 1, 20___ ("Effective Date"), by and between JOE EYEDOCTOR, an individual residing in the state of _____ ("Eyedoctor"), and SEYMOUR CLEARLY, an individual residing in the state of _____ ("Clearly").

## Recitals

A. Eyedoctor owns and operates the certain optometry practice known as Eye Center Optometry. Immediately before the Effective Date, Clearly purchased an undivided fifty percent (50%) interest in all the tangible and intangible assets of Eyedoctor's business (excluding certain of Eyedoctor's personal property) pursuant to that certain Agreement for Purchase and Sale of Assets of even date herewith. Clearly's obligation to pay Eyedoctor for the purchase of the assets is evidenced by a Promissory Note of even date herewith ("Promissory Note") and is secured by a Security Agreement of even date herewith.

B. Eyedoctor and Clearly desire to form a general partnership pursuant to the State Uniform Partnership Act for the purpose of engaging in the practice of optometry. Eyedoctor and Clearly each desire to contribute cash and their undivided interests in Eye Center Optometry to the capital of the Partnership on the terms and conditions set forth herein.

C. Unless the context otherwise requires, terms that are capitalized and not otherwise defined in context shall have the meanings set forth or cross-referenced in Article II of this Agreement.

NOW, THEREFORE, in consideration of the premises and the mutual covenants, terms and conditions hereinafter set forth, the parties hereto agree as follows:

## Agreement

### Article I: Formation

1.1  Formation. The Partnership shall be formed as of the Effective Date set forth above.

1.2  Name. The name of the Partnership is EYE CENTER OPTOMETRY.

1.3  Purpose. The purpose of the Partnership is to engage in the business of operating and managing an optometry practice and any and all activities related or incidental thereto. The Partnership shall engage in no other business unless agreed upon by the Partners. To enable the Partners to engage in the practice of optometry, the Partnership shall provide the Partners with all necessary facilities and equipment and complete office and technical service, including the keeping of files, books, records, preparation of professional and other reports and correspondence; making appointments for patients; handling all arrangements for laboratory work and services; and hiring and paying for laboratory, secretarial, and clerical personnel required and all expenses incurred by the parties in the conduct of the practice, with the exception of licenses, malpractice and other personal insurance, and professional memberships and dues.

1.4  Representations of the Partners. Each of the Partners represents that he is duly licensed to practice optometry under the laws of the State of _____ and agrees that he will conduct his practice according to the standards set by the American Optometric Association. The Partners shall engage in the practice of optometry solely under the true name of each Partner as that name is set forth in the license granted to the Partner by the State Board of Optometry.

1.5  Place of Business. The principal office and place of business of the Partnership is located at 123 Main Street, Anytown, USA, County of _____, State of _____. The Partners may change the location of the Partnership's principal office and may establish such additional offices of the Partnership as they may from time to time determine.

1.6  Term. The Partnership shall begin upon the Effective Date and shall end on December 31, 20___, unless sooner dissolved in accordance with the provisions of this Agreement.

### Article II: Definitions

The following terms have the definitions hereinafter indicated whenever used in this Agreement with initial capital letters:

2.1  Act. The State Uniform Partnership Act as amended from time to time.

2.2  Affiliate. With respect to any Person; (i) any Person directly or indirectly controlling, controlled by or under common control with such Person; (ii) any Person owning or controlling ten percent (10%) or more of the outstanding voting interests of such Person; (iii) any officer, director, or general partner of such Person; or (iv) any Person who is an officer, director, general partner, trustee, or holder of ten percent (10%) or more of the voting Interests of any Person described in clauses (i) through (iii) of this sentence. For purposes of this definition, the term "controls," "is controlled by," or "is under common control with" shall mean the possession, direct or indirect, of the power to direct or cause the direction of the management and policies of a person or entity, whether through the ownership of voting securities, by contract or otherwise.

2.3  Agreement. This Agreement of Partnership, as it may be amended from time to time.

2.4  Assets. The assets listed on Exhibit A attached hereto and incorporated herein.

2.5  Bankruptcy. The Bankruptcy of a Person shall be deemed to have occurred or a Person shall be deemed "bankrupt" upon the happening of any of the following: (i) the filing of an application by such Person for, or a consent to, the appointment of a trustee of its or his assets; (ii) the filing by such Person of a voluntary petition in bankruptcy or the seeking of relief under Title 11 of the United States Code, as now constituted or hereafter amended, or the filing of a pleading in any court of record admitting in writing its or his inability to pay its or his debts as they come due; (iii) the making by such Person of a general assignment for the benefit

*Continued*

# Agreement of Partnership of
# Eye Center Optometry—cont'd

of creditors; (iv) the filing by such Person of an answer admitting the material allegations of, or its or his consenting to, or defaulting in answering, a bankruptcy petition filed against it or him in any bankruptcy proceeding or petition seeking relief under Title 11 of the United States Code, as now constituted or as hereafter amended; or (v) the entry of an order, judgment or decree by any court of competent jurisdiction adjudicating such Person as bankrupt or appointing a trustee of its or his assets, and such order, judgment or decree continues unstayed and in effect for a period of ninety (90) consecutive days.

2.6  Capital Account. The Partnership shall maintain a separate Capital Account for each Partner in accordance with federal income tax accounting principles and Regulation.

2.7  Capital Contribution. The total amount of money or property contributed by the Partners to the Partnership pursuant to the terms of this Agreement.

2.8  Code. The Internal Revenue Code of 1986, as amended, and any successor statutory provisions.

2.9  Disabled Partner shall have the meaning set forth in Section 5.6(b).

2.10  Dissolution Event shall have the meaning set forth in Section 10.1.

2.11  Fiscal Year. The taxable year of the Partnership which, except in the case of a short taxable year, shall be the calendar year.

2.12  Interest. The ownership interest of a Partner in the Partnership at any particular time including the right of such Partner to any and all benefits to which such Partner may be entitled as provided in this Agreement and in the Act, together with the obligations of such Partner to comply with all the terms and provisions of this Agreement and of the Act.

2.13  Managing Partner. The Person set forth in Section 5.1 (b).

2.14  Net Cash Flow. The total net cash revenues generated by the Partnership less the portion thereof used to pay or establish reserves for all Partnership expenses, debt payments, purchases of investment assets, capital improvements, replacements and depreciation as determined by the Partners in their reasonable discretion. With regard to Net Cash Flow, the Partners shall make a determination, in accordance with their duty of care and loyalty to the Partnership, as to the need for cash in the operation of the Partnership business, considering both current needs for operating capital and prudent reserves for future operating capital, as well the amounts of any Partnership debts and the necessity or advisability of paying such debts or at least reducing them within the limits of the Partnership's credit, all in keeping with the Partnership's purposes. Any cash derived from income shall, to the extent deemed unnecessary for Partnership purposes by the Partners under the foregoing standards, be deemed Net Cash Flow under this Agreement.

2.15  Net Income or Net Loss. The net income or net loss of the Partnership, as the case may be, for federal income tax purposes, determined annually by the Partnership or its accountants in accordance with the rules of Code §703 and Regulation §1.703-1.

2.16  Partners. Eyedoctor and Clearly and any other Person who becomes a partner of the Partnership in accordance with the terms hereof.

2.17  Partnership. The partnership created by this Agreement, as said partnership may from time to time be constituted; and any partnership which shall continue the business of the Partnership in accordance with the provisions of Article X.

2.18  Partnership Value shall have the meaning set forth in Section 7.3(a).

2.19  Percentage Interest. A Partner's percentage interest in the Partnership as reflected in the then Capital Account of such Partner relative to the then Capital Accounts of all Partners: The initial Percentage Interest of each of Eyedoctor and Clearly shall be fifty percent (50%).

2.20  Person. Any individual, partnership, corporation, limited liability company, trust, estate, association, custodian, nominee or any other individual or entity in its own or any representative capacity.

2.21  Prime Rate shall mean the prime interest rate announced by Bank of America, N.T.& S.A. or its successor, as such rate may be changed from time to time by Bank of America, N.T.& S.A. or its successor.

2.22  Regulations. The Treasury Regulations promulgated under the Code, including proposed regulations.

2.23  Valuation Date shall have the meaning set forth in Section 7.3(a).

### Article III: Partnership Interests and Capital

3.1  Initial Capital Contributions. As of the date hereof, Eyedoctor and Clearly shall each contribute to the capital of the Partnership cash in the amount of Ten Thousand Dollars ($10,000) and their undivided equal interests in the Assets described on Exhibit A attached hereto and incorporated herein, which consist of the tangible and intangible assets of that certain business known as Eye Center Optometry. Based on the contribution of the cash and Assets as described in the preceding sentence, and the Partners' respective interests therein, the initial Percentage Interests of each of the Partners shall each be fifty percent (50%).

3.2  Additional Capital Contributions. As and when further funds are required to meet cash needs of the Partnership not met by the Capital Contributions described in Section 3.1 and revenues of the Partnership, the Partners may solicit additional Capital Contributions from the Partners; provided, no Partner shall be required to make additional contributions to the capital of the Partnership, except as required by law.

3.3  Loans by Partners to the Partnership. Any Partner may, upon the approval of all the Partners, advance monies to the Partnership for use in the Partnership's operations. The aggregate amount of such advances shall be an obligation of the Partnership to the Partner who advanced the monies and shall bear interest at the Prime Rate plus one percent (1%) per annum or at the highest rate permitted by the applicable usury law, whichever is less. Such advances shall be deemed a loan by the Partner to the Partnership and shall not be deemed a Capital Contribution. Any such advances which are unpaid, together with accrued and unpaid interest, shall be payable out of the first Net Cash Flow.

## Agreement of Partnership of
## Eye Center Optometry—cont'd

3.4  No Withdrawal of Capital Contributions. Except upon dissolution and liquidation of the Partnership, no Partner shall have the right to withdraw or reduce its Capital Contribution.

3.5  Interest. Interest earned on Partnership funds shall inure to the benefit of the Partnership. The Partners shall not receive interest on their Capital Contributions or Capital Accounts.

3.6  No Priority. Except as expressly set forth in Article IV, no Partner shall have priority over any other Partner as to return of Capital Contributions, allocations of income, gain, losses, credits, deductions, or as to distributions.

### Article IV: Profits, Losses, and Distributions

4.1  Allocations of Net Income and Net Losses. Net Income or Net Losses for any Fiscal Year shall be allocated to the Partners in proportion to their relative Percentage Interests.

4.2  Partnership Adjustments. In the event of a transfer of all or any part of the Interest of a Partner or the death, dissolution or liquidation of a Partner or the distribution of property, the remaining Partners may elect, on behalf of the Partnership to adjust the basis of the Partnership assets pursuant to Code ß754. Any increase or decrease in the amount of any item of income, gain, loss, deduction or credit attributable to an adjustment to the basis of Partnership assets made pursuant to a valid election under Code ß754, and pursuant to corresponding provisions of applicable state and local income tax laws, shall be charged or credited, as the case may be, to those Partners entitled thereto under such laws.

4.3  Allocations with Respect to Transferred Interests. Net Income or Net Losses allocable to an Interest assigned during a Fiscal Year shall be allocated to each Person who was the holder of such Interest during such Fiscal Year, in proportion to the number of days that each such holder was recognized as the owner of such Interest during such Fiscal Year or by an interim closing of the books or in any other proportion permitted by the Code and selected by the Partners in accordance with this Agreement, without regard to the results of Partnership operations or the date, amount or recipient of any distributions which may have been made with respect to such Interest. The effective date of the assignment shall be (i) in the case of a voluntary assignment, the actual date the assignment is recorded on the books of the Partnership, or (ii) in the case of involuntary assignment, the date of the operative event.

4.4  Cash Distributions. Except as otherwise provided in Section 5.4(a) and Section 10.2 hereof, Net Cash Flow, if any, shall be distributed to the Partners in proportion to their relative Percentage Interests at such times and in such amounts as determined by the Partners. If any distributions are made to a Partner during the Fiscal Year, such distribution shall be charged against that Partner's share of the Net Income for the Fiscal Year in which made, and if the total distributions to any Partner during any such Fiscal Year exceeds that Partner's share of the Net Income for that year, the Partner shall be entitled to no further distributions until the deficiency has been repaid to the Partnership.

4.5  Tax Allocations. Income, gains, losses and deductions with respect to any property (other than money) contributed to the capital of the Partnership shall, solely for tax purposes, be allocated among the Partners so as to take account of any variation between the adjusted basis of such property to the Partnership for federal income tax purposes and its initial value in accordance with Code §704(c) and the applicable Regulations promulgated thereunder.

### Article V: Rights and Obligations of the Partners

5.1  Management.

   a. Major Decisions. The Partners shall manage and control the affairs of the Partnership to the best of their abilities and promote the interests and carry out the business of the Partnership. Each Partner shall have an equal voice in the management and conduct of the Partnership business with respect to any major decisions; no major decision shall be made without the unanimous consent of the Partners. "Major decisions" shall include, but shall not be limited to, the following:

      (i)  confessing a judgment against the Partnership;

      (ii)  borrowing money in the Partnership name for any purpose or utilizing collateral owned by the Partnership as security for such loans;

      (iii)  assigning, transferring, pledging, compromising or releasing of any of the claims of, or debts due the Partnership;

      (iv)  making, executing or delivering any assignment for the benefit of creditors or any mortgage, deed, guarantee, indemnity bond, surety bond, or contract of sale in any way relating to the property of the Partnership;

      (v)  entering into any lease (except as expressly provided in Section 5.4);

      (vi)  incurring any expense in excess of Five Hundred Dollars ($500);

      (vii)  employing, engaging or discharging any employee or agent of the Partnership; and

      (viii)  entering into any contract for special service in excess of Five Hundred Dollars ($500).

   b. Managing Partner. The Managing Partner shall be responsible for the day-to-day management and ministerial acts of the Partnership. In this connection, and not by way of limitation, but subject to Section 5.l(a) above, the Managing Partner shall have the duty and is authorized to do all things and execute all documents necessary to (i) carry out the purpose of the Partnership; (ii) implement decisions relating to general management and professional policy; (iii) purchase supplies, furniture and equipment; (iv) maintain such insurance coverage necessary or appropriate to the business of the Partnership, in such amounts and of such types, as the Managing Partner shall determine from time to time; (v) retain legal counsel, auditors, and other professionals in connection with the Partnership business and to pay therefor such remuneration as the Managing Partner may deem reasonable and proper; (vi) ensure good patient relations; and (vii) supervise the clerical,

*Continued*

# Agreement of Partnership of
# Eye Center Optometry—cont'd

administrative, and other employees of the Partnership. Eyedoctor shall initially serve as Managing Partner until such time as all of Clearly's obligations under the Promissory Note have been satisfied; thereafter, no person shall serve as Managing Partner, and the Partners shall jointly be responsible for the day-to-day management of the Partnership, unless the Partners designate a Managing Partner.

5.2   Authority. The Partners may bind the Partnership, by execution of documents or otherwise, to any obligation not inconsistent with the provisions of this Agreement. Except as otherwise provided in Sections 5.3 and 5.4, the Partners may contract or otherwise deal with any Person for the transaction of the business of the Partnership, which Person may, under supervision of the Partners, perform any acts or services for the Partnership as the Partners may approve.

5.3   Limitations on the Partners. The Partners shall not have any authority or be entitled to, and each Partner covenants and agrees that it shall not:

    a. perform any act in violation of any applicable law or regulation thereunder, including applicable federal and state securities laws;

    b. perform any act in violation of the Act or this Agreement; or

    c. cause the Partnership to make loans to a Partner or the Affiliates of a Partner.

5.4   Dealing with the Partnership. The Partners and any of their Affiliates shall have the right to contract or otherwise deal with the Partnership for the sale of goods or services after obtaining the consent of the Partners in respect of such transaction. Any contract with a Partner or an Affiliate for goods and services shall be in writing and shall contain a clause allowing termination by the Partnership without penalty on sixty (60) days' notice or immediately in the event of the Bankruptcy, withdrawal, removal or dissolution of the Partner or Affiliate. Notwithstanding the foregoing, Clearly acknowledges and agrees that the leasehold interest covering the premises in which the business of the Partnership is located is subject to a lease agreement of which Eyedoctor, as owner of the building in which such premises are located, is a party, and the rights and obligations under such lease agreement have been assigned to and assumed by the Partnership contemporaneously herewith, and such lease agreement shall be enforceable in accordance with its terms.

    a. Allocation of Compensation to Partners. It is anticipated that both partners shall devote approximately equal time to patient care. It is also anticipated that the senior partner may wish to spend less time in the future. To the extent that either partner makes less time available for patient care and that the same partner is thus less productive (as measured by the number of examinations performed) the distribution of income shall be modified. The modification shall be calculated as a percentage by using whichever disparity is less (days or number of patients) as a numerator and the other partner's comparable days or number of patients as a denominator.

5.5   Partnership Bank Accounts. The Partnership shall maintain one or more bank accounts in such banks or institutions as the Partners from time to time shall designate, and such account or accounts shall be drawn by check signed by the Managing Partner, unless otherwise designated by the Partners. All monies of the Partnership and all instruments for the payment of monies to it shall be deposited in the bank account or accounts of the Partnership and all debts and obligations of the Partnership shall be paid by check, except petty expense items.

5.6   Devotion to Partnership Business; Disability; Outside Activities.

    a. Devotion to Partnership Business. No Partner shall be required to devote his full time or attention to the business of the Partnership, provided, however, each Partner shall be required to devote as much time to the business of the Partnership as is necessary for the proper performance of the Partners' duties hereunder and the Partnership's reasonable success.

    b. Disability of a Partner. If any Partner, in the opinion of any medical doctor duly licensed to practice in the State of _____, becomes unable because of any physical or mental disability to devote the time and attention to the Partnership to fulfill his regular office hours, such Partner (the "Disabled Partner") shall, subject to the following terms and conditions, be excused from devoting any time or attention to the Partnership business during the continuance of such disability:

      (i) During the first six (6) months of disability, the Disabled Partner shall continue to be entitled to receive his full share of Net Income, if any, as provided herein.

      (ii) During the following six (6) months of disability, the Disabled Partner shall be entitled to receive seventy-five percent (75%) of his share of Net Income, if any, as provided herein.

      (iii) During the following twelve (12) months of disability, the Disabled Partner shall be entitled to receive fifty percent (50%) of his share of Net Income, if any, as provided herein.

      (iv) Notwithstanding subparagraphs (i) through (iii) above, if the Disabled Partner is able to devote to the Partnership at least fifty percent (50%) of his regular office hours performing his professional duties, he shall be entitled to receive his full share of Net Income, if any, as provided herein for a period of three (3) years from the date of disability.

      (v) Notwithstanding subparagraphs (i) through (iv) above, if the Disabled Partner is unable to devote the necessary time and attention to the Partnership to fulfill his regular office hours, then three (3) months after the Disabled Partner's disability, the Partnership may hire an optometrist to cover the normal work days of the Disabled Partner and such optometrist's salary shall be paid out of the distributions which the Disabled Partner otherwise would have been entitled to receive. Notwithstanding the preceding sentence, if the Disabled Partner is able to devote to the Partnership at least

## Agreement of Partnership of
## Eye Center Optometry—cont'd

fifty percent (50%) of his regular office hours performing his professional duties, the Partnership shall not hire another optometrist until at least six (6) months after the Disabled Partner's disability, and such optometrist shall be hired only on a part-time basis to cover the normal work days of the Disabled Partner. Such optometrist's salary shall be paid out of the distributions which the Disabled Partner otherwise would have been entitled to receive.

   (vi) For the purpose of calculating Net Income as applicable in Sections 5.6(b) i, ii, iii, and iv Section 5.4(a) shall not be applicable.

  c. Partners' Outside Activities. No Partner shall engage in any other optometric business or hold any professionally related office or appointment without the consent of the other Partners; provided, however, any Partner may accept teaching or research appointments at _____.

5.7  Insurance, Malpractice, Indemnification.

  a. Insurance. Each Partner shall personally keep in force, at the Partner's own expense, adequate and reasonable amounts of professional liability insurance, general liability and property insurance, and automobile insurance as mutually agreed by the Partners to be reasonable, and shall name the Partnership as an additional insured under such policies of insurance. In no event shall the amount of professional liability insurance coverage for each Partner be less than One Million Dollars ($1,000,000) per occurrence and Three Million Dollars ($3,000,000) in the aggregate.

  b. Malpractice, Indemnification. Each Partner shall indemnify the Partnership for all damages and expenses for which the Partnership may become liable as a result of any alleged act of negligence or professional malpractice on the part of such Partner to the extent that the damages and expenses are not paid or reimbursed under a policy of insurance carried by the Partnership or in which the Partnership is named as an additional insured.

5.8  Compensation and Reimbursement of Expenses. No Partner, including the Managing Partner, shall receive any salary, fee, or draw for services rendered to or on behalf of the Partnership without the consent of all the Partners provided, however, the Partnership shall reimburse each Partner, including the Managing Partner, for any out-of-pocket expenses reasonably incurred by such Partner on behalf of the Partnership.

5.9  Covenant Not to Compete. No Partner nor any of its Affiliates, successors or assigns may, without the written consent of the remaining Partners, either directly or indirectly, engage in the practice of optometry within a radius of five (5) miles of Eye Center Optometry, Anytown, County of _____, State of _____, during the term of this Agreement and for a period of two (2) years after the date such Partner sells, transfers, or assigns his Interest as a Partner or withdraws or retires as a Partner.

### Article VI: Withdrawal and Removal of Partner

6.1  Assignment or Withdrawal by a Partner. No Partner may sell, transfer, or assign his Interest as Partner, in whole or in part, or withdraw from the Partnership, except with the consent of all the remaining Partners.

6.2  Removal of Partner. Any Partner may be removed by the remaining Partners for cause (including any act of fraud, bad faith, willful misconduct, or gross negligence). The remaining Partners shall serve the removed Partner with a written notice stating the grounds for and effective date of the removal and bearing all such Partners' signatures.

### Article VII: Transfers of Partner Interests

7.1  Transfers. No Partner may sell, assign, transfer, give, or otherwise dispose of or pledge, hypothecate, mortgage, grant a lien on, or otherwise encumber, whether voluntarily or by operation of law, at judicial sale or otherwise (any of the foregoing, a "Transfer"), his Interest in the Partnership or any part thereof except as permitted in this Article VII, and any such Transfer in violation of this Article VII shall be null and void as against the Partnership, except as otherwise provided by law.

7.2  Permitted Transfers.

  a. Notwithstanding Section 7.1, the following Transfers shall be permitted:

    (i) Any Transfer with the express written consent of all of the other Partners, which consent shall not be unreasonably withheld;

    (ii) Any Transfer by a Partner pursuant to Sections 7.3. 7.4 or 7.5;

    (iii) Any Transfer by a Partner on or after January 1, 20___, to any of his children who are licensed optometrists at the time of the transfer.

  b. Any permitted transferee shall execute an instrument satisfactory to the Partners accepting and adopting the terms and provisions of this Agreement.

  c. Notwithstanding the foregoing permitted Transfers, no Transfer of all or any partial Interest in the Partnership may be made except in compliance with the then applicable rules and regulations of any governmental authority and in compliance with applicable laws, including the laws governing the practice of optometry.

7.3  Retirement by Eyedoctor. Any time on or after January 1, 20___, Eyedoctor may either (i) transfer his Interest to any licensed optometrist with the consent of Clearly which shall not be unreasonably withheld, including any of his children, at such price and upon such terms as determined by Eyedoctor or (ii) require Clearly to purchase his Interest at the price and in the manner set forth below; provided, if Eyedoctor proposes to sell his Interest to any licensed optometrist other than his child, Eyedoctor shall first offer to sell his Interest to Clearly by giving written notice to Clearly setting forth the price for the Interest. Clearly shall exercise his option to purchase Eyedoctor's Interest by giving Eyedoctor written notice of intent to sell his acceptance within thirty (30) days

*Continued*

# Agreement of Partnership of
# Eye Center Optometry—cont'd

of his receipt of Eyedoctor's notice of intent to sell his Interest. If Clearly does not exercise his option to purchase the Interest within said 30 day period, Eyedoctor shall have the right to sell his Interest to such licensed optometrist at the price and on the terms set forth in the notice.

    a. Purchase Price. The purchase price for Eyedoctor's Interest shall be determined as follows:

        (i) The Partnership's average monthly gross receipts shall be determined by dividing the aggregate amount of the Partnership's gross receipts over the previous thirty-six (36) months, ending as of the last day of the month immediately preceding the date of Eyedoctor's notice to sell his Interest (the "Valuation Date") divided by 36; provided, if the Partnership has been operating its business less than 36 months, the Partnership's gross receipts shall be determined over the number of months the Partnership has been operating its business, and such amount of aggregate gross receipts shall be divided by the number of months in which the Partnership has been operating its business. The amount of the Partnership's gross receipts shall be determined from the Partnership's books and records as of the Valuation Date by the Partnership's accountants, which determination shall be binding and conclusive upon all parties hereto.

        (ii) The quotient determined in subparagraph (i) above shall be multiplied by 10 to determine the value of the Partnership (the "Partnership Value");

        (iii) The Partnership Value shall be multiplied by two-thirds ($\frac{2}{3}$) of Eyedoctor's Percentage Interest to which shall be added Eyedoctor's average annual draw (over 36 months or as in (i) above) to determine the value and purchase price of Eyedoctor's interest.

    b. Payment of the Purchase Price. The purchase price payable by Clearly shall be paid in equal annual installments over a period of ten (10) years commencing thirty (30) days after the date of sale. Clearly's obligation to pay the purchase price shall be evidenced by a promissory note bearing interest at the Prime Rate plus one percent (1%) per annum or at the highest rate permitted by the applicable usury law, whichever is less. Such promissory note shall be secured by Clearly's Interest and the Partnership Assets and Clearly shall execute any and all instruments reasonably requested by Eyedoctor to adequately secure payment of the purchase price.

7.4 Sale of Disabled Partner's Interest. A Disabled Partner may transfer his Interest to any licensed optometrist with the consent of the other Partner, which consent shall not be unreasonably withheld, at such price and upon such terms as determined by Disabled Partner; provided the Disabled Partner shall first offer to sell his Interest to the other Partner by giving written notice to the other Partner setting forth the price for the Interest determined in the manner set forth below; provided, further, this right of first refusal shall not apply if the disabled Partner is Eyedoctor and Eyedoctor wishes to transfer his Interest to any of his children who are then licensed optometrists. The other Partner shall exercise his option to purchase the Disabled Partner's Interest by giving the Disabled Partner written notice of his acceptance within thirty (30) days of his receipt of the Disabled Partner's notice of intent to sell his Interest. If the other Partner does not exercise his option to purchase the Interest within said 30 day period, the Disabled Partner shall have the right to sell his Interest to any other Person at any price and on any terms he desires.

    a. Purchase Price. The purchase price for the Disabled Partner's Interest shall be ninety percent (90%) of the Partnership Value (determined as of the last day of the month immediately preceding the date of the Disabled Partner's notice to sell his Interest) multiplied by the Disabled Partner's Percentage Interest.

    b. Payment of the Purchase Price. The purchase price payable to the Disabled Partner by the other Partner shall be paid in equal annual installments over a period of ten (10) years, commencing sixty (60) days after the date of the Disabled Partner's notice to the other Partner of his intent to sell his Interest. The other Partner's obligation to pay the purchase price shall be evidenced by a promissory note bearing interest at the Prime Rate plus one percent (1%) per annum or at the highest rate permitted by the applicable usury law, whichever is less. Such promissory note shall be secured by the other Partner's Interest and the Partnership Assets and such other Partner shall execute any and all instruments reasonably requested by the Disabled Partner to adequately secure payment of the purchase price.

7.5 Disabled Partner's Obligation to Sell Interest. Notwithstanding Section 5.6(b) above, two (2) years after the disability of a Disabled Partner, the other Partner shall have the option to purchase the Interest of the Disabled Partner by delivering written notice to the disabled Partner of his intention to purchase the Disabled Partner's Interest.

    a. Purchase Price. The purchase price of the Disabled Partner's Interest shall be ninety percent (90%) of the Partnership Value (determined as of the last day of the month immediately preceding the date of the disability) multiplied by the Disabled Partner's Percentage Interest.

    b. Payment of the Purchase Price. The purchase price payable to the Disabled Partner by the other Partner shall be paid in equal annual installments over a period of ten (10) years, commencing sixty (60) days after the date of the other Partner's notice of intent to purchase the Disabled Partner's Interest. The other Partner's obligation to pay the purchase price shall be evidenced by a promissory note bearing interest at the Prime Rate plus one percent (1%) per annum or at the highest rate permitted by the applicable usury law, whichever is less. Such promissory note shall be secured by the other Partner's Interest and the Partnership Assets and such other Partner shall execute any and all instruments reasonably requested by the Disabled Partner to adequately secure payment of the purchase price.

# Agreement of Partnership of
# Eye Center Optometry—cont'd

### Article VIII: Life Insurance

8.1  Agreement to Insure. On execution of this Agreement each Partner shall apply for and thereafter during the term of this Agreement carry insurance in the amount of One Hundred Fifty Thousand Dollars ($150,000) on the life of the other Partner.

8.2  Additional Insurance. Each Partner shall, during the term of this Agreement, apply for and carry such additional insurance on the life of the other Partner as may be determined by the Partners.

8.3  Ownership of Policies. Each Partner shall own any insurance policies he applies for insuring the life of the other Partner pursuant to this Agreement, shall hold full legal title to the insurance policy, and shall have the exclusive right to exercise any rights, options, or privileges provided for in the policy or permitted by the insurance company issuing the policy, provided no Partner shall exercise any right, option, or privilege without giving the other Partner thirty (30) days' written notice of the intention to do so.

8.4  Payment of Premiums. During the term of this Agreement, each Partner shall pay, as they become due, all premiums on policies owned pursuant to this Agreement and shall give proof of each payment to each other Partner whose life is insured by the policy on which the premium became due within thirty (30) days after the due date of the premium. If any premium is not paid within thirty (30) days after its due date, the Partner whose life is insured by the policy on which such premium is due shall have the right to pay the premium and be reimbursed for the payment by the owner of the policy. The insurance company issuing any policy required by this Agreement is authorized and directed to furnish the insured Partner any information he may request in writing pertaining to the status of any insurance policy.

8.5  Survivor's Option to Purchase Policies: Termination of Option.

    a. Survivor's Option to Purchase Policies. On any Partner's death, the surviving Partner shall have the right to purchase from the deceased Partner's estate and the executors or administrators of the estate shall sell to the surviving Partner, any or all policies owned by the deceased Partner insuring the life of the surviving Partner. The purchase price for the policy or policies shall be equal to the interpolated terminal reserve of the policy or policies as of the date of the deceased Partner's death, less any existing indebtedness charged against the policies, plus the proportionate part of the gross premiums last paid thereon before the date of the deceased Partner's death that cover a period extending beyond that date.

    b. Termination of Survivor's Option. If the surviving Partner fails to pay the purchase price (determined as provided in Section 8.5(a) above) for any insurance policy insuring that Partner's life to the executors or administrators of the deceased Partner's estate within sixty (60) days after their appointment and qualification, the right to purchase that policy shall terminate and the executors or administrators of the deceased Partner's estate may take any action with respect to the policy as they desire.

### Article IX: Death of a Partner; Cross Purchase

9.1  Mandatory Purchase and Sale of Interest on Death of Partner. On any Partner's death, the surviving Partner shall purchase from the deceased Partner's estate, and the executors or administrators of the decedent's estate shall sell to the surviving Partner, the decedent's Interest at the price and on the terms and conditions specified in this Article.

9.2  Purchase Price of Interest. On any Partner's death, the surviving Partner shall pay to the deceased Partner's estate in the manner set forth below as the full purchase price for the decedent's Interest, an amount equal to the greater of (i) the Partnership Value (as of the last day of the month immediately preceding the Partner's death) multiplied by the decedent's Percentage Interest or (ii) the amount of the policy owned by the surviving Partner on the life of the deceased Partner.

9.3  Payment of Purchase Price. Each Partner agrees that on the death of a Partner the proceeds of any policies subject to this Agreement owned by any Partner on the deceased Partner's life shall be applied toward payment of the purchase price payable by him pursuant to Section 9.2 above. If the purchase price payable by the surviving Partner exceeds the proceeds of the insurance policies subject to this Agreement owned by him on the life of the deceased Partner, the balance of the purchase price shall be paid by the surviving Partner in equal annual installments over a period of five (5) years, commencing sixty (60) days after the date of the deceased Partner's death. The surviving Partner's obligation to pay the purchase price shall be evidenced by a promissory note bearing interest at the Prime Rate plus one percent (1%) per annum or at the highest rate permitted by the applicable usury law, whichever is less. The promissory note shall be secured by the surviving Partner's Interest and the Partnership Assets and the surviving Partner shall execute any and all instruments reasonably requested by the executors or administrators of the decedent's estate to adequately secure payment of the purchase price.

9.4  Execution of Instruments. On receipt of an amount equal to the proceeds of any insurance policies owned by the surviving Partner on the life of the deceased Partner and any promissory note required to be executed by the surviving Partner pursuant to Section 9.3 above, or on receipt of the insurance proceeds and cash in lieu of the promissory note, the executors or administrators of the decedent's estate shall execute and deliver to the surviving Partner any instruments necessary to transfer to the surviving Partner full title to the portion of the deceased Partner's Interest purchased by the Surviving Partner.

9.5  Partnership Profits after Death. All profits earned by the Partnership business after the date of the deceased Partner's death shall belong to the surviving Partner. The deceased Partner's estate shall have no right or claim to profits or interest on profits earned after the deceased Partner's death.

*Continued*

# Agreement of Partnership of
# Eye Center Optometry—cont'd

9.6  Assumption of Partnership Obligations. On the death of any partner, the surviving Partner shall assume all Partnership obligations and shall protect and indemnify the decedent's estate, the executors or administrators of that estate, and the property of that estate from liability of any Partnership obligation.

9.7  Purchase of Policies on Termination. If this Agreement terminates before the death of a Partner, each Partner shall be entitled to an assignment of any insurance policy on his own life. An assignment of a policy insuring a Partner's life shall be made when he pays to the owner of that policy within sixty (60) days after termination of this Agreement, an amount equal to the interpolated terminal reserve of the policy or policies as of the date of transfer, less any existing indebtedness charged against the policy, plus the proportionate part of the gross premiums last paid thereon before the date of transfer that covers a period extending beyond that date.

## Article X: Dissolution and Liquidation

10.1  Dissolution. Unless sooner terminated in accordance with its terms, the Partnership shall be dissolved upon the occurrence of any one of the following (each a "Dissolution Event"):

   a. an election to dissolve the Partnership is made by all of the Partners;
   b. the cessation of the Partnership's business;
   c. the death, incapacity (except as provided in Section 5.6 with respect to any Disabled Partner), bankruptcy, dissolution, removal or withdrawal of a Partner unless the remaining Partners shall vote to continue the Partnership;
   d. the expiration of the term of the Partnership as set forth in Section 1.6;
   e. revocation of the license or termination of the right of a Partner to practice as a doctor of optometry;
   f. during the first two years of this Agreement, either Partner may, upon reasonable cause, dissolve the Partnership by giving ninety (90) days' prior written notice to the other Partner;
   g. if a Partner either fails to pay the premiums on or assigns, surrenders, borrows against, changes the beneficiary of, or alters the payment provisions of any life insurance policy which he owns pursuant to Article VIII, the other Partner may elect to dissolve the Partnership by giving ninety (90) days' prior written notice to the Partner breaching the provisions hereof with respect to the life insurance policy; or any other event causing dissolution of the Partnership under the Act.

10.2  Winding up and Liquidation of the Partnership.

   a. Upon dissolution of the Partnership, the Partners or the remaining Partner, as the case may be, shall diligently proceed to wind up the affairs of the Partnership. The Partnership shall be continued during its winding up and the liquidating Partners shall have all the rights and powers of the Partners under this Agreement and shall have the right to do all acts authorized by law and this Agreement for the purpose of winding up the affairs of the Partnership.
   b. Before the payment of the final liquidating distribution, a full accounting of the assets and liabilities shall be taken, all liabilities and obligations of the Partnership shall be paid or provided for (whether by such reserve as the Partners shall deem appropriate) all gains, profits, losses, deductions, and credits shall be allocated pursuant to Article IV. The assets of the Partnership shall then be distributed in accordance with the Partners' respective Capital Account balances.

10.3  Acceleration of Obligations Under Promissory Note. Upon dissolution of the Partnership, Clearly's obligations under the Promissory Note shall not be affected unless otherwise agreed in writing.

## Article XI: Accounting, Inspection Rights, and Reports

11.1  Books and Records. The Partners shall maintain at the office of the Partnership full and accurate books of the Partnership showing all receipts and expenditures, assets and liabilities, profits and losses, and all other books, records, and information required by the Act or necessary for recording the Partnership's business and affairs. Books of account of the Partnership shall be kept on a cash basis by or under the direction of the Partners. An auditor's review of the Partnership's books of account may be made, at the Partnership's expense, as of the close of any Fiscal Year if requested in writing by any Partner.

11.2  Inspection Rights. Each Partner shall, at all times, have access to, and may inspect and copy, any Partnership books and records.

11.3  Reports to Partners. As soon as practicable after the end of each Fiscal Year, and in all events not later than the March 15 next succeeding the end of each Fiscal Year, the Partnership shall furnish or cause to be furnished to each Partner by each March reports containing at least the following information:

   a. a copy of the Partnership's federal income tax return for the Fiscal Year, including supporting profit and loss statements;
   b. estimates of the Partner's allocation of income, gain, loss, deduction, or credit of the Partnership for the Fiscal Year; and
   c. IRS Form K-1, or any similar form as may be required by the Internal Revenue Service, stating the Partner's allocation of income, gain, loss, deduction, or credit of the Partnership for the Fiscal Year.

## Article XII: Miscellaneous

12.1  Title to Partnership Property. All property owned by the Partnership, whether real or personal, tangible or intangible, shall be deemed to be owned by the Partnership as an entity, and no Partner, individually, shall have any ownership of such property. The Partnership may hold any of its assets in its own name or in the name of a nominee, which nominee may be one or more individuals, corporations, partnerships, trusts, or other entities.

12.2  Severability. Each provision of this Agreement shall be considered separate and, if for any reason, any provision which is not essential to the effectuation of the basic purposes of this Agreement is determined to be invalid, illegal, or unenforceable,

# Agreement of Partnership of
# Eye Center Optometry—cont'd

such invalidity, illegality, or unenforceability shall not impair the operation of or affect those provisions of this Agreement that are otherwise valid.

12.3  Applicable Law. This Agreement, and the application or interpretation thereof, shall be governed exclusively by its terms and by the laws of the State of _____, excluding the conflicts of law provisions thereof.

12.4  Amendment. This Agreement may be amended only by a written instrument executed by all of the Partners.

12.5  Arbitration. All claims and disputes between or among the Partners relating in any way to this Agreement or its performance, interpretation, validity, or breach, or to any other rights, duties, or obligations between the Partners, whether or not arising under this Agreement, shall be settled by final and binding arbitration in accordance with the then current Commercial Arbitration Rules of the American Arbitration Association. Demand for arbitration shall be made within six (6) months after the dispute in question has arisen or be forever barred. Arbitration shall be in Anytown, USA, before a single neutral arbitrator from the Association's panel. Judgment on the award rendered by the arbitrator may be entered in any court having jurisdiction. Each party shall bear its own costs and attorneys' fees and one-half of the cost of arbitration, regardless of which party is determined to be the prevailing party.

12.6  Binding Agreement. This Agreement and all terms, provisions, and conditions hereof shall be binding upon the parties hereto, and shall inure to the benefit of the parties hereto and, except as otherwise provided herein, to their respective heirs, executors, personal representatives, successors, and lawful assigns.

12.7  Headings. All Section headings in this Agreement are for convenience of reference only and are not intended to qualify the meaning of any Section. Unless otherwise specifically stated, references to Sections, Subsections, Articles or Schedules refer to the Sections, Subsections, Articles, or Schedules of this Agreement.

12.8  Notices. Any notice, payment, demand, or communication required or permitted to be given by any provision of this Agreement shall be in writing and sent by overnight courier, or by telephone or facsimile, if such telephone conversation or facsimile is followed by a hard copy of the telephone conversation or facsimile communication sent by overnight courier, charges prepaid and addressed as follows, or to such other address as such Person may from time to time specify by notice to the Partners:

    a. If to the Partnership, to the Partnership at the address set forth in Section 1.5 hereof; and
    b. If to a Partner, to the address set forth on the signature page below. Any such notice shall be deemed to be delivered, given, and received for all purposes as of the date so delivered.

12.9  Counterparts. This Agreement may be executed in one or more counterparts, each of which shall be considered to be an original, but all of which together shall constitute one and the same instrument.

IN WITNESS WHEREOF, this Agreement has been executed as of the date first set forth above.

_____
JOE EYEDOCTOR
Address: _____

_____
SEYMOUR CLEARLY
Address: _____

# Exhibit A

## Assets Contributed to Partnership

Except for the personal property noted below, the assets contributed to the Partnership consist of all the tangible and intangible property as of the close of business on December 31, 20___, of that certain business known as Eye Center Optometry, including but not limited to the following:

- Ophthalmic equipment
- Leasehold improvements
- Leasehold interest, including options
- Frame and contact lens inventory
- Office supplies
- Office furniture and equipment
- Prepaid taxes, insurance, and other expenses
- Current accounts receivable
- Patient files and records
- Goodwill

Assets contributed to the Partnership do not include Eyedoctor's personal property located at the business of Eye Center Optometry, including the following:

- Personal library
- Personal diagnostic equipment and tools
- Antique collection of frames, equipment, etc.
- Artwork
- Projectors, slide trays, and films

# Agreement for Purchase and Sale of Assets

THIS AGREEMENT is made as of January 1, 20___, by and between JOE EYEDOCTOR, an individual residing in the State of _____ ("Seller"), and SEYMOUR CLEARLY, an individual residing in the State of _____ ("Buyer").

## Recitals

A. Seller owns and operates that certain optometry practice known as Eye Center Optometry located at 123 Main Street, Anytown, USA.

B. Seller desires to sell and Buyer desires to purchase an undivided one-half interest in all the inventory, equipment, supplies, furniture, leasehold improvements, goodwill, and other tangible and intangible property of Eye Center Optometry (excluding certain personal property of Seller).

C. Immediately after the purchase and sale of the assets as described herein, Buyer will contribute such assets to Eye Center Optometry, a general partnership to be formed between Buyer and Seller (the "Partnership") pursuant to the certain Agreement of Partnership of even date herewith (the "Partnership Agreement").

NOW, THEREFORE, in consideration of the mutual covenants, agreements, representations and warranties contained in this Agreement, the parties agree as follows:

## Agreement

1. Purchase and Sale of Assets.
   a. Purchase and Sale. Subject to the terms and conditions contained in this Agreement, Buyer shall purchase from Seller, and Seller shall sell, assign, transfer, and convey to Buyer, free and clear of all liens, claims, and encumbrances, an undivided one-half interest in the inventory, equipment, supplies, furniture, leasehold improvements, goodwill, and other tangible and intangible property of Eye Center Optometry (excluding certain personal property of Seller) as more particularly described in Exhibit A attached hereto and incorporated herein ("Assets"). In addition, Seller shall covenant not-to-compete with the Partnership on the terms and conditions described below.
   b. Condition of Assets. Except as expressly provided herein, Seller makes no representations or warranties concerning the condition of the Assets; Buyer acknowledges and agrees that such Assets are being sold "AS IS."

2. Purchase Price and Terms of Payment
   a. Purchase Price. The purchase price to be paid for the Assets and Seller's covenant not-to-compete as provided herein shall be $_____.
   b. Payment of Purchase Price. The purchase price shall be secured in accordance with the terms of that Security Agreement of even date herewith substantially in the form attached hereto as Exhibit B and shall be payable to seller in accordance with the terms of that Promissory Note of even date herewith substantially in the form attached hereto as Exhibit C.
   c. Allocation of Purchase Price. The purchase price for the Assets and the covenant not-to-compete shall be allocated as provided in Exhibit A. Each party agrees to prepare its federal and state income tax returns for all current and future tax reporting periods in a manner consistent with the allocations set forth in Exhibit A.

3. Representations and Warranties of Seller. Seller represents and warrants to Buyer that:
   a. Title to Assets. Seller hereby conveys full, absolute, good, and marketable title to the Assets, free and clear of all liens, claims, charges, debts, liabilities, security interests, or other encumbrances of any kind whatsoever.
   b. Brokers, Finders, and Consultants. Seller has not employed any brokers, finders, or consultants in connection with the transactions contemplated by this Agreement and no broker's, finder's, or consultant's fee is or will be payable by Seller with respect thereto. Seller shall indemnify Buyer and hold him harmless against any claims for any expenses, fees, or commissions of any broker, finder or consultant claimed to be retained by or working in Seller's behalf.

4. Representations and Warranties of Buyer. Buyer represents and warrants to Seller as follows:
   a. Inspection of Assets. Buyer acknowledges and agrees that he has had an opportunity to inspect the Assets, and in so purchasing the Assets he is relying solely on the results of his inspections and not relying on any representation or warranty of the Seller or any of his employees, agents, or representatives, except as expressly provided herein.
   b. Brokers, Finders, and Consultants. Buyer has not employed any brokers, finders, or consultants in connection with the transactions contemplated by this Agreement and no broker's, finder's, or consultant's fee is or will be payable by Buyer with respect thereto. Buyer shall indemnify Seller and hold him harmless against any claims for any expenses, fees, or commissions of any broker, finder, or consultant claimed to be retained by or working in Buyer's behalf.

5. Arbitration. All claims and disputes between or among the parties relating in any way to this Agreement or its performance, interpretation, validity, or breach, or to any other rights, duties, or obligations between the parties shall be settled by final and binding arbitration in accordance with the then current Commercial Arbitration Rules of the American Arbitration Association. Demand for arbitration shall be made within six (6) months after the dispute in question has arisen or be forever barred. Arbitration shall be in Anytown, USA, before a single neutral arbitrator from the Association's panel. Judgment on the award rendered by the arbitrator may be entered in any court having jurisdiction. The prevailing party shall be entitled to an award of costs and attorneys' fees.

*Continued*

# Agreement for Purchase and
## Sale of Assets—cont'd

6. Entire Agreement. This Agreement and the agreements referenced herein constitute the entire agreement between the parties hereto with respect to the subject matter hereof and supersede all prior and contemporaneous agreements, understandings, negotiations, and discussions, whether oral or written, of the parties with respect thereto.

7. Advice of Counsel. The parties hereby acknowledge that in connection with the negotiation and execution of this Agreement they have been represented by counsel of their own choice or, having reasonable opportunity to seek such representation, have voluntarily declined to do so. The parties acknowledge that they have read the entire contents of this Agreement and are fully aware of its contents and legal effect. The parties acknowledge that they have not been influenced nor did they rely upon any declarations, representations, or promises of the other party to this Agreement, including attorneys representing said party, which are not contained herein.

8. Governing Law. This Agreement and the respective rights and obligations of the parties hereto shall be governed by and interpreted in accordance with the laws of the State of _____.

9. Counterparts. This Agreement may be executed in one or more counterparts, each of which shall be considered to be an original, but all of which together shall constitute one and the same instrument.

IN WITNESS WHEREOF, the parties have executed this Agreement effective as of the date first above written.

SELLER                                      BUYER

_____            _____

JOE EYEDOCTOR                               SEYMOUR CLEARLY

# Exhibit A

## List of Assets and Purchase Price Allocation

Except for the personal property noted below, Buyer hereby purchases an undivided one-half interest in the Assets described below, and the purchase price allocated to each such asset, including Seller's covenant not-to-compete, is set forth immediately opposite such Asset:

| Asset | Purchase Price Allocation |
|---|---|
| Ophthalmic equipment | $ _____ |
| Leasehold improvements and leasehold interest, including options | $ _____ |
| Frame and contact lens inventory | $ _____ |
| Office supplies | $ _____ |
| Office furniture and equipment | $ _____ |
| Prepaid taxes, insurance, and other expenses | $ _____ |
| Current accounts receivable | $ _____ |
| Goodwill (including patient files and records) | $ _____ |
| Covenant not-to-compete | $ _____ |
| TOTAL | $ _____ |

Assets that are not included in the sale include Seller's personal property located at the business of Eye Center Optometry, including the following:

- Personal library
- Personal diagnostic equipment and tools
- Antique collection of frames, equipment, etc
- Artwork
- Projectors, slide trays, and films

# Exhibit B—Security Agreement

THIS SECURITY AGREEMENT is made as of January 1, 20___, by and between JOE EYEDOCTOR, an individual residing in the State of _____ (the "Secured Party"), and SEYMOUR CLEARLY, an individual residing in the State of _____ (the "Debtor").

## Recitals

A. Debtor and Secured Party entered into an Agreement for Purchase and Sale of Assets dated as of January 1, 20___ (the "Asset Agreement"), whereby Secured Party agreed to sell, and Debtor agreed to purchase, an undivided one-half interest in the inventory, equipment, supplies, furniture, leasehold improvements, goodwill, and other tangible and intangible property of Seller's optometry practice known as Eye Center Optometry (excluding certain personal property of Seller) as more particularly described in Exhibit A attached thereto ("Assets"), for the sum of $ _____. Immediately after the purchase of the Assets, Debtor will contribute his undivided interest in such Assets to Eye Center Optometry, a general partnership to be formed between Debtor and Secured Party ("Partnership") pursuant to the certain Agreement of Partnership of even date herewith ("Partnership Agreement").

B. Pursuant to the Asset Agreement, Debtor agreed to pay Secured Party the purchase price in accordance with the terms of that certain Promissory Note of even date herewith ("Note"), substantially in the form attached hereto as Exhibit A and made a part hereof.

C. As security for Debtor's payment of the amount owed under the terms of the Note, Debtor has agreed to give Secured Party a security interest in the Assets on the terms and conditions set forth herein.

NOW, THEREFORE, in consideration of the above recitals, and of the covenants and agreements set forth herein, the parties agree as follows:

## Agreement

1. Grant of Security Interest. Debtor hereby grants to Secured Party a security interest in the collateral described in Section 2 to secure the payment of the obligations described in Section 3 of this Agreement.

2. Collateral. Debtor's personal property serving as collateral and subject to the above security interest consists of Debtor's undivided one-half interest in the Assets (collectively, the "Collateral"). Secured Party's security interest includes all proceeds of the Collateral. This security interest in proceeds is designed to further secure the obligations subject to this Agreement and in no event shall be understood as an authorization to dispose of the Collateral other than as expressly permitted by this Agreement or the Partnership Agreement.

3. Obligations to Debtor. This Agreement secures that Note of even date herewith in the principal amount of $_____ Thousand _____ Hundred Dollars ($ _____), payments to be made in annual installments of not less than those reflected in 3(a) with interest thereon at the rate of nine percent (9%) per annum, the first payment commencing December 1, 20___. This Agreement also secures all other obligations of Debtor to Secured Party for which Debtor may become liable in any manner to Secured Party under this Agreement, including without limitation any expenses incurred in the protection of the Collateral and any expenses incurred in the enforcement of this Agreement.

    a. Payment Schedule.

| | |
|---|---|
| On 12-1-20__ | $ _____.00 |
| On 12-1-20__ | $ _____.00 |
| On 12-1-20__ | $ _____.00 |
| On 12-1-20__ | $ _____.00 |
| On 12-1-20__ | $ _____.00 |
| On 12-1-20__ | $ _____.00 |
| On 12-1-20__ | $ _____.00 |
| On 12-1-20__ | $ _____.00 |
| On 12-1-20__ | $ _____.00 |
| On 12-1-20__ | $ _____.00 |

4. Termination. Upon Debtor's payment of all sums due under the terms of the Note, this Agreement shall terminate and Secured Party shall release its security interest in the Collateral and terminate all of its UCC filings against Debtor.

5. Warranties and Commitments
    a. Security Interest Outstanding. Debtor warrants that there are no outstanding security interests in the Collateral (including filed financing statements).
    b. Negative Pledge. Debtor agrees that during the course of this Agreement and as long as any obligation that is subject to this Agreement remains outstanding, Debtor will not grant a security interest in the Collateral to any person without the prior written consent of Secured Party.
    c. Liens and Encumbrances. Debtor agrees that during the course of this Agreement, Debtor will keep the Collateral free from any and all liens, encumbrances, and the like.
    d. Sale of Collateral. Except for Debtor's contribution of his undivided interest in the Assets to the Partnership, Debtor will not otherwise sell, offer for sale, transfer, or dispose of the Collateral in a manner prohibited by law or in any manner inconsistent with Secured Party's security interest.

# Exhibit B—Security Agreement—cont'd

6.  Financing Statements. Debtor agrees to execute one or more financing statements in a form satisfactory to Secured Party who is authorized to file a financing statement in any location deemed necessary or advisable to perfect Secured Party's security interest in the Collateral or proceeds. Debtor expressly agrees to sign the financing statements on request of Secured Party. Debtor also agrees to cooperate fully with Secured Party in executing additional financing statements, amendments to financing statements, and the like as may be deemed necessary or advisable by Secured Party to maintain and continue the security interest created by this Security Agreement.

7.  Default. It is agreed that the following events shall constitute a default under this Agreement:

   a. Nonpayment. Any failure of Debtor to pay when due any obligation secured by this Agreement shall constitute a default. This includes, but is not limited to, any failure to pay principal or interest under the Note when due.

   b. Nonperformance. Any failure of Debtor to perform or observe fully and in a satisfactory manner the terms of this Agreement shall constitute a default.

   c. Levy and Attachments. Seizure, attachment, or levy of the Collateral shall operate as a default under this Agreement.

   d. Insolvency and the Like. It shall operate as a default under this Agreement if for any reason: (i) Debtor becomes insolvent; (ii) Debtor becomes subject to any proceeding under the bankruptcy or insolvency laws, including an assignment for the benefit of creditors; or (iii) Debtor has its property placed under the custody of a receiver or trustee.

   e. Unauthorized Use of Collateral or Proceeds. The sale, transfer, or use of the Collateral or its proceeds except as authorized in this Agreement or the Partnership Agreement shall operate as a default under this Agreement.

8.  Acceleration on Default. In the event of any default under this Agreement, the entire indebtedness secured by this Agreement shall become immediately due and payable.

9.  Secured Party's Remedies. On default or acceleration, Secured Party shall have the following rights and remedies, which are cumulative in nature and are immediately available to Secured Party: (i) all rights and remedies provided by law, including but not limited to those provided by the _____ Uniform Commercial Code; (ii) all rights and remedies provided in this Agreement; and (iii) all rights and remedies provided in the Note.

   a. Cure of Default for Nonpayment or Nonperformance. A default by Debtor for reason of nonpayment or nonperformance may be cured only upon mutual agreement by Secured Party and Debtor. Secured Party will allow Debtor sufficient time, not to exceed sixty (60) days, to cure a default for reason of nonpayment or nonperformance provided that Debtor submits a plan satisfactory to Secured Party within ten (10) days of any such default.

10. Waiver of Rights. All rights and remedies of Secured Party as provided in this Agreement, or as found in the Note or any other instrument executed in connection with this Agreement, or arising by operation of law shall continue in full force and effect during the full course of this Agreement unless specifically waived by Secured Party in a signed writing to that effect. Forbearance, failure, or delay on the part of Secured Party in the exercise of any right or remedy shall not constitute a waiver of that right or remedy. The exercise or partial exercise of any right or remedy shall not preclude the further exercise of the right or remedy.

11. Attorney's Fees and Costs. If any action at law, suit in equity, or special proceeding be brought by Debtor or Secured Party to enforce any rights hereunder or under the Note, the prevailing party shall be entitled to recover whatever attorney's fees and costs the court shall allow.

12. Arbitration. All claims and disputes between or among the parties relating in any way to this Agreement or its performance, interpretation, validity or breach, or to any other rights, duties, or obligations between the parties shall be settled by final and binding arbitration in accordance with the then current Commercial Arbitration Rules of the American Arbitration Association. Demand for arbitration shall be made within six (6) months after the dispute in question has arisen or be forever barred. Arbitration shall be in Anytown, USA, before a single neutral arbitrator from the Association's panel. Judgment on the award rendered by the arbitrator may be entered in any court having jurisdiction. Unless the arbitrators provide otherwise, the prevailing party shall be reimbursed for its reasonable fees and expenses, including attorneys' fees, incurred in connection with such dispute.

13. Successors and Assigns. This Agreement shall inure to the benefit of and bind the successors and assigns of the parties hereto.

14. Severability. If any provision of this Agreement shall be found to be unenforceable in any legal proceeding, the remaining provisions shall remain in force and effect.

15. Entire Agreement. This Agreement and the agreements referenced herein constitute the entire agreement between the parties hereto with respect to the subject matter hereof and supersede all prior and contemporaneous agreements, understandings, negotiations and discussions, whether oral or written, of the parties with respect thereto.

16. Governing Law. This Agreement and the respective rights and obligations of the parties hereto shall be governed by and interpreted in accordance with the laws of the State of_____.

17. Counterparts. This Agreement may be executed in one or more counterparts, each of which shall be considered to be an original, but all of which together shall constitute one and the same instrument.

IN WITNESS WHEREOF, the parties have executed this Agreement effective as of the day and year first above written.

DEBTOR:                    SECURED PARTY:

_____     _____
JOE EYEDOCTOR                   SEYMOUR CLEARLY

# Exhibit C—Promissory Note

Anytown, USA
January 1, 20__

FOR VALUE RECEIVED, receipt of which is hereby acknowledged, the undersigned does hereby promise to pay to JOE EYEDOCTOR the sum of _____ THOUSAND _____ HUNDRED DOLLARS ($_____) in cash, in annual installments with interest payable in annual installments on the unpaid principal balance at the rate of _____ percent (____%) per annum, the first payment of principal and interest commencing December 1, 20___.
Principal and interest shall be payable in lawful money of the United States. This Note may be prepaid in whole or in part at any time without penalty.

At the option of the holder of this Note, irrespective of any agreed maturity, the entire indebtedness evidenced hereby shall immediately become due and payable, and without the necessity of presentment, demand, protest, notice, or other formalities of any kind, all of which, together with any and all lack of diligence or delays that may occur in connection with the collection of this Note, are hereby expressly waived by the undersigned, upon the happening of any of the following events: (a) failure of the undersigned to keep or perform any of the terms and provisions of this Note; (b) default on the payment of the indebtedness evidenced hereby or any part thereof when due; (c) the levy of any attachment, execution, or any other process against the undersigned, and said lien is not released within fifteen (15) days; (d) the insolvency, commission of an act of bankruptcy, general assignment for the benefit of creditors, filing of any petition in bankruptcy or for relief under the provisions of any federal or state bankruptcy or related law, of, by, or against the undersigned; or (e) the dissolution of that certain partnership known as "Eye Center Optometry," a general partnership between the undersigned and the holder of this Note created pursuant to an Agreement of Partnership of even date herewith.

In the event of default, the holder hereof shall also be entitled to receive all costs of collection incurred by such holder, including, without limitation, reasonable attorneys' fees.

This Note is secured by a pledge of the undersigned's undivided one-half interest in the inventory, equipment, supplies, furniture, leasehold improvements, goodwill, and other tangible and intangible property of that certain optometry practice known as Eye Center Optometry pursuant to that certain Security Agreement of even date herewith between the maker and the holder hereof.

_____
SEYMOUR CLEARLY

# Optometric Group Partnership Agreement

THIS AGREEMENT OF PARTNERSHIP ("Agreement") is entered into by and among the Partners, JOE ONE, OD, A PROFESSIONAL Optometric Corporation, and JOHN TWO, OD (comprising one Partner, henceforth "ONE-TWO"), JOHN THREE, OD, and RICHARD FOUR, OD (comprising one Partner, henceforth "THREE-FOUR"), ROBERT FIVE, OD, and ROSEMARY FIVE, OD (comprising one Partner, henceforth "FIVE"), KURT SIX, OD, and LINDA SEVEN, OD (comprising one Partner, henceforth "SIX-SEVEN") (All collectively the "Partners") and is effective as of January 1, 20___. The Partners desire to set forth the provisions of their Partnership agreement and reduce their agreement to a writing agreement. Thus this agreement will supersede any other previous agreements made by _____ OPTOMETRIC GROUP.

## Article I. Nature of Partnership
### Definition of Partnership
1.01  They hereby form a General Partnership ("Partnership") pursuant to the provisions of Chapter 1, Title 2 of the Corporations Code of the State of California ("Uniform Partnership Act").

### Definition of Partner
1.02  A Partner may be comprised of one or more individuals.

### Name of Partnership
1.03  The name of the Partnership shall be _____ OPTOMETRIC GROUP.

### Purpose of Partnership
1.04  The Partnership shall engage in the business of providing working premises; owning and leasing common property, equipment, and supplies for the optometric offices of the Partners; hiring employees for the common purposes of the optometric practices of the Partners; billing for individual patients accounts; and pursuing all activities incident or related thereto. However, the specification of the particular business shall not be deemed a limitation on the general power of the Partnership.

### Principal Place of Business
1.05  Principal place of business of the Partnership shall be located at 123 Main Street, Anytown, USA or such other places as the Partners may designate.

### Terms of Partnership
1.06  The Partnership shall commence formal existence on the execution hereof, although the Partnership commenced existence without the benefit of a written Partnership agreement on January 1, 20__.

### Powers
1.07  The Partnership is empowered to do any and all things necessary, appropriate, or convenient for the furtherance and accomplishment of its purposes, and for the protection and benefits of the Partnership and its properties, including but not limited to the following:
   a. Entering into and performing contracts of any kind;
   b. Acquiring, constructing, operating, maintaining, owning, transferring, renting, or leasing any property.
   c. Borrowing money and issuing evidences of indebtedness and securing any such indebtedness by mortgage, deed of trust, pledge, lien, or other security interest in or on any properties of the Partnerships;
   d. Applying for and obtaining government authorizations and approvals;
   e. Bringing and defending actions at law or equity; and
   f. Subject to the express provisions of this Agreement, they may purchase the interest of any Partner.

## Article II: Statutory Filings
### Fictitious Business Name Statement
2.01  The Partners, or any one of them on the Partnership's behalf, shall sign and cause to be filed and published an appropriate fictitious business name statement under the _____ Fictitious Business Name Law, within 40 days after any subsequent change in its membership and before the expiration of any previously filed statement. The Partnership must also file and or renew the fictitious business name statement with the State Board of Optometry. Each Partner appoints Perry Mason Esq. as their agent and attorney-in-fact to execute on their behalf any such fictitious business name statement relating to this Partnership.

*Continued*

# Optometric Group Partnership
# Agreement—cont'd

### Address and Agent for Services

2.02  The Partnership may execute and file with the California Secretary of State a statement pursuant to California Corporations Code Sections 24003 in which the location and complete address of the Partnership's principal office in California, as set forth above, is designated and in which an agent of the Partnership for service of process is designated.

## Article III: Members of Partnership
### Amended Partners

3.01  The name and mailing address of each Partner follows:

### Name Address

JOE ONE, OD, & JOHN TWO, OD,
JOHN THREE, OD, & RICHARD FOUR, OD,
ROBERT FIVE, OD, & ROSEMARY FIVE, OD,
KURT SIX, OD, & LINDA SEVEN, OD,
123 Main Street, Anytown, USA

### Admission of Additional Partners

3.02  Subject to any other provisions of this Agreement, after the formation of the Partnership a person or persons may be admitted as a Partner with the written consent of all the Partners on the execution of an amendment to this original Partnership Agreement. Admission of a new Partner or Partners shall not cause dissolution of the Partnership.

### Admission of Substituted Partners

3.03  Subject to any other provision of this Agreement, after the formation of the Partnership a person or persons may be admitted as a substituted Partner with the written consent of all the Partners, except his, her, or their predecessor in interest, on the execution of an amendment to this original Partnership Agreement. Admission of a substituted Partner shall not cause dissolution of the Partnership.

### Additional Partners Bound by Agreement

3.04  Notwithstanding any other provisions of this Agreement, before any person or person is admitted to this Partnership as an additional or substituted Partner, he, she, or they shall agree in writing to be bound by all of the provisions of this Agreement.

## Article IV: Finances of Partnership
### Initial Capital Contributions of Original Partners

4.01  The Partners will contribute capital to the Partnership in the percentage or amount following their respective names:
**Name Amount/Percentage**
ONE-TWO: 25%
THREE-FOUR: 25%
FIVE: 25%
SIX-SEVEN: 25%

### Additional Capital Contributions of Partners

4.02(a)  On the first day of each month during the term of this Agreement each Partner will contribute a percentage of the monthly overhead of which the amount will be determined by the managing Partners, for each Partner's contribution to operating expenses incurred by the Partnership ("Overhead Contribution"). The balance of the Overhead Contribution must be deposited by the 18th of the month. The amount of the monthly Overhead Contribution is to be adjusted to reflect any changes in the operating cost of the Partnership.

4.02(b)  In addition to a Partner's monthly Overhead Contribution, each Partner shall be charged any direct expenses associated with such Partner's optometric practice, which expenses shall be paid by the due date of the month after the billing of such expense to the Partner. These may include but are not limited to the following: Partner's lab expenses, Partner's individual equipment purchases and maintenance, etc. These are not the liability of the Partnership.

4.02(c)  Other than the above-described further capital contributions, no Partner may make any voluntary contributions of capital to the Partnership without the consent of the Partners whose combined capital interest is 51% or more.

4.02(d)  If the overhead contribution is not paid by the Partner by the allotted due date, a penalty of 3% will be assessed the delinquent Partner if late by more than three days. The penalty assessment will be up to the discretion of the remaining Partners.

# Optometric Group Partnership Agreement—cont'd

### Interest on Capital Contributions
4.03  No Partner shall receive any interest on his or her contributions to the Partnership capital.

### Loans to Partnership
4.04  No Partner shall lend or advance money to the Partnership or for the Partnership's benefit without the approval of the Partners whose combined capital interest is 51% or more. If any Partner, with the requisite consent of the other Partners, lends any money to or for the benefit of the Partnership in addition to his or her required contributions to its capital, the loan shall be a debt of the Partnership to that Partner and shall be on such terms as agreed by the Partners whose combined capital interest is 51% or more. The liability shall not be regarded as an increase in the lending Partner's capital, and it shall not entitle the lending Partner to any increased share of the Partnership's profit.

### Withdrawal of Capital
4.05  No Partner may withdraw any portion of the capital of the Partnership and no Partner shall be entitled to the return of his or her contribution to the capital of the Partnership except on dissolution of the Partnership or by prior agreement of the Partners, or as otherwise provided herein.

## Article V: Division of Profits and Losses
### Partner's Share
5.01  The net profits and losses of the Partnership, which are to be determined after subtracting ordinary and necessary operating expenses related to the Partnership business.

### Assumption of Liability
5.02  The Partnership specifically agrees to assume only those liabilities as shown on Exhibit A attached hereto and made a part hereof.

## Article VI: Distribution to Partners
### Annual Distribution Based on Profit
6.01  At the end of the fiscal year of the Partnership, there shall be distributed in cash to the Partners, as determined pursuant to Section 6.02 hereinafter, in proportion to their respective shares in the Partnership's profit for that fiscal year as computed under this Agreement.

### Overall Limits on Distributions
6.02  Notwithstanding anything in this Agreement to the contrary, the aggregate amount distributed to the Partners from the Partnership's profits shall not exceed the amount of cash available for distribution, taking into consideration the Partnership's reasonable working capital needs as determined by 51% in capital interest of the Partners.

## Article VII: Accounting
### Fiscal Year
7.01  The fiscal year of the Partnership shall be the calendar year.

### Method of Accounting
7.02  The Partnership books shall be kept on a cash basis unless the Partnership accountant determines otherwise.

### Capital Account
7.03  An individual capital account shall be maintained for each Partner consisting of his or her contribution to the initial capital of the Partnership, any additional contributions to the Partnership capital made pursuant to this Agreement, and any amounts transferred from his or her income account to his or her capital account pursuant to this Agreement. A capital account shall be maintained in accordance with Treasury Regulations, Section 1.704-1 (b)(2)(iv). No additional share of profits or losses shall inure to any Partner because of changes or fluctuations in such Partner's capital account.

*Continued*

# Optometric Group Partnership
# Agreement—cont'd

### Increase in Capital Accounts

7.04  The capital account for each Partner shall be credited with or increasing by the following:

    a. The Partner's initial capital contribution into Partnership;

    b. Any additional capital contributions authorized by a majority of the Partnership from time to time shall be equally shared by all the Partners.

### Reduction of Capital Accounts

7.05  The capital account for each Partner shall be debited with or reduced by the following:

    a. The Partner's share under this Agreement of the Partnership's losses and of any items then required under the applicable tax laws, rules, and regulations to be debited to the capital accounts of the Partners, to the extent and in the manner so required; and

    b. On the Partnership's dissolution and its winding up, the debits authorized by the provisions of this Agreement that relate to adjustments of capital accounts in connection with liquidation.

### Capital Account Adjustments on Liquidation

7.06  In connection with the actual liquidation of assets of the Partnership on its dissolution and winding up, the capital account shall be adjusted to reflect the following:

    a. The results of operations for the fiscal period then ended;

    b. The results of transactions in connection with the liquidation;

    c. Unrealized gain or loss on property of the Partnership that is to be or has been transferred to creditors on account of their claims or distributed to Partners on account of their interest in the Partnership. The amount of such unrealized gain or loss shall be computed by comparing the fair market value of any such property to its adjusted basis for federal income tax purposes. Such unrealized gain or loss shall be allocated to the Partner's capital accounts in the same manner such as the gain or loss from the actual sale of such property would have been allocated; and

    d. The distribution of cash or property to the Partners made on liquidation. If there is a deficit in any Partner's capital account after the capital accounts have been adjusted as provided in this Agreement in connection with the Liquidation of the assets of the Partnership, the Partner (the Partner at the time and not any predecessor) shall contribute the amount of such deficit to the Partnership before the end of the taxable year of the liquidation or by such earlier date as may be required to complete the liquidation in accordance with the duly adopted plan on liquidation. Amounts thus contributed shall be distributed to any among the creditors and the Partners in accordance with the then applicable provisions for distribution of Partnership property and dissolution, winding up, and liquidation.

### Determination of Profit and Loss

7.07  The Partnership's net profit or net loss for each fiscal year shall be determined as soon as practicable after the close of that fiscal year in accordance with the accounting principles used in the preparation of the federal income tax returns filed by the Partnership for that year. "Profit" and "Loss" for all purposes of this Agreement shall be determined in accordance with the accounting method followed by the Partnership for federal income tax purposes and otherwise in accordance with generally accepted accounting principles and procedures applied in a consistent manner. However, the calculation of Profit and Loss shall take into account Partnership income exempt from federal income tax and Partnership expenses and costs not deductible or properly chargeable to capital for federal income tax purposes. Every item of income, gain, loss, deduction, credit, or tax preference entering into the computation of Profit or Loss shall be considered as allocated to that Partner for any year in which the Partnership operates at a Loss. Any increase or reduction in the amount of any such item of income, gain, loss, or deduction attributable to an adjustment to the basis of the Partnership property made pursuant to a valid election under Section 754 of the Internal Revenue Code of 1986, as amended (or any successor statute corresponding to that Section) and pursuant to the corresponding provisions of the applicable state and local income tax laws, shall be charged or credited, as the case may be and any increase or reduction in the amount of any item of credit or tax preference attributable to any such adjustment shall be allocated, to the capital accounts of those Partners entitled to them under such code or laws.

## Article VIII: Records and Reports, Banking Expenditures, and Services Rendered to Partners
### Maintenance of Books, Records, Reports, and Accounts

8.01  At all times the Partnership shall maintain or cause to be maintained true and proper books, records, and reports in which shall be entered fully and accurately all transactions of the Partnership.

### Location of Books, Records, Reports, and Accounts

8.02  All books, records, reports, and accounts, together with this Agreement and any amendments thereto, shall at all times be kept and maintained at the principal place of business of the Partnership or at the offices of the Partnership's accountants. Copies of Partnership amendments and agreements are to be held by all Partners.

# Optometric Group Partnership Agreement—cont'd

### Inspection of books, Records, Reports, and Accounts
8.03  All books, records, reports, and accounts shall be open to inspection by any Partner or a duly authorized representative, on reasonable notice, at any reasonable time during business hours, for any purposes reasonably relating to his or her respective interest as a Partner, and said Partner or representative shall have the further right to make copies or excerpts therefrom.

### Financial Statements
8.04  The books shall be closed and balanced as needed and there shall be delivered to each Partner a balance sheet and a profit and loss statement, together with a statement showing the accounts of each Partner, the distributions to each Partner and, in the case of the December 31 statement, each Partner's share of profit or loss from the Partnership for the year just ended reportable for state and federal income tax purposes.

### Banking
8.05  The Partnership shall open and thereafter maintain a separate bank account in the name of the Partnership in which there shall be deposited all funds of the Partnership. No other funds shall be deposited in the account. The funds in said account shall be used solely for the business of the Partnership, and all withdrawals for such purpose may be made on checks signed by one of the Partners, except as provided below.

### Expenditures
8.06  All expenditures of Partnership funds may be made upon the approval of all Partners, however, any and all Partnership checks may be signed by only one (1) Partner.

### Services Rendered to Partners
8.07  In the event that the Partnership renders services to the Partners on a nonequal basis, whether such services be the use of equipment, facilities, supplies, or personnel, the Partnership shall have the right to establish a schedule of fees to be charged to the Partner or Partners using such services to compensate the Partnership fairly for such services provided.

## Article IX: Rights, Powers, Duties, and Restriction of Partners
### Partner's Efforts
9.01  Persons routinely performing administrative duties may be reimbursed for their time by an amount agreed upon by a majority vote of all Partners. An administrative duty shall be defined as an ongoing business-related function that directly affects the maintenance of the normal overhead expenses. A majority vote by all Partners shall determine if a given duty shall be considered as an administrative function.

### Decision
9.02  Policies, decisions, purchases, etc., will be based on a simple majority vote of the Partners, unless authority has been given by the Partnership to a specific Partner to render decisions in his or her administrative field. However, no Partner shall have the right to obtain a loan (commercial, business, personal, or otherwise) on behalf of the Partnership, without a majority vote of the Partnership.

## Article X: Transfer of Partnership Interests
### Restriction of Sale of Partnership Interests
10.01  No Partnership, nor his or her heirs, personal representatives, successors, or assigns, shall have the right, at any time, to sell or transfer all or any portion of his or her interest in this Partnership without the written consent of the remaining Partners.

## Article XI: Disability, Retirement, Withdrawal, Bankruptcy, Insolvency, and Expulsion
### Partnership Continues on Disability, Withdrawal, Retirement, Death, or Expulsion
11.01  The Partnership shall not dissolve or terminate on any Partner's death, permanent physical or mental disability, retirement, voluntary withdrawal, or expulsion from the Partnership.

### Expulsion of a Partner
11.02  The expulsion of a Partner or an individual that comprises a portion of a Partner as defined in section 1.02.

*Continued*

# Optometric Group Partnership
# Agreement—cont'd

### Criteria for Expulsion of a Partner

11.02(a) The following are criteria for expulsion of a Partner from the Partnership. One or more of these criteria may be grounds for, but not limited to, immediate expulsion.

    (i) Use of non prescribed drugs or alcohol on the job

    (ii) Insurance fraud

    (iii) Moral turpitude

    (iv) Theft

    (v) Mental incompetence

All allegations must be proven. Decision will be based on a majority vote of the Partners, less the vote of the involved doctor.

### In the Event of an Expulsion

11.02(b) In the event of an expulsion, the expelled Partner will not be allowed to take their accounts receivable, their original patient records, or any equipment, and said items shall become the property of Gigantic Optometry Group. The expelled Partner has the right to copy expelled Partner's records at the expelled Partner's expenses. The expelled Partner will be absolved of all Partnership debt and thus shall relinquish all interest in capital accounts of the Partnership. The expelled Partner shall be responsible for their own lab bills, personal debt, and other personal incidental expenses related to the Partnership. The expelled Partner may sell his, her, or their practice to a qualified licensed optometrist agreed upon by the remaining Partners. The Partnership and its Partners are under no obligation to purchase the practice.

### Disability of a Partner

11.03 In the event of a disability of a partner, these events would need to be examined. This would apply only if a Partner is comprised of one individual or if all of the individuals of a Partner were simultaneously disabled.

### Temporary Disability

11.03(a) Each Partner shall be allowed a period of no longer than six (6) months for any sickness or disability, during which time he or she may arrange for and pay a qualified and licensed optometrist to take his or her place. The able Partners must agree with the disabled Partner's choice of replacement. During this temporary disability period the disabled Partner must continue to make the required monthly Overhead Contribution and other required contributions set forth in Article 4.02 for twelve (12) months.

### Permanent Disability

11.03(b) If after six (6) months (or sooner if need be) it is decided on the basis of medical evidence or by mutual agreement of all Partners that a Partner is no longer able to contribute to the development of the optometric practice, the Partnership or its Partners are under no obligation to purchase the practice. The disabled Partner may sell his or her practice to a licensed, qualified optometrist agreed upon by the remaining Partners.

### Overhead Protection Insurance

11.03(c) As a benefit to each of the Partners, in the event of a disability, the Partnership shall purchase on behalf of the Partners, an overhead insurance policy containing coverage and benefits as agreed upon by all of the Partners. The premium cost for the overhead insurance policy shall be paid by each individual Partner and shall be considered an operating expense of each individual Partner.

### Retirement or Withdrawal

11.03(d) Any Partner shall have the right to retire or withdraw from the Partnership at any time upon giving written notice of his or her intention to the remaining Partners. Said notice shall be presented at least six (6) months prior to the retirement date. If less than six (6) months notice is given, the balance of that six months Overhead Contribution is due on the date of withdrawal or retirement. In addition the withdrawing Partner forfeits their accounts receivable and owes the Partnership, an additional three (3) months overhead, if he, she, or they cannot find a buyer for their share of the Partnership. The withdrawing Partner pays for the copying of the charts. In the case of the retiring Partner, they forfeit their accounts receivable and owe the Partnership an additional three (3) months overhead, if he, she, or they cannot find a buyer for their share of the Partnership. The retiring or withdrawing Partner will be absolved of all Partnership debt, and thus shall relinquish all interest in capital accounts of the Partnership. The retiring or withdrawing Partner shall be responsible for their own lab bills, personal debt, and other personal incidental expenses related to the Partnership. The retiring or withdrawing Partner shall relinquish their equipment to the practice. The retiring Partner shall leave their equipment and pay their lab bills. The retiring or withdrawing Partner may sell his, her, or their practice to a qualified licensed optometrist agreed upon by the remaining Partners. The Partnership and its Partners are under no obligation to purchase the practice.

# Optometric Group Partnership
# Agreement—cont'd

### Death, Bankruptcy, or Insolvency

11.04  In the event of the death, bankruptcy, or insolvency of any Partner, the Partnership interest belonging to such deceased, bankrupt, or insolvent Partner shall be purchased by the remaining Partner or Partners, and the representatives of the deceased, bankrupt, or insolvent Partner shall be required to sell said Partnership interest to the remaining Partners according to the following terms and provisions: The Purchase price for any Partnership interest belonging to a deceased, bankrupt, or insolvent Partner shall be equal to the fair market value of the equipment used in such Partner's practice and the value of the accounts receivable attributable to such Partner less fifty percent (50%) to allow for collection of the Partner's accounts receivable by the Partnership. The payment terms shall minimize disruption for the remaining Partners and enhance the probability of success for any incoming Partner. In the event of the purchase of a deceased Partner's interest, where life insurance policy obtained by the Partnership for the purpose of funding the buyout of a deceased Partners' interest, payment shall be immediate.

### Bankruptcy or Insolvency

11.05  In the event of the bankruptcy or insolvency of any Partner, the Partnership interest belonging to such bankrupt or insolvent Partner shall be purchased by the remaining Partner or Partners, and the representatives of the bankrupt or insolvent Partner shall be required to sell said Partnership interest to the remaining Partners according to the following terms and provisions: The Purchase price for any Partnership interest belonging to a bankrupt or insolvent Partner shall be equal to the fair market value of the equipment used in such Partner's practice and the value of the accounts receivable attributable to such Partner less fifty percent (50%) to allow for collection of the Partner's accounts receivable by the Partnership. The payment terms shall minimize disruption for the remaining Partners and enhance the probability of success for any incoming Partner.

### Death

11.06  In the event of the death of a Partner, the following provisions shall apply to pay the personal representative or designated beneficiary of the deceased Partner the agreed payments for the deceased Partner's interest in the Partnership.

11.06(a)  It is the intention of the Partners to acquire life insurance policies on the life of each Partner and that the proceeds of the policies shall be paid to the personal representative or designated beneficiary of the deceased Partner in full payment for and satisfaction of the deceased Partner's interest in the Partnership.

11.06(b)  The Partners agree that the premiums on this policy shall be paid by the Partnership and charged as a Partnership expense for income tax purposes to guarantee enforcement of this policy.

11.06(c)  The Partners further agree that the proceeds of this policy shall pay to the Partnership in the amount of $100,000.00, in the event of a death of a Partner.

11.06(d)  Finally, the Partners agree that the balance of the proceeds will go to the deceased Partner's heirs as full payment for and satisfaction of the deceased Partner's interest in the Partnership.

11.06(e)  If a Partner comprises two or more individuals, then the individual Partner agreement must have a detailed life insurance buyout in the event of a death of any individual comprising the Partner. All life insurance policies for the individuals that comprise the Partner will have the premiums of this policy paid by the Partnership and charged as a Partnership expense.

11.06(f)  If for any reason life insurance is not in existence on the life of a Partner at the time of the Partner's death, then in such event the deceased Partner shall relinquish their interest in the Partnership to the Partnership, and the deceased Partner's heir will forfeit all interest in the Partner's assets in the Partnership.

### Dissolution of Partnership by Death, Withdrawal, or Bankruptcy of All Partners

11.07  On dissolution of the Partnership by the withdrawal, death, or bankruptcy of all of the Partners, the Partnership shall be wound up and dissolved as provided herein. This will be decided by majority vote of all the Partners. The number of votes allotted each Partner shall be equal to their capital accounts. On any dissolution of the Partnership under this Agreement or applicable law, except as otherwise provided in this Agreement, the continuing operation of the Partnership's business shall be confined to those activities reasonably necessary to wind up the Partnership's affairs, discharge its obligations, and preserve and distribute its assets. Promptly on dissolution, a Notice of Dissolution shall be published under the applicable Corporations Code Section or any equivalent successor statute then applicable.

### Distributions of Liquidation

11.08  On the dissolution of the Partnership, its business shall be wound up and its properties liquidated and the net proceeds of the liquidation, together with any property to be distributed in kind, shall be distributed as follows:

11.08(a)  First, to the payment of the Partnership's debts and obligations that are then due, including any loans or advances that may have been made by any of the Partners (such advances that may have been made by any of the Partners having priority over debts and obligations to Partners and the expenses of winding up and liquidation;

*Continued*

# Optometric Group Partnership Agreement—cont'd

11.08(b)  Second, to the establishment of any reserves that the Partners may consider necessary, appropriate, or desirable for any future, contingent or unforeseen liabilities, obligations, or debts of the Partnership, which reserves may but need not be deposited with an independent escrow holder with instructions to disburse them in payment of those liabilities, obligations, and debts and, at the expiration of such period as the Partners may have specified, to distribute the balance remaining as provided in this Agreement; and

11.08(c)  Third, to the Partners in proportion to the balances in their respective capital accounts after giving effect to the adjustments of capital accounts in connection with liquidation authorized by this Agreement, but if all capital accounts then have zero balances such distributions to Partners shall be made in proportions to the allocations of profit from the sale of Partnership property applicable under this Agreement as of the date of such distributions.

## Article XII: Office Hours, Office Days, Holidays, and Days Doctors Can Work

### Office Hours, Office Days, and Holidays

12.01  Office hours, office days, and holidays will be stated on Appendix A.

### When a Partner Can Work

12.02  A Partner is allowed to work no more than the established office hours and office days established in Appendix A. If a Partner consists of two or more doctors they may not work on the same day, unless approved by a majority vote of the Partners.

### Changes to Office Hours, Office Days, and Holidays

12.03  From time to time changes may be made to the established office hours, office days, and holidays. Thus Appendix A may be updated from time to time by a majority vote of the Partnership. If changes are made to Appendix A, changes must also be made to the employee and office policy manual.

## Article XIII: Miscellaneous Clauses and Representatives

### Notices

13.01  All notices provided for in this Agreement shall be directed to the parties at the addresses hereinabove set forth opposite their respective names, or at such other places as the Partnership shall be so notified, in writing, by the Partner and the Partnership, at its principal office by registered or certified mail.

### Governing Laws

13.02  All questions with respect to the construction of this Agreement and the rights and liabilities of the parties hereto shall be governed by the laws of the State of _____.

### Binding on Heirs and Successors

13.03  Subject to the restrictions against assignment as herein contained, this Agreement shall inure to the benefits of and shall be binding upon the assigns, successors in interest, personal representatives, estates, heirs, and legatees of each of the parties hereto.

### Counterparts

13.04  This Agreement may be executed in counterparts and all so executed shall constitute one agreement which shall be binding on all the parties hereto, notwithstanding that all of the parties are not signatory to the original or the same counterpart.

### Entire Agreement

13.05  This Agreement contains the entire understanding among the Partners and supersedes any prior written oral agreements between them respecting the subject matter contained herein. There are no representations, agreements, arrangements, or understandings, oral or written, between and among the Partners relating to the subject matter of this Agreement that are not fully expressed.

### Amendments

13.06  This Agreement is subject to amendment only with the unanimous consent of all of the Partners.

### Litigation Costs

13.07  In the event of any dispute or litigation arising hereunder, the prevailing party in any related litigation shall be entitled to an award of reasonable attorney's fees and court costs, including costs of discovery.

### Indemnification

13.08  Each Partner shall indemnify and hold harmless the Partnership, each of the other Partners, and the individuals that make up each Partner from any and all expenses and liability resulting from or arising out of any negligent acts or omissions or misconduct on his, her, or their part to the extent that the amount is not covered by the applicable insurance carried by the Partnership.

## Optometric Group Partnership Agreement—cont'd

### *Severability*

13.09  If any term, provision, covenant, or condition of this Agreement is held by a court of competent jurisdiction to be invalid, void, or unenforceable, the remainder to this Agreement shall remain in full force and effect and shall in no way be affected, impaired, or invalidated.

EXECUTED ON FEBRUARY _____, 20___, at Anytown, USA

By
Partner ONE-TWO
JOE ONE, OD, JOHN TWO, OD
Partner THREE-FOUR
JOHN THREE, OD, RICHARD FOUR, OD
Partner FIVE
ROBERT FIVE, OD, ROSEMARY FIVE, OD
Partner SIX-SEVEN
KURT SIX, OD, LINDA SEVEN, OD

# Office Manual

The office manual is an essential document in each office. It sets the tone for the doctor-employee relationship and enumerates the policies and procedures that need to be followed in the office. Each manual has several sections that should be placed in a binder and labeled appropriately. A copy of the manual is given to each employee for his or her reference. It needs to be returned to the office if employment is terminated.

Below are examples of the sections that should be included in the office manual. Often several examples for each section are given; you can choose the one that seems to fit your situation the best. Not all sections need to be used depending on the size of your office and the number of employees you have.

So that you can get a rapid start on developing your office manual, we encourage you to copy and paste the sections you want to use and then modify them to apply to your office.

# Introduction

## Example #1

We would like to take this opportunity to welcome you to Dr. Seymour Clearly's office. We hope your new job will live up to your expectations and that your stay with us will be a rewarding one. If you have been working for us, we wish to express our sincere appreciation for your valued service.

We are pleased to provide you with this Employee Handbook, which outlines the personnel policies and practices in effect at Dr. Clearly's office. The handbook applies to all employees and will be a helpful reference. We encourage you to ask questions of your managers and co-workers. By doing so you will learn your job more quickly.

Early in your employment with us you will realize that we have set very high standards for you. These are necessary if we are to sustain our growth and achievement in a highly competitive industry. At the same time, we are committed to providing you challenge, recognition, and appropriate compensation and benefits to help you reach your goals and objectives, as well as the goals of our office. By working together in this way, we are confident that the future will be both productive and prosperous for all of us.

This handbook provides answers and guidance to most of the questions you may have about the office's benefit programs, as well as policies and procedures. If anything is unclear, please discuss the matter with your manager. You are responsible for reading and understanding this Employee Handbook. Compliance with the office's policies and procedures is a condition of employment. This handbook is designed to familiarize you with our major policies. We hope it answers most of the questions you may have, but please understand that it cannot cover every possible situation. Your manager or any other manager will be happy to answer any questions you may have.

Because our business atmosphere and economic conditions are always changing, the contents of this handbook may be changed at any time. Dr. Clearly, at his option, may change, amend, delete, suspend, or discontinue any part or parts of the policies in this handbook at any time without prior notice. Dr. Clearly also reserves the right to interpret the policies in this handbook and to deviate from them when, in his discretion, he determines it is appropriate. Dr. Clearly will notify employees of any significant changes that affect them.

This handbook is not a binding contract between Dr. Seymour Clearly and his employees, and it is not intended to alter the at-will employment status.

Best wishes for your success and happiness here at Dr. Clearly's office.

## Example #2

### Welcome to New Employees

Dr. Seymour Clearly and all the staff extend a sincere and hearty welcome to you. Starting something new may be difficult and frustrating, but everyone on our staff started out the same way. We understand if you are a little nervous at first, and we are here to help you get off to a great beginning. If you are in doubt about anything, **always ask.**

Always try to look neat and well groomed. Be conscious of your telephone voice, and address patients by name whenever possible. Patients remember good manners and a nice smile. **You** are now an important representative of this office. Try to learn your way around the office quickly, as well as the names of each of your fellow staff members.

Carefully read this entire office manual. Be especially sure to read the section entitled "Personnel Policies and Guidelines," which describes your rights, privileges, and responsibilities as an employee.

Criticism is meant only in a positive way and as an aid in helping your performance. The potential for learning and increasing your skills is unlimited. **Don't rush.** Learn the simple basics of running this office as efficiently as possible. You are going to make some mistakes at first. We will be surprised if you don't. Do not be discouraged by your mistakes, but learn from them so that you will not repeat them. The simplest duties can seem enormous when times are hectic or when impatient patients confront you. Develop your own system for handling the routines, and always remember that you are doing all that is humanly possible in a given situation.

Staff meetings are held weekly so that we may discuss potential problem areas and provide solutions. Your participation makes our office an even better place of employment for every staff member. Any grievances should immediately be brought to the attention of Dr. Clearly.

Be patient with everyone, especially with yourself. Always speak with a warm and friendly tone of voice, and **smile.** Remember, we chose you to be part of our staff because we see in you many special qualities that will contribute to the success of our practice. Try to aim everything you do toward achieving the highest quality of care for our patients.

## Example #3

Welcome to Anytown Optometric Center. You are now part of a team that is dedicated to providing the finest possible family optometric eye care at a fair and reasonable cost.

You are expected to be an advocate for the patients you serve, providing and offering the best care possible. The Anytown Optometric Center practice is designed to serve the patient, not the employee. Your ability to communicate and empathize with the patients in the most efficient method possible is very important to your success at Anytown Optometric Center.

This practice was established as a separate business in August 1988 to allow the expansion and emphasis of family optometric, optical, contact lens, and therapeutic eye care services.

# Mission Statement (Orientation)

## Example #1
### *Staff Philosophy*
Our office is dedicated to serving our patients with the maximum quality of care. Every decision and every action by our employees should be aimed toward this goal. We believe that our patients are our friends; without them we would have no job, and without their friendship and confidence we would have no new patients. We place great importance on remembering our patients' names and on treating them with courtesy, fairness, and respect. We believe that our employees are the heart of our practice. The qualities that they convey to our patients have an impact many times greater than our office decor, our building, or our equipment. We have zero tolerance for rudeness by members of our staff. The ability to remain cheerful under pressure is equally important as attaining the maximum technical skill. We should strive at all times to be gracious and accommodating, both to our patients and our fellow employees. We want to have only staff members who will work together with a sincere spirit of cooperation and teamwork. We believe this is a key ingredient in the success of our practice and in promoting a pleasant and rewarding work environment for our employees. We want our practice to be at the forefront of our profession. If we are not the best optometry office in our state, then why not?

## Example #2
### *Mission Statement*
Anytown Optometric Center's mission is to offer our patients the most comprehensive eye care available by providing excellent service and quality products in an atmosphere of friendliness and respect. As a team, we will stay at the forefront of technology in our profession and strive to maximize patient education to help them understand all aspects of their vision and preventive eye care.

## Example #3
### *Orientation*
Employees should become familiar with the guidelines in this handbook. The handbook attempts to outline the current policies concerning wages, working hours, and other general office policies.

This handbook is not a contract of employment and is only a highlight of general policies to aid your understanding. From time to time the policies will be modified, deleted, or expanded. Anytown Optometric Center reserves the right to make these changes as needed.

Several forms, including W-2, Proof of Citizenship, and Emergency Information, will be requested from you for the completion of your employee file.

# Profile of Doctors

**Example**

Seymore Clearly, OD, FAAO

Education:

**Diploma,** DeAnza High School, 1961, Richmond, CA
**Associates of Arts,** Menlo College, 1963, Menlo Park, CA
**Bachelor of Science,** Biological Sciences (Bacteriology), University of Southern California, 1966, Los Angeles, CA
**Bachelor of Science,** Visual Science, Los Angeles College of Optometry, 1968, Los Angeles, CA
**Doctor of Optometry,** Los Angeles College of Optometry, 1970, Los Angeles, CA
Note: Los Angeles College of Optometry moved to Fullerton in 1971 and became Southern California College of Optometry.

Professional:

Fellow of the American Academy of Optometry
Beta Sigma Kappa, Optometric Honor Fraternity
California Optometric Association, San Fernando Valley Optometric Society (Society President 1998)
Southern California College of Optometry Trustee (Chairman of the Board of Trustees 2001-present)

Community:

Anytown Jaycees, Past President
Anytown Kiwanis Club, Past President
Anytown Planning Commission, Past Chairman

Employment:

1970-72, Faculty, SCCO
1970-72, Partnership, Partner #1, OD, and Partner #2, OD
1973-88, Anytown Eye Medical Group
1988-97, Anytown Eye Optometric Center
1997-Present, Anytown Optometric Center

# Personnel Policies and Guidelines

## Acknowledgment of Receipt of Employee Handbook and Employment At-Will Statement

This will acknowledge that I have received a copy of the Company employee handbook, which contains important information on the Company's policies, procedures, and benefits, including the policies on Anti-Harassment/Discrimination, Substance Use and Abuse, and Confidentiality. I understand and agree that I am responsible for carefully reading and familiarizing myself with the policies in this handbook, for referring to it whenever questions arise, and for complying with all rules applicable to me.

I understand and agree that the policies described in the handbook are intended as guidelines only and do not constitute a contract of employment. I understand that the Company reserves the right to modify, rescind, or amend its policies, procedures, or benefits at any time at its sole discretion. I further understand that the Company reserves the right to interpret its policies or vary its procedures as it deems necessary or appropriate.

I specifically understand and agree that my employment is terminable at will, with or without cause or notice either by myself or the Company, regardless of the length of my employment or the granting of benefits of any kind. I understand and agree that nothing in this handbook is intended to modify the Company's policy of at-will employment. The at-will employment relationship may not be modified except by a specific written agreement signed by me and the president of the Company.

My signature below certifies that I understand that this is the entire agreement between the Company and me concerning the duration of my employment and the circumstances under which my employment may be terminated. It supersedes all prior or contemporaneous inconsistent agreements, understandings, and representations concerning my employment with the Company. However, the at-will employment agreement can be modified only in the manner specified above. If I have an individually negotiated written employment agreement with the Company, then the terms and conditions of that agreement will prevail to the extent it differs from the policies in this handbook (including the at-will employment policy).

Date Issued: _____

I have received the Company's Employee Handbook. I have read (or will read) and agree to abide by the policies and procedures contained in the handbook.

Employee Signature _____    Employee Printed Name _____    Date _____

Manager Signature _____    Manager Printed Name _____    Date _____

The signed original copy of this agreement must be given to your manager. It will be filed in your personnel file.

## At-Will Employment

Employees are divided into three classifications. The rights and obligations of each classification are defined below. The ending of the waiting period, described below, does not grant or imply "permanent" employment status. All employment and compensation with Dr. Clearly is "at will," in that it can be terminated with or without cause, or with or without notice, at any time at the option of Dr. Clearly. No contract of employment other than "at will" has been expressed or implied. In all instances where this handbook refers to "employee" without designating that employee's status, the provision is applicable to all employees.

The employment relationship is completely voluntary on your part and on the part of Anytown Optometric Center. No promise can or will be made to you concerning the length and/or continued status of your employment. Anytown Optometric Center reserves the right to terminate the employment relationship at any time and for any reason deemed appropriate.

All employment and compensation with the Company is "at will" unless otherwise specified in a written employment agreement. This means employment with the Company can be terminated with or without cause, and with or without notice, at any time at the option of either the Company or you. Nothing in this handbook, or in any document or statement, creates or is intended to create a promise or representation of continued employment of any kind. No contract of employment other than "at will" has been expressed or implied, and no circumstances arising out of your employment including, but not limited to, changes in compensation, title, location/length of employment, and so forth, will alter the "at-will" employment relationship. Only the president of the Company has the authority to make any such agreement and then only in writing. In connection with this policy, the Company reserves the right to modify or alter an employee's position, at its sole discretion, with or without cause or advance notice, through actions other than termination, including demotion, promotion, transfer, reclassification, or reassignment. In addition, the Company reserves the right to exercise its managerial discretion in imposing any form of discipline it deems appropriate.

## Equal Opportunity Employment

The Company has a policy to provide equal employment opportunities to all employees and employment applicants without regard to unlawful considerations of race, religion, color, national origin, sex, sexual orientation, age, disability, marital status, or any other classification protected by applicable local, state, or federal laws. This policy applies to all aspects of employment, including, but not limited to, hiring, job assignment, compensation, promotion, benefits, training, discipline, and termination. Reasonable accommodation is available for qualified individuals with disabilities, upon request.

*Continued*

## Personnel Policies and Guidelines—cont'd

### Discrimination

As required by law, Anytown Optometric Center prohibits discrimination on the basis of race, color, religion, sex, national origin, age, or handicap in any matter affecting employment. As an employee, you will be expected to follow this policy in your dealing with patients, visitors, and fellow employees.

### Sexual Harassment

#### Example #1

Anytown Optometric Center prohibits sexual harassment of any kind. Sexual harassment includes, but is not limited to, unwanted sexual advances; requests for sexual favors; and other verbal, graphic, or physical conduct of a sexual nature. Any employee who feels that he or she has been the victim of and/or observes or is aware of harassment should contact his or her supervisor or a Anytown Optometric Center doctor so that an investigation can be conducted immediately and appropriate corrective action can be taken.

#### Example #2

The Company is committed to providing a work environment free of sexual harassment or any form of unlawful harassment or discrimination. Harassment or unlawful discrimination against individuals on the basis of race, national origin, religion, sex, sexual orientation, disability, or any other classification protected by state or federal laws is illegal and prohibited by Company policy. Such conduct by or toward any employee, contract worker, or anyone who does business with the Company will not be tolerated. Any employee or contract worker who violates this policy will be subject to disciplinary action, up to and including termination of his or her employment or engagement.

### Resignation/Dismissal

Although you are an at-will employee, the Company would appreciate at least 2 weeks' advance notice of your resignation. This gives us time to find a proper replacement and complete the resignation process. The process includes turning in Company property, completing required forms, obtaining appropriate clearances, and participating in an exit interview.

### Exit Interview

In most cases, when you leave the Company you will have an exit interview with the Human Resources Administrator or a designated representative on or before your last day. This exit interview documents the reasons you are leaving and solicits constructive feedback to improve the Company policies, procedures, and employee and public relations, as well as provides an opportunity to review your continuing confidentiality obligations, document all Company property you must return before leaving employment with the Company, and complete required forms.

### Resignations

All employees are expected to give timely notice before resignation. Timely notice, as used in this policy, is at least 2 weeks written notice before the employee's expected last day of work. Please keep in mind that this notice period may need to be longer depending on the circumstances. Once you consider leaving, knowing your intentions would be appreciated so that we may work something out in a mutually satisfying schedule.

### Reduction to Staff

If reductions to staff become necessary for financial or other reasons, consideration will be given to the employee's history of work performance, the employee's performance reviews, the employee's attitudes and enthusiasm, and other factors. Dr. Clearly has the discretion to keep the best employee for the job. Seniority is not a factor in deciding which employee to retain.

### Termination

Any employee who does not meet his or her performance standard may be counseled at any time. Such counseling can be formal or informal. A written record of the counseling session will be made, detailing the specific improvements needed. If the problem continues, employment may be terminated. Although identifying every possible cause for discipline or termination is impossible, the following is a partial list of causes for termination of employment or possible disciplinary action.

- Poor attitude
- Unsatisfactory job performance
- Frequent tardiness
- Unexcused absences
- Disloyalty
- Prolonged or continual absences that can constitute an abuse, at Dr. Clearly's discretion
- Frequently not following instructions and routines
- Not meeting the expected work habits as listed in this handbook.

## Personnel Policies and Guidelines—cont'd

The following items will result in immediate termination without prior counseling:
- Intoxication or use of nonprescribed prescription-type drugs on the job
- Theft
- Falsifying the time actually worked

### Dismissal

Certain practices are of such significance as to be the basis for dismissal. Some of these practices are:

1. Dishonesty, including falsification of Company records, employment applications, or timecards; unauthorized possession or use of property belonging to the Company or the doctors; the performance of unauthorized personal work on company time.
2. Disclosure of business or patient information without authorization.
3. Negligence severe enough to result in harm or threat of harm to a patient or co-worker.
4. Absences without notice.

A written statement of the reasons for dismissal will be provided to the employee by the supervisor and retained in the employee's personnel records. A discharged employee will be paid for all worked time and any benefit hours due as required by state wage and hour regulation.

### Overtime

All nonexempt employees must keep an accurate daily record of attendance and hours worked. Employees may be required to work beyond their regularly scheduled workday whenever that situation is deemed necessary or appropriate by their supervisor or Company management. The Company will attempt to provide reasonable advance notice, but that may not always be possible. Employees are expected to cooperate with such requests. Nonexempt employees will be paid an overtime premium for all hours worked in excess of 8 per workday or 40 per workweek. Exempt employees are not eligible for overtime pay. Nonexempt employees may not work overtime without the prior approval of their supervisor. Employees who fail to comply with this policy may be subject to disciplinary action up to and including termination.

### Calculation of Overtime

Compensation for authorized overtime will be paid to nonexempt employees in accordance with applicable state and federal laws. In calculating eligibility for overtime compensation, only hours actually worked will be included.

For the purpose of calculating an employee's entitlement to overtime compensation, the "workday" means the 24-hour period that begins at 12:00 AM and ends at 11:59 PM. The "workweek" means the 7-day period that begins at 12:00 AM Sunday and ends at 11:59 PM the following Saturday.

All nonexempt employees will be paid a premium for overtime hours as follows:

1. One and one-half times their regular rate of pay for all hours worked in excess of 8 per workday, up to 12, or in excess of 40 in a workweek;
2. One and one-half times their regular rate of pay for the first 8 hours on the seventh consecutive day of work in a workweek; and
3. Double the regular rate of pay for all hours worked in excess of 12 in a workday and after 8 hours on the seventh consecutive day of work in a workweek.

All overtime work must be preapproved by Dr. Clearly. Overtime work without such preapproval will not be paid. Dr. Clearly reserves the right to amend these overtime provisions in accordance with the laws and regulations currently in effect.

From time to time situations will require overtime to meet the needs of Anytown Optometric Center. Every effort will be made to keep these demands to a minimum and consider the private time of employees. All overtime must be approved and noted in advance by the supervisor of the affected center.

*Continued*

## Personnel Policies and Guidelines—cont'd

### Performance Review
*Example #1*

The Company is continuously evaluating your job performance. Day-to-day interaction between you and your manager should give you a sense of how your manager perceives your performance. Performance reviews will be conducted every December for all employees, or as the Company deems necessary. New employees may be reviewed more frequently. A review may also be conducted in the event of a promotion or change in duties and responsibilities. During formal performance reviews, your manager will consider factors including the following:

- Your attendance, initiative, and effort
- Your knowledge of your work
- Your cooperation and willingness to work as part of a team
- The quality and quantity of your work
- Your attention to direction and detail

The primary reason for performance reviews is to identify your strengths and weaknesses, reinforce your good habits, and develop ways to improve your weak areas, if any. This review also serves to compare your job performances with the Company's goals, necessary skills, demands, and description of your job. In addition to individual job performance reviews, the Company may periodically conduct a review of job descriptions and make necessary adjustments in the duties and responsibilities of each position as it deems necessary at its sole and absolute discretion.

Employees must complete and submit an "Employee Self-Review" 1 week before meeting with their managers to discuss their performance reviews. After the review, employees will be required to sign the performance review evaluation report to acknowledge that it has been presented to them and discussed with them by their manager and that they are aware of its contents. Employees may also provide input to the review. The evaluation (and any employee response) will be maintained in the employee's personnel file.

In some instances, and at the sole discretion of the Company, employees may be placed on an evaluation or performance improvement program or given a reasonable time in which to cure deficiencies in performance. Failure to correct performance deficiencies may result in termination at any time as determined at the Company's sole and absolute discretion.

The Company does not award wage adjustments on an automatic basis, annual basis, or an employee's length of service for cost-of-living adjustments or at any preset interval. Wage adjustments, if any, are determined and awarded at the sole discretion of the Company.

### *Example #2*

Performance reviews will be conducted annually. Evaluations will be reviewed with the employee and will become part of the employee's written record. Despite the performance review, all employment is "at will" and may be terminated at any time by either the employee or Dr. Clearly.

The performance review is designed to provide an honest, open appraisal of the employee's strengths and areas needing improvement, as well as an opportunity for the employee to discuss problems or recommend improvements. Salary increases will be discussed when practical, such as once a year at the performance reviews. We try to make salaries commensurate with each employee's skills, job performance, and job description. Salary increases are entirely at Dr. Clearly's discretion and may be based on current economic conditions; the operation of the office; and/or the employee's merit, performance, attendance, attitude, and initiative. All salary increases are effective the first day of the next calendar month. Employees will receive pay bimonthly, every other Friday. Pay is calculated by the quarter hour according to time clock methods.

### Pay Period
*Example #1*

Payday for all employees is twice a month as follows: The first pay period begins on the first day of the month at 12:00 AM and ends at 11:59 PM on the fifteenth of the month. Thereafter, the second pay period begins on the sixteenth of the month at 12:00 AM and ends at 11:59 PM on the last day of the month.

Paychecks for all employees are distributed on the fifteenth and last day of the month. All employees are paid by check or direct deposit on the above-mentioned payday. Changes will be made and announced in advance whenever Company holidays or closings interfere with the normal payday.

The Company does not grant payroll advances.

### *Example #2*

Time cards are collected every other Tuesday. Payroll will be issued on the Friday after the collection of the time cards. Payroll will include the 2 weeks before the collection of time cards.

### Holidays
*Example #1*

Regular full-time employees are typically eligible for 10 paid holidays in each calendar year. Regular part-time and temporary employees are not eligible for paid holidays. Actual holidays may vary and will be posted in January of each year. Up to three additional holidays may be designated by Anytown Optometric Center at its sole discretion and will be posted in January of each year, if so designated.

# Personnel Policies and Guidelines—cont'd

*Paid*

| Holiday | Date Usually Observed |
|---|---|
| ✓New Year's Day | January 1 |
| ✗Presidents' Day | Third Monday in February |
| ✓Memorial Day | Last Monday in May |
| ✓Independence Day | July 4 |
| ✓Labor Day | First Monday in September |
| ✗Veterans' Day | November 11 |
| ✓Thanksgiving Day | Fourth Thursday in November |
| ✓Day after Thanksgiving | Fourth Friday in November |
| ✓Christmas Day + *Eve* | December 25 |
| ✗Day after Christmas | December 26 |

When a holiday falls on a Saturday or Sunday, it is usually observed on the preceding Friday or the following Monday. Holiday observances will be announced in advance. When a company holiday occurs during an eligible employee's paid vacation, an additional day off will be added either at the beginning or the end of the vacation period.

To receive holiday pay, eligible employees must be regularly scheduled to work on the day on which the holiday is observed and work their regularly scheduled working days immediately before and immediately after the holiday. Nonexempt employees required to work on a paid scheduled holiday will receive their wages at their straight-time rate for the hours worked on the holiday, plus holiday pay, which is calculated at the straight-time rate. Paid time off for holidays will not be counted as hours worked for the purposes of determining overtime.

The Company recognizes that some employees may wish to observe, as periods of worship or commemoration, certain religious days that are not included in the Company's holiday schedule. Employees may use accrued vacation for paid time off for this purpose. Otherwise, the time off will be without pay. The Company will make a reasonable effort to accommodate an employee's religious beliefs, consistent with the Company's operating requirements, provided such accommodation does not create an undue hardship for the Company. An employee who wishes to request time off for religious holidays should provide reasonable advance notice to his or her manager.

## Example #2
The Office will be closed for the following holidays, with exceptions specified:
- New Year's Day
- Presidents' Day (usually the third Monday in February)
- Memorial Day
- Fourth of July (only if on a workday, and always on the fourth itself)
- Labor Day
- Thanksgiving Day
- Day after Thanksgiving
- Christmas Day
- New Year's Eve

## Example #3
Anytown Optometric Center observes the following nine paid holidays:
- New Year's Day
- Memorial Day
- Independence Day
- Labor Day
- Thanksgiving (2 days)
- Christmas

Management establishes the additional two days in December of the preceding year. If one of the listed holidays falls on Sunday, the observed day will be established by the December staff meeting.

If a holiday falls on the normal day off for a nonexempt employee, the employee will receive a day's pay as additional compensation.

Employees will not be paid for sick leave the first workday before or after a holiday.

## Disability/Medical Leave of Absence
### Example #1
An employee's disability is between him or her and his or her medical physician. As long as the employee's medical doctor certifies he or she can no longer work because of an accident or illness that is not work related, he or she may collect state disability compensation. For more information, call your state's Disability Board.

If an employee is off work for a non-work-related injury and/or is under a physician's care, then Dr. Clearly must have a copy of the medical doctor's release when the employee returns to work.

*Continued*

## Personnel Policies and Guidelines—cont'd

No additional paid medical leave is given by Dr. Clearly beyond accrued sick leave and vacation days. An employee will receive no compensation once all accrued sick leave and vacation days are used.

During any disability or medical leave, no vacation, sick leave, benefit allowance, or any other benefits or compensation will accrue.

Dr. Clearly will use his best efforts to maintain an employee's position. An employee who is absent from work—as a result of a non-work-related illness, injury, or disability—for more than 8 weeks in a calendar year may be required to reapply for his or her position.

### Example #2

Employees are required to contact the supervisor before their scheduled start time on a daily basis while they are off sick. After completing the required probationary period, full-time employees will accumulate sick leave at a rate of 1.667 hours for each full pay period of employment. Computation of sick leave will be based on actual hours worked, not including sick time or overtime. You will accumulate 1 week (40 hours) of sick time after 12 months of employment. You may accumulate up to 3 weeks (120 hours) of sick leave.

Surplus, unused sick time in excess of 120 hours will be paid to you within a reasonable period after the end of each calendar year. If a sickness exceeds the accumulated sick time, the additional time will be charged to personal leave. If the sickness exceeds the accumulated personal and sick time, leave will be continued at no pay. Sick leave is intended for use of employees during a personal illness.

### Lunch and Rest Periods

Each Anytown Optometric Center employee is scheduled at least one half-hour lunch break. The supervisor arranges the time. An employee lounge is provided with a refrigerator, microwave, toaster oven, and coffee maker for employee use. Food should be eaten only in the lounge area, not in patient areas.

In addition to your lunch break, you are allowed a 15-minute break for each 3.5 hours worked. The break will be in the middle of each work period if practical. Employees working less than 3.5 hours in a day are not eligible for a break.

### Jury Duty/Witness Leave
### Example #1

As a citizen you have a civic duty to report for jury duty or as a witness in court whenever called. You must notify your manager of the need for time off for jury duty as soon as a notice or summons from a court is received. Employees will be paid for 5 days of jury duty; if their service is required for a longer period, they may use accrued vacation days or take a leave of absence without pay. Employees may be requested to provide written verification from the court clerk of having served. If work time remains after any day of jury selection or jury duty, employees are required to call in and report to work for the remainder of their work schedule. Any mileage allowance, fee, and so forth paid by the court for jury services are to be retained by the employee.

### Example #2

Full-time, non–waiting period employees shall receive their regular wages for 3 days while serving on jury duty or as a subpoenaed witness. After 3 days of jury duty or testifying as a subpoenaed witness, employees must use their accrued vacation time or sick time to be paid. Employees may take the time without pay. If an employee is dismissed from jury duty or as a subpoenaed witness before 1:30 PM, the employee shall return to work immediately.

### Example #3

Anytown Optometric Center does not pay for time away from the office for jury duty.

### Example #4

As with voting, jury duty service is a personal obligation and service that each of us, as good citizens, must complete from time to time. We ask that you provide us as much notice as possible of impending jury duty. We do not provide compensatory time or pay for your service to the community.

### Bereavement Leave
### Example #1

In the event of a death in the immediate family, all regular full-time employees may have up to 3 days of paid leave at their regular rate or base salary to handle family affairs and attend the funeral. Your manager may approve additional unpaid time off or use of vacation time. Immediate family is defined as parents, spouse, children, siblings, and grandparents.

### Example #2

Full-time, non–waiting period employees are allowed up to 3 days per year for deaths in the employee's family. Family, for the purpose of paid bereavement leave, is limited to parents, siblings, children, spouses, and the "steps" of each. All other bereavement leave shall be considered taken without pay. Bereavement leave may not be carried over from year to year.

## Personnel Policies and Guidelines—cont'd

The employee should make every effort to give Dr. Clearly as much notice as possible before taking such leave. All unpaid bereavement leave shall be at the sole discretion of Dr. Clearly. In certain cases, Dr. Clearly may, in his sole discretion, determine that an employee is unable to work and may grant a discretionary bereavement leave.

### Personal Leaves of Absence
#### Example #1
The Company provides one personal day off with pay in each calendar year to regular full-time employees to provide a cushion for incapacitation from illness or time off needed for sickness, bereavement, or other personal use only. The personal day must be scheduled with the prior approval of the employee's manager. In the event that the personal day is not used by the end of the calendar year, employees may carry the unused time forward to the next calendar year. If the total amount of unused personal time off reaches a maximum ("cap") of two personal days, the employee will no longer be eligible to earn any additional personal days off until the employee uses the time off and brings the available amount below the cap. Nonexempt employees may take personal time off in increments of one-half day; exempt employees may use personal time off in increments of a full day. Unused personal time off will be paid out upon termination of employment.

#### Example #2
If, for some unforeseen personal reason, an employee is required to be away from his or her job for an extended period, an unpaid leave of absence may be requested. Leaves of absence shall be requested in writing. Approval for a leave of absence will be at Dr. Clearly's sole discretion. Criteria for approval will include the reason for request, the employee's performance record, length of employment, and workload requirements for the rest of the staff. Leaves of absence are at the discretion of Dr. Clearly. They are not a matter of right. The employee cannot assume that any job will be available on return of any unpaid leave of absence. No vacation, sick leave, or other benefits will accrue during this period.

### Pregnancy Disability Leave
#### Example #1
All employees who are disabled on account of pregnancy, childbirth, or a related medical condition may request an unpaid leave of absence. Such leave will be granted for the period of disability, up to a maximum of 4 months. Time off may be requested for prenatal care, severe morning sickness, doctor-ordered bed rest, childbirth, and recovery from childbirth.

Any employee who wishes to take a pregnancy disability leave must notify her manager or the Human Resources Department of the date the leave is expected to commence and the estimated duration of such leave. Such notice should be given as indicated above and supported by a medical certification of disability. Before returning to work, the employee must provide a medical certification that she is able to resume her original job duties. Obtain appropriate forms from the Human Resources Department.

An employee who returns to work immediately after the expiration of an approved pregnancy disability leave generally will be reemployed in her former position or a comparable job, as required by law.

Pregnancy disability leave is unpaid. However, employees who are eligible to do so may use any accrued vacation but must use all accrued paid sick time during pregnancy disability leave. Such benefits, if used, will supplement any state disability insurance benefits the employee receives and will not extend the period of the approved leave.

Employees who are affected by pregnancy may also be eligible to transfer to a less-strenuous or less-hazardous position or duties if certain prerequisites are met. Reasonable accommodations may be requested with the advice of the employee's health care provider. For more information on pregnancy disability leave or transfer and its effect on the terms, conditions, or benefits of employment, please contact the Human Resources Department.

#### Example #2
Pregnant employees may work up to their due date as provided by their attending physician. A period of 6 weeks of leave from the due date or delivery date (whichever date is first) is the amount of anticipated leave from employment from Anytown Optometric Center. A job position will be held until that time pending, a meeting between the employee and supervisor before return. Alternate schedules can be discussed at that time, but management must reserve the right to require an employee to return to a full-time schedule, if necessary, to maintain the office operation. Failure of an employee to report to the supervisor before the end of the 6-week maternity leave will be interpreted as a resignation.

### Leave for Domestic Violence
Unpaid time off is available, as required by law, to employees who are victims of domestic violence for the purpose of appearing in court to obtain legal relief. Victims of domestic violence should provide reasonable advance notice when possible; otherwise, they must provide evidence from the court or prosecuting attorney regarding their court appearance within a reasonable time. Employees who are victims of domestic violence also may be eligible for additional unpaid leave under certain circumstances. Please contact the Human Resources Department for more information and eligibility requirements.

*Continued*

# Personnel Policies and Guidelines—cont'd

## Military Leave

Military leaves are available to eligible employees who enter the Uniformed Services of the United States, including the National Guard and the Commissioned Corps of the Public Health Service, or the state military forces, or the reserve components of the same, to participate in active or inactive duty or training. Time off is also permitted for an examination to determine one's fitness for duty in any of the federal military forces. Such leave will be granted in accordance with the applicable state and federal laws, provided all legal requirements are satisfied and the employee returns to work or applies for reemployment within the time prescribed by law. You must provide advance notice of the need for leave whenever possible. Please give the Human Resources Department as much advance notice as possible to allow the Company to make arrangements to cover your position.

Employees on federal military leave may be entitled to continue health insurance benefits, at the employee's expense, for up to 18 months.

To obtain further information about military leaves, please contact the Human Resources Department.

## Expense Reimbursement

Where attendance at training programs, seminars, conferences, lectures, meetings, or other outside activities benefiting Anytown Optometric Center is required or authorized by the Company, customary and reasonable expenses will be reimbursed upon submission of proper receipts in accordance with the Company's reimbursement policy. Customary and reasonable expenses generally include registration fees, materials, meals, transportation, lodging, and parking.

Reimbursement to employees for the use of their personal motor vehicles on authorized Company business will be at the current IRS-approved mileage rate. This mileage rate covers all operating costs, including depreciation, tires and repairs, gasoline, insurance, towing, and other similar expenditures. For more information, contact the Human Resources Department to obtain a copy of the Travel Expense Reimbursement Policy.

## Continuing Education

Employees will be compensated for the normal work time missed while attending continuing education that is encouraged and approved by Anytown Optometric Center. The cost of registration for approved education will be reimbursed. All travel, lodging, and meals will normally be the responsibility of the employee. In each calendar year, up to 3 days' time for preapproved education can be compensated at the normal rate of pay.

Exempt employees will be excused from normal office obligations but will not receive additional time as compensation. All education programs must be approved in advance and will be approved based on appropriateness for specific skills needed in your employment and convenience to the routine operation of the office.

## Keys

Each employee who is given a key shall be responsible for its safekeeping. If a key is lost, stolen, or missing, the employee shall notify Dr. Clearly immediately. Upon termination or resignation, the employee must surrender the key by the end of his or her final day worked.

## Personal Standards
### Example #1

Dress, grooming, and personal cleanliness standards contribute to the morale of all employees and affect the business image the Company presents to the community. During business hours or when representing the Company, you are expected to present a clean, neat, and tasteful appearance. You should dress and groom yourself according to the requirements of your position and accepted social standards. Clothing must be neat, clean, tasteful, and professional when necessary for meetings or business gatherings. Avoid clothing that can create a safety hazard in your work area. Managers may issue more specific guidelines. Your manager or department head is responsible for establishing a reasonable dress code, from the following guidelines, appropriate to the job you perform. If your manager feels your personal appearance is inappropriate, you will be asked to leave the workplace until you are properly dressed or groomed. Consult your manager if you have questions regarding what constitutes appropriate appearance.

### Business Casual and Relaxed Casual Days

The Company has adopted a business casual approach to office dress for Mondays through Thursdays. This is a welcome alternative to the formality of typical business attire. Business casual wear should be clean, neat, and professional. Stained, wrinkled, frayed, or revealing clothing is never appropriate in the workplace. If you are considering wearing something and you are not sure if it is acceptable, err on the side of caution and choose something else. Traditional business attire may be worn in lieu of business casual or relaxed casual wear at your option.

Listed below is a general overview of acceptable business casual wear as well, as a listing of some of the more common items that are not appropriate for the office. Obviously, neither group is intended to be all inclusive. Rather, these items should help set the general parameters for proper business casual wear and allow you to make intelligent judgments about items that are not specifically addressed. Examples of acceptable business casual business wear include:

- Polo-style shirts
- Oxford shirts

# Personnel Policies and Guidelines—cont'd

- Blouses
- Knit tops
- Sweaters/cardigans
- Blazers/sport coats
- Casual pants/slacks (Dockers are fine)
- Skirts/dresses

Examples of inappropriate clothing items that should not be worn on business and relaxed casual days include:

- Jeans (except as discussed below)
- Shorts (except as discussed below)
- T-shirts (except as discussed below)
- Sweatshirts (except as discussed below)
- Sweat suits
- Miniskirts
- Spandex
- Bared midriffs, halter tops, or spaghetti strap and tank tops
- Flip-flops (such as the ones you wear at the beach) or sloppy sandals
- Noisy clothing (may include some shoes, bracelets, and anklets)

Fridays are designated relaxed casual days for all employees. Month-end closing days are also designated relaxed casual days for those who participate. Other days, such as certain holidays or days proceeding holidays, may be designated as relaxed casual days with prior notification from your manager. However, not all relaxed casual clothing is appropriate for the office. Stained, wrinkled, frayed, or revealing clothing is never appropriate in the workplace.

Listed below is a general overview of acceptable relaxed casual business wear. This list is *not* intended to be all inclusive. Examples of acceptable relaxed casual business wear include:

- Jeans that are not excessively worn, frayed, or faded
- Shorts (in warmer months) that are not excessively worn, frayed, or faded
- T-shirts that do not contain offensive messages or images (refer to the Anti-Harassment and Conduct policies)
- Sweatshirts that do not contain offensive messages or images (refer to the Anti-Harassment and Conduct policies)

There may be times when you will be asked to dress in typical business attire. Management will notify you before an event requiring such attire.

## Example #2

Difficult as it may be to define good taste in dress standards, as an employee of a professional office you are expected to dress in a professional manner. Clothes should be neat and clean. Casual attire is not appropriate for the office. Women are requested to wear hosiery to work and not to wear denim/jean fabric clothes or clothes that are so sheer as to be out of place in a professional office. Male employees should wear a shirt, tie, and slacks on weekdays and collared shirts with slacks on Saturday.

## Example #3

No visible tattoos or extreme hair colors are allowed. Piercings are limited to women—one hole per ear. For men trimmed mustaches are allowed but no other facial hair.

## Office Decorum

Nonalcoholic beverages may be consumed at an employee's workstation. Food may only be consumed in the lounge. Gum chewing is not permitted. Nonperishable food may be stored in an employee's workstation if it is in an airtight container and stored in a drawer where it is not visible to patients.

Leisure reading and other personal projects may be performed only in the lounge. Notices of fundraisers, tickets, catalogues, or other items for sale may be kept in the lounge only. Your work area is expected to be maintained and organized.

For health and safety reasons, as well as compliance with state laws and regulations, smoking is not permitted in the entire office. Employees who smoke should take extreme care to prevent hair, clothing, breath, and hands from smelling of smoke.

## Discipline

At Anytown Optometric Center we are in a type of business that requires a high level of maturity and judgment from all employees. In this regard, you are expected to follow the instructions of the doctors and supervisors and comport yourself in a manner that is acceptable in our setting. Failure to meet this expectation may result in discipline ranging from verbal warning to termination of employment, depending on the severity of the failure.

Breaking any of the following rules shall be considered grounds for disciplinary action. Note that this list is illustrative only and contains examples of some, but not all, of the rules and regulations that are considered grounds for disciplinary action. Other offenses in the following list may also be grounds for discipline, up to and including discharge if appropriate.

1. Failure to provide service to a patient or fellow employee that is within the usual and normal scope of your duties, or could be reasonably and appropriately rendered, or is required by reason of emergency.

*Continued*

## Personnel Policies and Guidelines—cont'd

2. Lack of responsibility in completing work assignments, as may be indicated by:
   - Repeated tardiness
   - Excessive absences
   - Misuse of work time or sick time
   - Failure to follow instructions of doctors or supervisors
   - Violation of Anytown Optometric Center policies
   - Insubordination
   - Acting disrespectfully toward any patient or co-worker
   - Misuse of equipment or instruments that belong to the doctors of Anytown Optometric Center.
3. Disregard of personal grooming, cleanliness, hygiene; the use of profane, unrestrained, or abusive language; disorderly conduct; smoking in unauthorized areas.

   Anytown Optometric Center reserves the right to deviate from this policy when it feels that circumstances warrant such deviation.

### Amendments
*Example #1*

This handbook may be amended from time to time. Employees shall be given a copy of the amendments for their reference. Employees shall also sign a copy acknowledging receipt of the amendments. This signed copy shall become a part of the employee's employment file and, once signed, said policy shall be adhered to by the employee.

*Example #2*

Revisions in Anytown Optometric Center policy are announced by memorandum, by bulletin notices, and as announcements at staff meetings by supervisors or doctors.

### Staff Meetings

Periodic staff meetings are held for all employees to keep them informed. These meetings should be used to communicate among various departments in a timely fashion. All meetings will specifically schedule time for employee comments.

# Conditions of Employment

### Classification of Employees
*Example #1*

Employees are divided into three classifications. The rights and obligations of each classification are defined below. The ending of the waiting period, described below, does not grant nor imply "permanent" employment status. All employment and compensation with Dr. Clearly is "at will," in that it can be terminated with or without cause, or with or without notice, at any time at the option of Dr. Clearly. No contract of employment other than "at will" has been expressed or implied. In all instances where this handbook refers to "employee" without designating that employee's status, the provision is applicable to all employees.

**Waiting Period Employee**

The first 180 days (6 calendar months) of employment is a waiting period. During this time, all employees are considered to be waiting period employees. During this period a waiting period employee may be terminated without notice. Waiting period employees receive no benefits. Vacation time will accrue during this period but may not be used. Any employee who leaves during the waiting period will forfeit all accrued vacation time.

**Non–Waiting Period Employee/Full Time**

All non–waiting period/full-time employees are either hourly or salaried and are hired to work a full workweek of 40 hours per week.

**Non–Waiting Period Employee/Part Time**

A non–waiting period/part-time employee is an employee hired to work fewer than 40 hours per week. Part-time employees receive no benefits, including vacation and sick leave, unless stated otherwise in this handbook.

*Example #2*

The following terms are used to describe employees and their status.

**Regular Full-Time Employees**

Regular full-time employees are regularly scheduled to work 36 or more hours per week. Regular full-time employees are eligible for most employee benefits described in this handbook, subject to the terms and conditions of the applicable benefit plans and policies, or as specifically stated in this handbook.

# Conditions of Employment—cont'd

### Regular Part-Time Employees
An employee who is regularly scheduled to work fewer than 36 hours per week is a regular part-time employee. Regular part-time employees are not eligible for Company benefits, including, but not limited to, sick days or holiday pay, except to the extent required by law or as specifically stated in this handbook.

### Exempt Employees
Exempt status is determined by federal and state law. In general, exempt employees are those engaged in executive, managerial, high-level administrative, and professional jobs that are paid a fixed salary and perform certain duties. Exempt employees are not subject to the minimum wage and overtime laws.

### Nonexempt Employees
All employees who are covered by the federal or state minimum wage and overtime laws are considered nonexempt. Employees working in nonexempt jobs are entitled to be paid at least the minimum wage per hour and a premium for overtime.

Employees will be advised of their status at the time of hire and of any change in status. Regardless of their status, employees of the Company are employed "at-will" and their employment relationship can be terminated by the Company or the employee at any time with or without cause.

### *Example #3*
The following terms are used to describe employees and their status.

### Exempt Employees
Exempt employees are management personnel, such as supervisors and professional personnel. Exempt employees are salaried and do not receive overtime pay. A permanent record of the exact hours worked is necessary to aid in accounting for sick time, vacation time, and personal time. Exempt employees are expected to average a minimum of 40 hours per week over a 4-week period.

### Nonexempt Employees
All other employees are considered nonexempt. Nonexempt employees are required to complete time cards. Overtime payment will be calculated on the basis of time exceeding the average 40 hours per week over a 4-week period.

### Part-Time Employees
All employees working an average of fewer than 32 hours per week are considered part time and are paid on an hourly basis. Part-time employees are not eligible for fringe benefits.

### Probation Period
A probation period of 3 months after the date of hire allows both you and Anytown Optometric Center the opportunity to assess the appropriateness of the relationship. During this period you are not eligible for any fringe benefits. Completion of this probation period does not entitle you to employment for any specified term or imply any changes in the termination reasons as defined in this handbook.

### Inactive Status
Employees who are on any type of leave of absence, work related or non–work related, that exceeds 3 weeks will be placed on inactive status. During the time an employee is on inactive status, benefits (e.g., vacation, sick leave) will not continue to accrue, except as otherwise provided by law.

## Meal and Rest Periods
### *Example #1*
Nonexempt employees scheduled to work more than 5 hours in a workday are provided with a 1-hour, unpaid, duty-free meal period daily. Such meal periods normally are scheduled between 11:00 AM and 2:00 PM, as staffing permits, and as scheduled by an employee's manager.

Nonexempt employees are provided with a 15-minute break in the morning and afternoon. This time is counted and paid as time worked. Therefore employees must not be absent from their workstations beyond the allotted rest period time and may not leave the premises during such rest periods.

### *Example #2*
By law, one half-hour lunch break must be taken after a 5-hour work period if the employee plans to return to work. An employee may be required to work 6 scheduled hours of work without a lunch break, but that will complete the day's work for said employee.

Employees shall not be paid during or for lunch time. Employees usually take a 1-hour lunch break. A staff meeting is held each Wednesday for an hour after lunch.

*Continued*

## Conditions of Employment—cont'd

### Compensation
#### *Pay Periods and Hours*

Payday for all employees is twice a month as follows. The first pay period begins on the first day of the month at 12:00 AM and ends at 11:59 PM on the fifteenth of the month. Thereafter, the second pay period begins on the sixteenth of the month at 12:00 AM and ends at 11:59 PM on the last day of the month.

Paychecks for all employees are distributed on the fifteenth and last day of the month. All employees are paid by check or direct deposit on the above-mentioned payday. Changes will be made and announced in advance when Company holidays or closings interfere with the normal payday.

The Company does not grant payroll advances.

#### *Deductions from Paychecks*

The Company is required by law to make certain deductions from your paycheck each time one is prepared. Among these are your federal, state, and local income taxes and your contribution to Social Security as required by law. Deductions will also be made for the following:

- Federal and state income tax withholding
- Social Security (FICA)
- State disability insurance (SDI)

Other items designated by the employee may include:

- Health insurance premiums
- Dental insurance premiums
- Vision insurance premiums
- 401(k) and/or Cafeteria 125 plan deductions

These deductions will be itemized on your check stub. The amount of the deductions may depend on your earnings and on the information you furnish on your W-4 form regarding the number of dependents and exemptions you claim. Any change in name, address, telephone number, marital status, or number of exemptions must be reported to your manager immediately to ensure proper credit for tax purposes. The W-2 form you receive each year indicates how much of your earnings were deducted for these purposes. Any other mandatory deduction to be made from your paycheck, such as court-ordered wage assignments or attachments, will be explained if the Company is ever ordered to make such deductions.

### Hours of Operation
#### *Example #1*
##### Business Hours/Schedules

The Company is normally open for business between the hours of 7:00 AM and 5:00 PM, Monday through Friday. The Company may assign work to employees on Saturday and Sunday as needed. Your manager will assign your individual work schedule. Some employees will have work schedules that start before, or end after, normal business hours. In no event may the starting time for nonexempt employees be earlier than 7:00 AM, nor the ending time later than 7:00 PM, without the department manager's and/or manager's approval.

All employees are expected to be at their desks or workstations at the start of their scheduled shifts, ready to perform their work. Exchanging work schedules with other employees requires a manager's approval. Work schedule exchanges will not be approved for mere convenience or if the exchange will result in disruption of or interference with normal operations or excessive overtime. All work schedule changes must be approved by your manager in advance.

#### *Example #2*
##### Office Hours

The office operates approximately 9 hours per day, 8:30 AM to 5:30 PM, on Monday, Tuesday, Thursday, and Friday and from 10:00 AM to 7:00 PM on Wednesday. Each employee has his or her designated starting time and finishing time. This time is not to be manipulated for an employee's convenience.

### Work Hours and Wages

The employees of Anytown Optometric Center have elected to establish a flexible work schedule. The schedule requires many full-time employees to work three of each four Saturdays. Many employees will be off Sundays and one other day during the Monday to Friday week. The day off during the week will be determined by the management of Anytown Optometric Center and will depend on the needs of the patient load and job description demands. Because many employees are entitled to one of every four Saturdays off, the total time worked will average 40 hours over a 4-week period. To substantially alter this flexible time schedule will require a majority vote of the employees, as noted in the California Labor Relations Bulletin.

#### *Saturdays Are Special*

With the high number of families in which all adults work, Saturday is often the only day they may avail themselves of eye care without losing wages. To serve our patients during this premium time, we will attempt to provide the full scope of our professional

## Conditions of Employment—cont'd

services every Saturday. By allowing many full-time employees to take one Saturday off each month, a special shorthanded condition exists for many Saturday schedules.

To reduce the impact on this very busy day, Saturday vacation or personal leave days will often be allowed only as part of a full week of vacation or personal leave. Employees may use their vacation or personal time on Saturdays as less than a full week subject to the approval of the supervisors.

### Employee Scheduling and Cooperation

On occasion an employee will need to work with a patient during the employee's lunch hour. If this employee's late return from lunch will leave the area understaffed for more than 5 minutes, the other employees in the area must decide how to rearrange their schedules to ensure proper staffing. Employees may decide among themselves how to redistribute their time so that one employee is not continually covering for other employees without receiving proper compensation.

### Time Cards/Records
#### Example #1

Each nonexempt employee is required to maintain an accurate record of time worked. Exempt employees are required to complete an attendance record to track absences, including leave time, and use of personal days. Time cards are official business records and may not be altered without your manager's approval nor falsified in any way.

The following guidelines pertain to nonexempt employees' time cards:

- Each employee is responsible for clocking in and out on his or her time card. Do not punch another employee's timecard or permit another to punch your time card.
- All time worked must be accurately recorded on the time card on a daily basis. The start and end of the workday as well as the start and end of the meal period and any personal time off must be recorded.
- All time cards must be signed in ink by you and your manager, attesting to the accuracy of the time card.
- Punch in no more than 12 minutes early; punch out no more than 12 minutes after the end of your scheduled workday. Any addition, correction, or change on your time card must be made and initialed by your manager.
- Time records are the property of the Company and must remain in the time card racks.
- All overtime must be preapproved by your manager; if you must leave work early for any reason, notify your manager.
- Time cards are to be submitted to the director of Human Resources. The employee is responsible for submitting time cards on time.

#### Errors in Pay

Every effort is made to avoid errors in your paycheck. If you believe an error has been made, tell the Human Resources Department immediately. He or she will take the necessary steps to research the problem and make a proper and prompt correction, if necessary.

#### Example #2
##### Reporting Pay

If an hourly employee is required to report to work and is furnished with less than one-half of his or her scheduled day's work, the employee is entitled to 2 hours pay or pay for one-half of his or her scheduled day's work, whichever is greater. If an employee is asked to leave early or when the employee's immediate supervisor asks for volunteers to leave early, the employee must use a sick day or vacation day for the remainder of the day if he or she wishes to be paid. Dr. Clearly is excused from providing reporting pay when the failure to provide work is caused by circumstances beyond Dr. Clearly's control or when the employee who is requested to work is on paid stand-by basis.

##### Time Recording

All employees will keep electronic time cards. If the automated system is not available, manual time cards must be kept on a daily basis. Time cards must be completed daily and submitted by the end of work on the Tuesday collection day.

### Reduction to Staff

If reducing staff becomes necessary for financial or other reasons, consideration will be given to the employee's history of work performance, performance reviews, attitudes and enthusiasm, and other factors. It is at Dr. Clearly's discretion to keep the best employee for the job. Seniority is not a factor in deciding which employee to retain.

# Benefits

## 401(k) and Profit Sharing Plan

The Company has established a 401(k) savings plan to provide employees the potential for future financial security for retirement. All regular full-time employees who have more than 3 months of service after their date of hire and have attained the age of 21 years are eligible to participate in the 401(k) and profit sharing plan.

The 401(k) savings plan allows you to elect how much salary you want to contribute and direct the investment of your plan account, so you can tailor your own retirement package to meet your individual needs. The Company also contributes an additional matching amount to each employee's 401(k) contribution.

Complete details of the 401(k) savings plan are described in the Summary Plan Description provided to eligible employees. Contact the Human Resources Department for more information about the 401(k) plan.

## Profit Sharing Plan

At the end of each calendar year, a profit, if any, will be declared and paid into an approved account as provided by the government-approved plan. The amount applied to each employee's account depends on vesting and salary level as noted in the plan. The program administrator will provide a periodic accounting to each employee.

## Health Insurance
### Example #1

Dr. Clearly provides to each full-time employee, other than waiting period employees, group medical and health insurance. After the waiting period has expired, employees become eligible for health benefits beginning on the next "first" of the month that occurs. Dr. Clearly provides coverage for the employee only. If the employee wishes to obtain coverage for other dependents, the employee may do so at the employee's cost and expense. Dr. Clearly makes no representations that the insurance he provides will allow for dependent coverage. The employee, by electing dependent coverage, authorizes Dr. Clearly to deduct the increased premium amounts from the employee's wages. Employees should refer to the plan's booklets for additional information on coverage. Employees may elect not to accept health insurance benefits.

### Example #2

The current policy requires a $750 annual medical deductible. After the first $250 is paid by the insured employee, Anytown Optometric Center will pay the remainder of the approved deductible as determined by the insurer. Spouses and children of employees may optionally be covered by the health insurance and be paid by payroll deduction.

## Childcare Benefits

The Company provides childcare assistance to all regular full-time employees. Given below is a brief description of childcare assistance that may be provided when feasible. For more detailed information, please contact the Human Resources Department.

## Flexible Spending Accounts
### Cafeteria Plan/Flexible Spending Account

Employees choose benefits (including childcare) from a list of options and contribute a part of pretax wages to a flexible spending account. This option allows employees to minimize the federal tax they must pay.

## Life Insurance

A fully funded $25,000 life insurance policy is provided by Anytown Optometric Center for each full-time employee.

## Sick Leave
### Example #1

Paid sick leave is available to regular full-time employees to use when they must be absent from work because of illness or injury or medical appointments of their own or their child, parent, spouse, or domestic partner. Paid sick leave is earned on a pro rata basis, as work is performed, at the rate of 1.667 hours per pay period or 5 days per year. Once this benefit is exhausted, further approved time off is without pay unless the employee has other paid leave available. Unused sick leave does not carry over to the next calendar year.

Employees may use sick leave pay only when they are on an approved absence because of an illness, injury, or medical appointment of their own or of their child, parent, spouse, or domestic partner. A medical certification may be required to verify eligibility for this benefit. Unused sick leave is not paid out upon termination of employment.

### Sick Leave Benefits

Employees may use accrued sick leave benefits in the event of the illness of a child. (See Sick Leave policy.)

# Benefits—cont'd

## Example #2

Sick leave is granted to full-time employees. Sick leave days begin accruing from an employee's first day of employment at the rate of approximately one-half day per month (i.e., generally 6 days per year). However, sick leave days cannot be used until after the employee has completed the waiting period.

Sick leave is not accrued during disability and medical leaves of absence or unpaid leaves of absence. An employee may not accrue more than 6 days of sick leave time. A maximum of 6 days may be used at one time. After 6 days, the sick leave is considered a disability leave. The employee may then use vacation time or take the time as an unpaid leave of absence.

If an employee knows he or she will not be able to work that day or the next day because of an emergency, that employee must notify Dr. Clearly. Upon return to work, the employee shall provide Dr. Clearly with medical proof of illness lasting more than 4 days.

Employees who come to work ill may be sent home by any of the doctors at his or her sole discretion. The employee's absence will be considered a sick leave day if the employee has accrued such time or as an unpaid leave of absence.

## Example #3

Employees are required to contact the supervisor before their scheduled start time on a daily basis while they are off sick. After completing the required probationary period, full-time employees will accumulate sick leave at a rate of 1.667 hours for each full pay period of employment. Computation of sick leave will be based on actual hours worked, not including sick time or overtime. You will accumulate 1 week (40 hours) of sick time after 12 months of employment. You may accumulate up to 3 weeks (120 hours) of sick leave.

Surplus, unused sick time in excess of 120 hours will be paid to you within a reasonable period after the end of each calendar year. If a sickness exceeds the accumulated sick time, the additional time will be charged to personal leave. If the sickness exceeds the accumulated personal and sick time, leave will be continued at no pay. Sick leave is intended for use of employees during their personal illness.

## Vacations

### Example #1

Only regular full-time employees are eligible for paid vacation benefits. Temporary and regular part-time employees do not accrue paid vacation benefits.

Our vacation plan is designed to provide eligible employees with the opportunity to rest and get away from the everyday routine. Eligible employees will earn paid vacation on a pro rata basis. The paid vacation accrual rate is based on length of employment, as follows:

| Years of Employment | Pay Period Accrual Rate (in Hours per Pay Period) | Total Accrual per Year (in Days) |
|---|---|---|
| 1 year | 1.667 | 5 |
| 2-4 years | 3.334 | 10 |
| 5+ years | 5.000 | 15 |

Eligible employees shall continue to earn vacation according to the above schedule until the employee has accrued the equivalent of twice his or her annual rate. Once this cap is reached, no further vacation benefits will accrue until some paid vacation time is used, thereby reducing the total amount of accrued vacation below the permitted maximum. When some paid vacation time is used, vacation compensation will begin to accrue again. Vacation benefits will cease to accrue during the portion of a leave of absence that extends beyond 3 weeks from the initial date on which the leave of absence began.

Vacation time may be used only if it is earned. Eligible nonexempt employees may take vacation time in minimal increments of one-half vacation day; exempt employees must use vacation time in increments of a full day. Employees are encouraged to take vacation during the year in which vacation benefits are earned. Vacation schedules must be coordinated with and approved by your manager with reasonable advanced notice. Accordingly, each eligible employee should submit vacation plans to his or her manager for approval 1 month before the requested vacation or as far in advance as possible. If circumstances compel a change in plans, the employee must give notice to his or her manager.

Although the Company will make reasonable efforts to accommodate employee requests in scheduling vacations, except as otherwise required by law, all vacations are scheduled subject to the Company's business needs and may have to be deferred. Moreover, the Company reserves the right to schedule an employee's vacation dates if an employee fails to take vacation during the year in which vacation benefits are earned.

Vacation credits will cease to accrue while an employee is on any unpaid leave of absence. Upon termination of employment, employees will be paid for unused vacation time that has been earned through the last day of work.

*Continued*

# Benefits—cont'd

## Example #2

Vacation time and the accumulation of vacation time is calculated by regularly scheduled hours worked and not by calendar days. Overtime hours are not included in the calculation of vacation day accrual. For purpose of computing the amount of vacation time earned, a "year" is defined as 2,080 regularly scheduled hours worked.

Paid "sick days" and vacation days and holidays from the office are counted as hours worked toward a year. All of each employee's regularly scheduled hours worked, beginning with his or her first day on the job, are included toward his or her year regarding vacation.

Full-time employees earn:

After completing 1 year of service: 5 days to be taken in the following year

With 2 through 5 years of service: 10 days to be taken in the following year

With 6 through 10 years of service: 15 days to be taken in the following year

With 10+ years of service: 20 days to be taken in the following year

Vacation time is granted on the anniversary of the hire date of the employee each year. Vacation time is not earned during a disability or time off without pay; therefore a prorated number of vacation days will be subtracted in a given year for disabilities and time off without pay.

A vacation schedule will be posted on the first of each year. Time off requests are made in order of seniority until February 15 of each year. Requests after February 15 are on a first-come, first-served basis. Requests should be made at least 2 weeks in advance.

Employees must get prior approval from Dr. Clearly for times already requested by other staff members.

The maximum amount of vacation customarily taken at one time is 1 week. Vacation days in excess of 1 week at a time must be approved by Dr. Clearly.

Employees earn vacation days proportional to the number of days they customarily work per week. For example, an employee who works 5 days per week earns 10 vacation days per year for years 2 through 5 of employment.

Employees must work at least 6 months before taking vacation days beginning in year 2.

Paid vacation days are intended to provide employees with a period of relaxation away from the work environment. Therefore employees should plan to use their vacation days during the year after which they are earned. Vacation days may not be "carried over" to the next year.

Dr. Clearly reserves the right to amend the vacation policy for new employees to allow for the accrual of vacation days at different rates and allow the new employee the ability to use vacation days before completing 1 year.

On an employee's last day of employment pursuant to timely written notice, as defined in the "Resignations" section, or upon termination, the employee shall be compensated for earned, unused vacation time.

Employees shall give 2 weeks written notice prior to taking two or more consecutive vacation days. Scheduling an employee's vacation time is at the discretion of Dr. Clearly. Generally only one employee at a time per division may be on vacation. Vacation scheduling is on a first-come, first-served basis, and requests shall be first submitted in writing to Dr. Clearly.

## Example #3

Vacation days are accumulated at a rate of 3.25 hours for each 2 weeks of employment. In 12 months 84.5 hours of vacation will be accumulated. For purposes of vacation compensation, employees will be paid for 8 hours leave for each week day and 4 hours for each Saturday.

Because of the importance of vacation time to maintain the highest performance and positive attitude on the job, employees are encouraged to schedule all their vacation or personal leave in segments of 1 week or more. A maximum of 3 weeks of paid vacation or personal leave time will be permitted each year. To further encourage the use of vacation or personal leave, a maximum of 40 hours of vacation can be carried from one year to the next. Additional unused vacation will be lost.

Small offices have special problems in attempting to schedule vacations and personal leave. Each employee is critical in the operation of the practice, and a combination of sickness and vacations can be devastating to the scheduling of patients. Vacation and personal time are most easily absorbed during the times of lowered activities in the office. Doctors will be asked to publish their vacation time by the second week of January each year. Employees can request their vacation time after the posting of the proposed doctor vacations. The granting of vacation time will be based on the convenience of the office schedule and the order in which the supervisors receive the requests.

## Personal Leaves of Absence

The Company provides one personal day off with pay in each calendar year to regular full-time employees to provide a cushion for incapacitation from illness or time off needed for sickness, bereavement, or other personal use only. The personal day must be scheduled with the prior approval of the employee's manager. In the event that the personal day is not used by the end of the calendar year, employees may carry the unused time forward to the next calendar year. If the total amount of unused personal time off reaches a maximum ("cap") of two personal days, the employee will no longer be eligible to earn any additional personal days off until the employee uses the time off and brings the available amount below the cap. Nonexempt employees may take personal time off in increments of one-half day; exempt employees may use personal time off in increments of a full day. Unused personal time off will be paid out upon termination of employment.

## Benefits—cont'd

### Uniform Allowance

If your position requires you to wear a uniform or lab coat, a uniform allowance is provided for you. After 6 months of continual employment, you may purchase two uniforms or lab coats. After each calendar year of employment based on the anniversary date of employment, you will be entitled to one additional uniform or lab coat. Authorization to purchase uniforms or lab coats must be obtained from your supervisor and purchased at a designated store.

### Professional Courtesy for Staff

Anytown Optometric Center offers a 100% professional courtesy on professional eye care services and cost charges for materials used in optical corrections and contact lenses for employees, spouses, and their children. Subject to approval of management, one free pair of glasses will be provided for employees of Anytown Optometric Center yearly based on the anniversary date of the employment.

Additionally, other family members of employees (parents, stepparents, brothers, sisters, and in-laws) will receive a 50% professional courtesy on professional eye care services, retail optical fees, and cost plus 20% on contact lenses and supplies. Extended family members may be eligible for a 30% discount on professional services and optical materials. (Please confirm this discount with management in advance.)

### Credit Union

As an employee of Anytown Optometric Center you may become a member of Vision One, the California Optometric Credit Union. The credit union can provide a variety of different services, including checking, savings accounts, credit cards, and loans. Details can be obtained from your supervisor.

### Costco Membership

Anytown Optometric Center will pay the yearly membership fee to Costco for full-time employees if requested.

# Job Descriptions

## By Area Worked
### When Working at the Front Desk

You are responsible for greeting all patients with smile on your face and a pleasant voice when they enter the office. Patient demographic information needs to be filled out and the information entered into the computer. Insurance information needs to be collected and eligibility needs to be verified. The patient's chart needs to be prepared with all the forms in the correct location. The other staff members or the doctor needs to be notified when the patient is ready to begin the examination.

Answering the telephone is a major responsibility of the staff at the front desk. This person must have excellent diction and language skills because this is the first impression that new patients will have of our office. The telephone must be answered by the third ring with a pleasant voice. Making appointments, changing appointments, canceling appointments, and calling to remind patients of appointments are all handled by the front desk personnel. Staff answering the telephone must have a good grasp of all the services available in the office and the expertise of the doctor. In this way they will be able to answer all the questions patient and phone shoppers may have.

Front desk personnel are responsible for the financial dealings in the office. They prepare fee slips, log the financial information into the computer, and handle monetary transactions with the patients. They should be intimately familiar with what insurance plans the office accepts and does not accept. Information to answer questions about eligibility, deductibles, coverage, and so forth is helpful to have on hand immediately. Front desk personnel are responsible for credit card transactions, check payments, and cash. Balancing the day sheet at the conclusion of business is mandatory.

Saying goodbye to each patient is important. Make sure they understand what was done for them while they were in the office, what is going to be done next and by whom, and when they are expected back in the office. Making appointments in advance is important and should be done whenever possible before the patient leaves. Notes should be kept in the chart and computer about the flow of future activities.

The front office staff are also responsible for maintaining the patient records (attaching loose papers to the sheets, filing, making sure that all the work for a patient has been completed before the chart is filed), billing (insurance companies and patients), collections (insurance companies and patients), and routing the chart to the laboratory area to make sure that materials (glasses and contact lenses) are ordered in a timely manner.

General responsibilities include keeping the area clean and neat, ordering supplies for various office machines, straightening up the reception room during the day, and making sure the bathroom is clean and fully stocked.

### When Working in the Style Center

Staff working in the style center are to assist patients in selecting the proper lenses and frames for their new glasses. They need to be familiar with all the frames that are carried in the office and all the different kinds of lens materials and options available. Multiple-pair dispensing is in the best interest of the patient and the office, so specialty eyewear should be suggested and the benefits to the patients emphasized. Contact lenses should be discussed with the patient when appropriate to see if some of their visual needs might best be served with contact lenses.

Often other options such as refractive surgery should be discussed or patient handouts provided. All these needs, as well as second pairs, sunglasses, and additional testing, should be discussed by the doctor, patient, and style center staff at an appropriate time, usually immediately upon completion of the examination but in some cases after special testing is complete. This "hand off" is essential to ensure that the patient knows exactly what recommendations are being made by the doctor. The staff person who is responsible for assisting the patient and for follow-through must be aware of what the recommendations are. The patient and the staff member assisting the patient must both hear the same thing at the same time and any questions either has can be addressed with the doctor at that time.

## Job Descriptions—cont'd

Working in the style center requires a complete knowledge of the fees and the insurance plans carried in the office. Fee slips are produced and presented to the patient for payment at the completion of the frame selection process. Payment can be processed by either style center staff or by another staff member working at the front desk. Before transitioning the patient to another staff member, be sure that staff member knows when the patient is to be seen next. This further "hand off" of the patient between staff members is also very important.

Frame inventory is the responsibility of the staff working in the style center. Each frame must be entered into the computer's inventory system and have a temple tag before it is placed in the frame display. Frames should or organized in an esthetically pleasing manner (so the frames "show" well) and so that the staff can easily find a particular frame or manufacturer. Specialty display cabinets should be decorated to accentuate the frames being displayed. These displays should be changed often to feature new frames and materials. Nonprescription sunglass displays should be easily accessible to contact lens patients and be stocked with frames of every style and for every age. Do not forget to mention the importance of ultraviolet protection, especially for infants and small children, and then direct the patient's attention to the children's sunglass area.

General responsibilities include keeping the frames dusted and the lenses cleaned and free of fingerprints. Glass cases, lens cleaning fluid, and microfiber clothes should be restocked as needed. Inventory should be managed on a weekly (or more often if needed) basis. Frames should be ordered in a timely manner so "good sellers" are fully stocked on the frame displays. The staff should work with the frame representatives for suggestions of frame displays and point-of-purchase materials.

### When Working in the Data Collection Room (Pretesting)

Staff working in this area are involved in direct patient contact and collection of clinical data necessary for the visual health and performance of the patient. Accuracy and attention to detail are very important. This individual will be responsible for collecting clinical data in the following areas:

- Visual fields
- Autorefraction and auto Ks
- Digital fundus photography
- Case history
- Visual acuity distance and near
- Stereopsis
- Color vision

Before the patient enters the room, the staff member is responsible to ensure that all the equipment and instruments to be used are present and calibrated. If electronic medical records are used in the office, all the clinical data you collect must be entered into the program in real time. When the data collection is completed, the patient is escorted into the examination room.

The examination room must be set up as the doctor has instructed. The instruments must be cleaned with alcohol, all the clinical supplies should be checked to make sure they are in place (contact lens cases, fluorescein strips, pens, paper, patient education materials, etc.), and the patient's personal belongings should be placed on a chair and not where the doctor needs to stand or sit. Make sure the patient is comfortable and state that the doctor will be there shortly. Notify the doctor that the patient is waiting. Doctors should also be alerted if any of the findings during the pretesting were abnormal or if anything unusual occurred during the testing.

General responsibilities include keeping the pretesting area and the examination room clean and neat. After each patient, the instruments should be placed in their original positions, trial lenses and the trial frame should be cleaned and put away, the chair and stand should be placed in the "ready" position, and the trash should be emptied. Any instruments needing to be sterilized should be cleaned and packaged for sterilization. Staff working in pretesting should make sure that all the professional supplies are ordered in a timely manner so shortages do not occur.

### When Working in the Contact Lens Area

Hygiene is of utmost importance when working in the contact lens area. Always make sure your hands are clean and the area is kept neat and hygienic. You are responsible for working with contact lens patients to place lenses on their eyes when instructed to do so by the doctor. When appropriate, contact lens trainings are done to teach new contact lens wearers how to properly insert, remove, and care for their contact lenses. This person must be familiar with all the contact lenses that are used in the office, the manufacturer, the available parameters, and their clinical uses. The proper contact lens solutions are very important for proper contact lens care. Always recommend the solutions prescribed by the doctor and give the patient the appropriate handouts and coupons for their use.

This staff member must be familiar with the contact lens fees in the office so the patient can be charged the correct amount for the contact lens services, contact lenses, and solutions. Always be sure you know when the doctor has requested to see the patient next and make that appointment for the patient before dismissing him or her. Follow-up is important to be sure that the patient's contact lenses were ordered (either revenue lenses or diagnostic lenses) in the right quantity and from the correct manufacturer.

General responsibilities include keeping the diagnostic contact lens inventory up to date. An ample supply of diagnostic lenses must be kept to be sure the doctor has the proper selection of lenses to fit the patients. Contact lens solution inventory must be kept up to date, including all the cleaners and rewetting drops. A good working relationship with the contact lens representatives is an important part of this job.

*Continued*

# Job Descriptions—cont'd

### When Working in the Laboratory

Staff working in the laboratory must be very detail oriented. From here all the materials (lenses and frames) are ordered from the laboratory. The orders to the laboratories must be checked and double-checked to ensure the glasses prescription is correct (no transcription errors), it is being ordered from the right laboratory, the lens type and frame have been specified, and all the "extras" (tints, coatings, special instructions) have been included. All the lens measurements must be checked to be sure all the necessary measurements are given to the laboratory so the glasses can be correctly fabricated (segment height, monocular PD). All contact lens orders come from here as well. The correct lens type and all of its specifications must be ordered correctly with the correct instructions regarding where the lenses are to be shipped. While ordering these materials, the fee slip must be checked to be sure that the patient has been charged for and has paid for all the materials being ordered.

When the jobs come back from the laboratory all the parameters must be checked to be sure the materials are "on spec" before the patient is called to come pick up his or her glasses. Remember, the office policy is "the laboratory made a mistake until proven otherwise." When the glasses are ready for dispensing, the patient should be called and an appointment set to come to the office to pick up the glasses and have them adjusted. Staff working in the laboratory are responsible for delivering glasses to the patients, adjusting glasses, and performing all glasses repairs.

A good working relationship is necessary with the laboratory manager of each of the laboratories the office deals with so you have a "go to" person in each laboratory if a problem occurs. Turnaround time is an important issue that has to be managed by the laboratory staff. Each job sent to a laboratory needs to be followed closely to ensure that it is delivered back to the office in a timely manner. Follow-up phone calls to the laboratories asking the status of a job are a daily occurrence.

Interaction with the other staff in the office is critical in this position. Good communication is necessary to ensure that frame inventory is correctly ordered, that contact lens inventory is kept up to date, and that the inventory management system for the frames and contact lenses is correct. This staff member is also responsible for managing the returns in the office. Frames and contact lenses that need to be returned to the manufacturers must be done so in a timely manner so the appropriate credits are issued to the office account.

Each month when the bills from the laboratories arrive, the laboratory staff is responsible for matching up invoices to be sure the office has been billed only for the materials ordered and that the proper credits have been issued. The preciseness of this process is critical to the financial health of the office (and your job).

In general terms, the work area needs to be kept neat and clean. Follow-up in this position is important. Myriad details need to be remembered about each job that leaves the office; systems must be put in place to track them and make sure that each pair of glasses delivered to a patient is "just what the doctor ordered."

## By Title

### Office Manager

The office manager is the most versatile employee in the office. He or she has been in the office for long enough to understand the office philosophy and the vision of the doctor and can perform all the functions required in the office. The office manager should have a daily meeting with the doctor to facilitate good communication between the doctor and the staff. He or she is the problem solver in the office. If any issues arise with interactions between patients and staff, the manager's task is to resolve them. If other employees have problems or questions, the office manager is the "go to" person.

The office manager coordinates the work schedules and assignments for the other staff. He or she is in charge of ensuring that the patient flow through the office is smooth and that patients are informed if delays will occur. The office manager must oversee the work of all the other employees. That task includes, but is not limited to, making sure of the following:

- Patients are greeted properly when they arrive at the office
- Telephone calls are answered promptly and handled efficiently and with the proper information about the office
- Patient "hand offs" between doctor/staff and staff/staff are consistent and properly completed
- Frame selections are efficient and proper efforts are being made for multiple-pair purchases
- Fee slips are written up correctly
- Materials such as frames, lenses, contact lenses, and cases are ordered correctly and in a timely manner
- Check-in of ophthalmic materials is maintained at a high level of accuracy
- Money is being handled accurately
- Billing is being done in a timely manner
- The day sheet is balanced
- Reports for the doctor are created so he or she can manage the finances of the office efficiently
- Weekly staff meetings have active participation (and leading them when called on to do so)
- All "problem patients" in the office are appropriately handled

Some offices are not large enough to have a separate office manager. This person is usually the front office person as well and therefore has to perform all these management duties in addition to all the functions of the front desk (see p. 256). This is a very important and responsible position.

Most of all, in addition to having all these skills, the office manager needs to be able to manage people. He or she has to be able to keep the patient flow in the office smooth by delegating various duties to other staff members as needed, all with a smile and a pleasant demeanor.

# Job Descriptions—cont'd

## Ophthalmic Technician

Ophthalmic technicians (OTs) provide many services in the office, including functions involving direct patient care and ophthalmic materials. Because of their training (and certification) they can be a valuable asset to the office. OTs are responsible for frames and lens selections with patients in the style center and subsequent ordering of those materials from the laboratory. They also work with frame representatives to manage the stock in the dispensary. OTs work with patients on all aspects of contact lens insertion, removal, and handling. They are also knowledgeable about contact lens solutions and other contact lens care products.

OTs are responsible for checking in all the jobs that return from the laboratory to be sure that the specifications are exact. They have a relationship with the laboratory managers, so they can handle problems with the laboratories independently. Their special training allows them to deliver all eyewear to the patient, instruct them on use, and triage problems patients may have in adapting to new prescriptions. They also handle all frame adjustments and repairs.

OTs are trained to perform all pretesting functions, including:

- Visual fields
- Autorefraction and auto Ks
- Fundus photography
- Color vision testing
- Visual acuity testing
- Stereopsis testing
- Case history
- Measuring the PD

They can also assist the doctor in performing diagnostic and therapeutic procedures. Most OTs are familiar with vision insurance and billing and can provide valuable assistance in those areas as well.

## Optometric Assistant

Optometric assistants perform many of the same functions as OTs but they do not have the same education or certification. Their work therefore must be supervised more closely by the doctor or an OT. As their skills improve and they gain experience working with patients, they can be allowed to work more independently.

California, as well as other states, regulates what duties can be performed by optometric assistants. The law requires that the office have a written policy concerning these limitations. The California Code reads:

An optometric assistant is an individual working in the office of an optometrist and acting under the optometrist's direct responsibility and supervision.

Supervision by an optometrist of an optometric assistant means the supplying or providing of direction, control, instruction, and evaluation, to include personal review of, and responsibility for, the results of testing.

Before the assignment of a task or procedure, an optometric assistant must first demonstrate to the satisfaction of the supervising optometrist that he or she possesses the necessary understanding of and ability to perform such tasks that may lawfully be assigned in a safe manner. These tasks may include:

- Measurement of visual acuity
- Keratometry
- Automated visual fields
- Retinal photography
- Non-contact tonometry

There shall be a written policy outlining what procedures can be done and by whom that is approved by the supervising optometrist and is to be maintained in his or her office. THE WRITTEN POLICY MUST ALSO STATE THAT NO PROFESSIONAL JUDGMENT OR INTERPRETATION OF DATA IS ALLOWED IN ANY SITUATION BY AN OPTOMETRIC ASSISTANT.

# Office Procedures

Office procedures should be in place for each of the following topics. Exactly what the procedures are and who is to perform those duties are very office specific. Having the staff contribute to this section is often helpful because they know best exactly how each task is to be performed. You should then edit their contributions to be sure what they are doing is what you want done in the office.

- Appointment scheduling
- Appointment delays
- Cleaning the office
- Closed door policy
- Closing the office
- Patient induction system
- Referrals and thank-yous
- Telephone etiquette
- Telephone (patient phone call) policy

# Office Policies

Office policies is a broad category that covers many activities in the office about which the staff must be knowledgeable. Often these policies refer to financial matters such as payment at the time services are rendered, accepted credit cards, accepted insurance companies, and refund policy.

Each staff member must be intimately familiar with these policies because they guide what the staff says to patients. The following is a list of some of the topics that should be considered when writing your office financial policies.

- Extended payment plan (request for credit)
- Collection and billing
- Refund policy (for glasses and contact lenses)
- Insurance processing
- How to choose the fees you charge

Other office policies do not involve financial matters and are more general in nature. Following are some examples of nonfinancial office policies.

## Fires and Emergencies

In case of emergency, dial 911. Exits, fire extinguishers, and first-aid kits are located throughout the facility. Employees must familiarize themselves with the location of Company emergency exits and equipment. Exits and areas around fire extinguishers must be kept clear at all times.

## Injury and Illness

Employee health and safety are extremely important. The Company is committed to providing a safe workplace. Accordingly, the Company emphasizes responsibility to take steps to promote safety in the workplace and work in a safe manner. To achieve the Company's goal of a safe workplace, everyone must be safety conscious at all times. All employees are expected to observe the safety policies of each area of our business, as further described below.

In keeping with its safety commitment, the Company has established an Injury and Illness Prevention Program. A copy of the program is available for your review, on request, from the Human Resources Department.

If you are aware of an unsafe situation, advise your manager or management of the problem. Employees are expected to promptly report all unsafe working conditions, accidents and injuries, regardless of how minor, to their managers and/or the Human Resources Department. No matter how insignificant an on-the-job injury may seem when it occurs, notify your manager or the Human Resources Department immediately. Failure to immediately report workplace injuries and/or accidents may result in disciplinary action.

## Ergonomics

The Company has developed an ergonomics program to minimize repetitive motion injuries (RMIs) in the workplace. The primary elements of the ergonomics program include (1) worksite evaluations, (2) control of exposures that may have caused RMIs, and (3) ergonomics training of employees. The ergonomics program also focuses on educating employees on their personal responsibility to ensure good work habits (such as posture and body mechanics) and adequate fitness for work.

RMIs are musculoskeletal injuries, identified and diagnosed by a licensed physician, that can result from a job, process, or operation in which employees perform the same repetitive motion tasks. Examples of repetitive motion tasks include, but are not limited to, sustained computer keyboard and mouse use; assembly of materials and products; and lifting, carrying, and loading objects. When an RMI has been reported at the Company that results from a job, process, or operation, a worksite evaluation will be conducted. The evaluation identifies potential exposures that may have caused RMIs and determines the methods the Company will use to control or minimize them. Affected employees will be informed of the potential exposures and trained in the control measures.

Every reasonable effort will be made to correct exposures in a timely manner that may have caused RMIs or, if the exposure is not capable of being corrected, minimize it to the extent feasible. In determining how to correct or minimize exposures, the Company will consider reasonable, cost-effective engineering or administrative controls. Employees are provided with training that includes an explanation of the ergonomics program, exposures that have been associated with RMIs, the symptoms and consequences of injuries caused by repetitive motion, the importance of reporting symptoms and injuries, and the methods used to minimize RMIs.

All employees are encouraged to immediately report to the Human Resources Department all suspected RMIs, RMI symptoms, or other ergonomic concerns. All employees are required to report to the Human Resources Department all workplace RMIs as soon as possible after they have been identified and diagnosed by a licensed physician.

## Safety Committee

This Company has a Safety Committee that is made up of a cross-section of our employees. The committee meets as needed to comply with our ongoing safety program. If there is something of concern to an employee regarding safety, it should be brought to the attention of one of the committee members so that it may be discussed at the next safety meeting. Minutes to all the meetings are available on request or may be posted.

# Part 5

# Office Policies and Procedures for Handling Managed Care Patients

# How to Use this Manual

This manual is a template you can use to customize for your particular situation, including description sheets with instructions on how to use the forms. Either you or a staff person can proceed through the manual; however, it may be highly educational for both you and your staff to do so together.

Before you begin, you may want to pull together all the information you now have on managed care plans so you can easily retrieve it when necessary for adding information to the manual.

## List of Plans Accepted by the Office

Often patients call asking if the office accepts their health plan. The patient may refer to the plan by the health maintenance organization (HMO) name, the vision plan, or the independent practice association (IPA). A list of typical names given to the plans by patients allows the staff to see quickly if the office accepts the plan. A phone number allows the staff to call the plan and check on patient eligibility.

Enter typical names used by patients to describe their plans on the form provided on the next page. Include the phone number and other possible names used by patients under the cross-reference section.

## List of Plans Accepted by the Office as of _____

| Name of Plan | Cross Reference | Phone |
|---|---|---|
| Aetna Senior Choice | See Vision Service Plan | (800) 776-0360 |
| Aveisis | Boeing | Patient bring form |
| Bankers Life | Medicare supplement | (800) 786-7557 |
| Block Vision Care | | (800) 879-6901 |
| Blue Shield-CPIF Life | MES | (800) 877-6371 |

## How to Use this Manual—cont'd

### List of Plans Accepted by the Office as of _____

| Name of Plan | Cross Reference | Phone |
|---|---|---|
|  |  |  |
|  |  |  |
|  |  |  |
|  |  |  |
|  |  |  |
|  |  |  |
|  |  |  |
|  |  |  |
|  |  |  |
|  |  |  |
|  |  |  |
|  |  |  |
|  |  |  |
|  |  |  |
|  |  |  |
|  |  |  |
|  |  |  |
|  |  |  |
|  |  |  |
|  |  |  |

### List of Plans Not Accepted by the Office

Sometimes it is quicker for the staff to check whether the patient is inquiring about a plan you are no longer accepting. You may initially be on a plan and then choose to leave. The patient may have your name on a list provided by the plan. Your staff will be required to explain to the patient why your name is listed although you no longer see patients on that plan.

Many successful offices like to refer the patient to a doctor who accepts their plan. The receptionist may say, "If you give me the name of your primary care doctor, I'll be happy to call and find out who is a provider for vision care on your plan."

A helpful receptionist can result in several scenarios: (a) the provider may be so far away that the patient decides to use your office and pay out of pocket; (b) the patient may not have vision coverage and choose your office because the staff have been so helpful; (c) in the future the patient's primary care doctor may switch to a plan accepted by your office; (d) the patient may switch to a plan accepted by your office; (e) the patient may have exam coverage through another doctor but no glasses coverage and choose to purchase their eyewear in your office; (f) the patient may have exam coverage through another doctor but may have glasses coverage through a plan you accept; (g) the patient may be unhappy with their vision care through their plan and come to your office instead; (h) the patient will tell his or her friends how well he or she was treated and recommend your office to them.

In any of the above cases, a patient who would not normally choose your office may become an enthusiastic supporter.

Enter common plans you do not accept on the next form. Include any notes that may be helpful to your staff. You may wish to discuss sample scripts to use with patient inquiries. An example of the form follows.

*Continued*

# How to Use this Manual—cont'd

**List of Plans Not Accepted by the Office as of** _____

| Name of Plan | Crossover Reference | Phone |
|---|---|---|
| Blue Cross Prudent Buyer | No vision coverage | (800) 333-0912 |
| Cole Vision | Send to Cal Oaks | 555-5144 |
| | 65 Plus Plan | |
| | Vision One Plan | |
| FHP Talbert Medical | Go to Hemet Eye | 555-8854 |
| Vision One Plan | Cole Vision | 555-5144 |
| Vision Plan of America | Send to Dr. Wong | 555-2020 |

**List of Plans Not Accepted by the Office as of** _____

| Name of Plan | Cross Reference | Phone |
|---|---|---|
| | | |
| | | |
| | | |
| | | |
| | | |
| | | |
| | | |
| | | |
| | | |
| | | |
| | | |
| | | |
| | | |
| | | |
| | | |
| | | |
| | | |
| | | |
| | | |

# Brief Summary of Accepted Managed Care Plans

After your staff has ascertained that the patient is a member of a plan that you accept, additional information on patient eligibility or plan coverage may be required. Tables with notes can provide a quick reference for a busy receptionist to find necessary information.

Enter summaries of each plan on the form:

## Summary of Managed Care Plans as of _____

| Name of Plan | Notes |
|---|---|
| AARP | Medicare supplement; patient pays refraction |
| Aetna Life Insurance, Co-Aetna Health Plan | HCFA form; patient pays difference from U&C and exam 30; Lenses 30, 40, 50; frame 30 |
| Aetna Senior Choice | Use Internet or call Vision Service Plan for eligibility;includes Primary Eyecare |
| AVP | Account # 957; call for authorization. We have forms; use CSC lab. |

## Summary of Managed Care Plans as of _____

| Name of Plan | Notes |
|---|---|
|  |  |
|  |  |
|  |  |
|  |  |
|  |  |
|  |  |
|  |  |
|  |  |
|  |  |
|  |  |
|  |  |
|  |  |
|  |  |
|  |  |
|  |  |
|  |  |
|  |  |
|  |  |

# Expanded Information Devoted to Each Plan

Each plan typically provides a guide to help determine eligibility, coverage, copayments, and authorization procedures. Include the appropriate pages from the guide in your Insurance Manual for review when additional information is necessary.

    Insert summary pages here.

### Telephone Call Summary Form

Unfortunately, many plans are changed without proper updating to the doctors. This often occurs at the beginning of the year. For example, many patients in the "baby boomer" generation are currently complaining to their plans that progressives are not adequately covered. A call to the plan's toll-free phone number may reveal that the plan now covers $95.00 of the total fee as opposed to last year's coverage of $85.00.

    If a patient has a managed care plan you do not see often, it may be best to call the plan and determine the coverage. Typically you will need to inquire about eligibility for exam, frames, and lenses. Ask about deductibles and record coverage for lens extras such as tints, photochromics, UV 400, progressives, and contact lens allowance. Office activities will flow more smoothly if this is accomplished before the actual patient visit.

    Use this form when inquiring about plans. You may wish to keep it in the patient's file or use it to update your manual. An example follows.

## TELEPHONE CALL SUMMARY

| Plan: | Patient: | Date: |
|---|---|---|
| Contact Person: | Phone: | Extension: |

Eligibility


Deductibles                              Exam                           Materials


Frame Charges


Lens Charges


Contact Lens Charges


Billing Information      Insurance Form      Super Bill      HCFA      Internet


*Comments:*

# Patient Price List

Most vision plans have a page summarizing the cost of lens extras and frame costs. Your optician will typically keep them in a drawer of the dispensing table. These summaries vary tremendously from plan to plan. If an optician cannot provide correct answers quickly, as opposed to guesses or estimates, the patient may view the office staff as not knowing what they are doing. This impression will make them less likely to purchase eyewear or recommend you to others.

Many offices look up fees by using a copy of the summaries provided by each plan at the dispensing table. Some plans are well outlined and charges are easy to find. More and more offices choose to transcribe their coverage to a standard format of their own design. This standard form is particularly helpful with plans you rarely see.

The benefit of using one standard format is that you can quickly determine costs without trying to find them on a form you are unfamiliar with. Your staff can quickly report the fees to the patient while appearing confident and efficient. Following is one possible standard format. Enter the fees of your managed care plans in the price lists and make copies to keep at the dispensing tables.

*Continued*

# Patient Price List—cont'd

**Patient's Price List for** _____

| Description | Single Vision | | Multifocal |
|---|---|---|---|
| **Materials** | | | |
| Polycarbonate | | | |
| Polaroid | | | |
| High-index plastic (<1.60) | | | |
| High-index plastic (>1.60) | | | |
| High-index glass | | | |
| Photochromics | | | |
| Low power aspheric | | | |
| Occupational lens | | | |
| **Multifocal Style** | | | |
| Blended | | | |
| Smart seg | | | |
| Progressive | | | |
| High-index plastic (<1.60) | | | |
| High-index plastic (>1.60) | | | |
| High-index glass | | | |
| Polycarbonate | | | |
| High-end progressives | | | |
| **Tints and coatings** | | | |
| Solid color | | | |
| Gradient | | | |
| Double gradient | | | |
| Mirror | | | |
| AR coating single layer | | | |
| AR coating multilayer | | | |
| Scratch-resistant 1 side | | | |
| Scratch-resistant 2 sides | | | |
| Edge treatment | | | |
| UV 400 | | | |
| **Others** | | | |
| Oversize | | | |
| Slab off | | | |
| Facet lens | | | |
| Rimless | | | |

Calculation of Frame Coverage:
Contact Lens Allowance:

# Scripts for Use by the Receptionist

One problem that doctors experience in the office is that their receptionists grow frustrated trying to handle all the different plans as well as with patients not knowing much about their own insurance coverage. Often the receptionist comes across as curt, abrupt, or even rude. Simple scripts can allow the receptionist to convey your desired image to your patients.

## Scheduling the Appointment

After scheduling an appointment, the receptionist asks, "Do you have any insurance we can help you with?" (this projects a helpful image).

When the patient then mentions the name of the plan, the receptionist turns to the insurance manual and tells the patient if preauthorization is necessary or a form or a card. If a form is necessary, the receptionist can volunteer to have it sent to the office for the patient. This allows you to keep control and further conveys a helpful attitude. For example, "Super Vision Plan requires a benefit form. Would you like me to obtain one for you? We are happy to help our patients. Often insurance can seem so confusing. I need your Social Security number, date of birth, and the name of your employer."

Sometimes the patient is not sure if he or she has vision coverage. A receptionist may say, "I believe Aetna Senior Choice provides vision insurance through the Vision Service Plan. I'll be happy to find out for you. What is your Social Security number?" The experience of many doctors has been that their patients often had coverage for many years and did not know it. Coverage increases the likelihood that the patient will return for examinations in a timely manner.

Many offices take complete responsibility for helping the patient with managed care plans. In the beginning, this may require several phone calls to medical health maintenance organizations (HMOs), preferred provider organizations (PPOs), and vision plans. Often the information received is contradictory. But after considerable effort, you will learn the vision coverage for specific managed care plans. When you hear a patient has Aetna Senior Choice, for example, you will know exactly what the vision coverage is. By controlling the situation, you provide a service to your patients and learn how to use the system to provide the best vision care.

Providing the best vision care may mean getting approval for a vision therapy program or authorization for a low vision evaluation. Learning the correct protocol can result in covered contact lenses for high anisometropes or high myopes. The first time you battle through the bureaucracy may be time consuming, but thereafter you will know exactly how to get things done.

## Greeting the Patient

If the patient has an insurance form that requires filling out, the patient can be asked to fill it out and sign it or the receptionist can fill it out so the patient need only sign it. For many patients, it is easier for the receptionist to complete. "I'm going to help you with your insurance by completing the form for you. You will simply be required to sign it." A second example statement by the receptionist to the patient may be, "Please show me your insurance coverage card and I'll determine the coverage for you."

Because what your receptionist says may be highly personalized, have staff create their own scripts and place them here. From time to time they may wish to review them and change them.

## Patient Sign-in Sheet

Some offices prefer to keep a record of patients entering the office by using a sign-in sheet. This also affords the receptionist time to become familiar with the patient's managed care plan before discussing it with the patient. The patient writes his or her name and health plan. If the plan is not recognized, the receptionist can look it up in the insurance manual and alert the staff about the coverage. Many offices believe the sign-in sheet improves efficiency.

Other offices, however, stress personal, friendly service. Rather than use a sign-in sheet, the staff is trained to greet the patient and identify by name if possible. For example, if the next scheduled patient is Mr. Ricardo Lopez, and a Hispanic gentleman approaches the front desk, the receptionist may say, "Welcome to Eye Center Optometry. You must be Mr. Lopez!" This can be warmer than a sign that says, "Sign in here," or a receptionist who says, "Sign in on that paper."

The following is an example of a sign-in sheet you may wish to use. Copy it onto your letterhead.

# Patient Sign-in Sheet

**Patients, please sign in:**
*Include your insurance provider's name.*

**Date** _____

| Patient's Name (Please Print) | Insurance Name | Patient's Name (Please Print) | Insurance Name | Time Arrived |
|---|---|---|---|---|
| | | | | |
| | | | | |
| | | | | |
| | | | | |
| | | | | |
| | | | | |
| | | | | |
| | | | | |
| | | | | |
| | | | | |
| | | | | |
| | | | | |
| | | | | |
| | | | | |
| | | | | |
| | | | | |
| | | | | |
| | | | | |
| | | | | |
| | | | | |
| | | | | |
| | | | | |
| | | | | |
| | | | | |
| | | | | |
| | | | | |
| | | | | |
| | | | | |
| | | | | |
| | | | | |
| | | | | |
| | | | | |

# Eligibility Guarantee

This form may be used to ensure payment in the event the managed care group does not pay for services or materials. There are times when authorization is unable to be given because of late hours or technological problems. Many offices include this in a packet of papers to be filled out by patients new to the office.

Sometimes a patient may make a late appointment and tell the receptionist he or she has no insurance only to later find out he or she may be covered through a spouse's insurance. He or she may say, "I found out I have insurance. My husband says it is Super Vision Insurance Plan."

The receptionist may reply, "I'm not familiar with that insurance. I'll be happy to call them for your coverage. Because it is after five o'clock, they will probably be closed until tomorrow. Please fill out this eligibility guarantee because you do have insurance. In case of insufficient coverage we will bill you for the difference. We do all we can to help our patients with their insurance. It can be so confusing!"

Presented in the correct manner, signing an eligibility guarantee can appear to be in the best interests of the patient. Have your staff compose sample scripts and place them here.

*Continued*

## Eligibility Guarantee—cont'd

I, _____, hereby certify that I am eligible for

NAME OF PATIENT/MEMBER/GUARDIAN

_____ effective _____.

           HEALTH PLAN               DATE

I have chosen _____

OFFICE OR OPTOMETRIST

to be my Medical Provider. I understand that if the above is not true or if I am not eligible under the terms of my health plan agreement, I am liable for all charges for services rendered. Also, if the above is not true, I agree to pay in full for all services received within 30 days of receiving a bill from the above noted provider.

_____

SIGNATURE OF MEMBER/GUARDIAN

_____

SUBSCRIBER NUMBER/SOCIAL SECURITY NUMBER

# Doctor's Plan Coverage Summary

Often the recommendations a doctor gives vary according to what the plan allows, or perhaps an additional explanation is necessary. Note on the file which plan the patient has. The doctor can use the following plan coverage summary form to recall which services require prior authorization and possible referral sources. Typically the summaries would be kept in the examination room. Below is a format used for this purpose. Complete plan coverage summaries. Make copies for the exam rooms. Below is a sample form.

## Doctor's Plan Coverage Summary

| Plan | Coverage |
| --- | --- |
| Aetna Senior Choice | Vision Service Plan primary eyecare coverage. Ophthalmologic referral to Dr. Cornea or Dr. Retina. Contact lens coverage for medical necessity. Prior authorization for anisometropia. from VSP. Low Vision with prior authorization. |
| AVP | Contact lens coverage of anisometropia 4.00 D or greater by prior authorization. |
| Pacificare | Vision training through PCP referral to Dr. Strabismus. |
| Sharp | Referral to/from Eye Care West IPA. Low vision consults covered. Aids not covered. |

*Continued*

## Doctor's Plan Coverage Summary—cont'd

| Plan | Coverage |
|------|----------|
|      |          |
|      |          |
|      |          |
|      |          |
|      |          |
|      |          |
|      |          |
|      |          |
|      |          |
|      |          |
|      |          |
|      |          |
|      |          |
|      |          |
|      |          |
|      |          |
|      |          |

# Managed Care Referral Request

More and more managed care plans allow services in addition to comprehensive eye examination based on referral from the primary care physician (PCP). One of the trends in managed care is the abolishment of "gag" clauses preventing the PCP from recommending alternative treatments. PCPs are approving visual therapy and low vision more often.

A Managed Care Referral Request form can simplify the paperwork involved in getting approval from the PCP. Copy the request form on your letterhead. Keep a supply in your manual.

*Continued*

## Managed Care Referral Request—cont'd

Primary Care Physician: _____     Date: _____

Patient: _____     DOB: _____

Insurance: _____     SSN: _____

I would like to see Dr. _____ for my eye problem. Please provide the required referral.


_____
Patient Signature

### Reason for Referral


### Services Requiring Authorization


Please call if you have any questions. You will be sent an examination and treatment summary for your files.


Referral # _____ Authorization Date _____

# Scripts for the Optician

A tendency for many opticians is to say to the patient, "Your plan covers any frame prices less than $45.00" or point to a display and say, "Your plan covers any of these frames." Or worse, they may say, "Your plan *only* covers frames less than $45.00." Most practice management experts will tell you not to prejudge what your patient can afford. Also, it is generally best not to belittle a plan as a "bad" or a "cheap" plan. Instead, stress the savings the plan provides.

Bring four to five frames to the patient, two of which are covered by their plan. After choosing a frame and lens options, say, "Without your insurance these glasses would cost $240.00, but your plan generously covers all except $50.00!"

Or you can say, "Your insurance plan covers the examination and a pair of general use glasses. This saves you $295.00. The doctor recommended you wear sunglasses to help prevent cataracts. These styles would look attractive in a sun lens." "Your plan allows you to upgrade to deluxe frames for only $25.00. That is a savings of $70.00!" "Your plan covers $40.00! That's fantastic. Let's get something special!" "Your plan allows you to upgrade your lenses to lenses with an ultraviolet light filter for only $12.00. This is a savings of $13.00!"

Some patients will be annoyed at deductibles, frame overcharges, or lens extras. They may initially insist on only getting whatever is covered by the plan. It is in the patient's interest and your interest to educate the patient as much as possible. If the patient says, "What does my plan cover? I want just what my plan covers," you may respond, "Your vision plan does cover some eyewear costs, but Dr. Clearly recommends a lens treatment that is more beneficial to you. I'll demonstrate to you what he recommends. Your vision plan greatly reduces your cost!" An optician who presents this in a cheerful, helpful tone will be able to communicate the benefits of the doctor's recommendations and the benefits of better frames. Or, similarly, "You have a great plan. It covers all our frames. The plan (name) specifies what to charge you for every frame, including the highest quality frames."

Educating the patient on products and benefits will result in increased patient compliance with doctor recommendations. In the past a private-paying patient may have had to pay $180 for something that only costs them $77 with their plan. Prescribing lens treatments should therefore be easier. For many offices, it is easier with managed care.

Write down scripts for your optician to use here. Remember to allow them to compose the script themselves.

# Scripts for Recall

Sometimes your patients will be more apt to come in for recall if the plan covers the annual exam. Other times their insurance may have changed and, for different reasons they think they must go to another doctor for vision care. Telephone recall allows you to educate the patient regarding coverage and whether the doctor also accepts the new insurance.

"The doctor recommended we see you this month to check for glaucoma. It has been one year since you were last examined. Do you still have Aetna Senior Choice Insurance?"

"No. I'm sorry I can't go to you anymore. I now have Secure Horizons."

"The Doctor also accepts patients with Secure Horizons. I will be happy to arrange an appointment for you that will be covered by your new insurance plan. Usually, when you have switched plans, you are immediately eligible for an eye examination and new glasses."

Occasionally your receptionist may be faced with the comment, "My vision plan only covers an exam every other year. I know I should come every year, but I can't really afford to." Some offices handle this by seeking other coverage, perhaps through a spouse's plan. More and more spouses are both working, and they often both have insurance coverage that extends to the spouse.

"We all have to make tough decisions when it comes to spending our hard-earned money. Of course, we see the need for annual eye examinations every day in this office. Sometimes a cataract or glaucoma just won't wait until your vision insurance kicks in. Because we recognize the need for regular eye examinations, there are two ways we can help you. More and more spouses are working. Sometimes both your insurance and your spouse's insurance provide vision coverage. Give me your husband's name, insurance company, and Social Security number and I'll determine whether you can be covered under his policy. If not, Dr. Clearly allows us to offer a courtesy fee waiver of 20% on all services when the need arises. Either way, I believe we can continue to take care of you and keep you seeing well."

Many offices offer a courtesy fee waiver to patients for the year that coverage is not available. The thrust of the receptionist's comments are targeting the need for regular vision care and the caring attitude of the office.

Decide on your office policy regarding patients who do not have annual exam coverage. Write it here.

Develop scripts for telephone recall and how to handle situations such as a change in managed care plans.

# Monitoring Payment

When checks are received from the managed care plan, make sure that they properly pay for each patient. Some doctors keep a log of patients and expected fees for each plan. These are checked off when the payment is received. Any discrepancies are pointed out to the plan administrators.

A vision plan may pay $20 more if billed correctly. Other times the doctor is allowed to charge the patient $20 more. If a plan reimburses $3 less per frame than agreed to, for example, the discrepancy can add up significantly over time. It is important to keep track of plan payments.

One method of keeping track is to arrange the doctor's copies of the billing forms in the order they are sent in. On the patient's file the date billed is noted. Once a month the staff can look over the billing forms and see which should have been paid by that date. They can follow up with the managed care plan regarding what is holding up payment.

If a patient calls inquiring about a billing form, the form can be found by looking up the billing date on the patient's file.

Another method to keep track of managed care payments is to enter billing data in a computer program. Accounts receivable can be reported according to 30-, 60-, or 90-day periods. Reports can be generated according to the specific managed care plan showing the date, patient name, and amount. As checks from the plan come in, these can be entered into the computer and discrepancies from billing can be detected.

Decide on a method for monitoring payments and write your protocol here.

# Staff Training Exercise

Below are possible scenarios that occur in practices with managed care patients. Distribute each case to the staff members it involves and discuss protocol and scripts in handling the situation. Time preparing today will save a great deal of time and grief tomorrow. You may wish to summarize the protocol and scripts here for easy review by your staff.

## Possible Scenarios that Occur in Offices with Managed Care Patients

As the number of managed care patients rises, eye care practitioners are experiencing frustration with handling some of the financial aspects of these patients. What policies and procedures do you use to handle the following situations?

1. A patient comes into the office for an appointment only to find out you do not accept her vision insurance. The patient leaves, causing a hole in your schedule.
2. A patient comes into the office for a scheduled examination but neglected to bring in the forms that demonstrate authorization of services and what is covered.
3. Your receptionist attempts to collect a deductible on the examination. The patient claims he should not have to pay any deductible.
4. A patient is upset because lens options are not covered by her plan.
5. A patient wants contact lenses instead of glasses and does not understand why he must pay extra.
6. A patient who is a high anisometrope and requires contact lenses asks, "Why doesn't the plan cover this if you say it is necessary?"
7. A patient requires a referral to an ophthalmologist. Who can see her under her plan?
8. You determine that an orthoptic evaluation or low vision evaluation is necessary. The patient asks, "If this is true, why doesn't the plan cover this necessary testing and treatment?"
9. A patient comes in for an appointment. His insurance requires a phone call to obtain authorization. The patient is presently not authorized for benefits.
10. Because glasses are only covered every 2 years, the patient does not want to change the prescription although a prescription change is indicated.
11. The patient is upset because only some of the frames are covered by her insurance.

# Capitation Plans

Capitation plans often place the doctor in the awkward situation that the better you are, the more the patient comes in, and the less income you net. Some doctors handle this by politely educating the patient that because of the policies inherent in his or her insurance plan, only a limited number of patients with that particular plan can be seen each week. "The next available time will be …" You risk the insurance company being unhappy with this arrangement, but this is better than the alternative of rushing exams, avoiding prescribing eyewear, and appearing to be rude and short with the patient. Capitated optometrists remember if the capitation plan covers materials, you not only lose the exam expense but also materials expense every time the patient comes in. Doctors handle this by allowing only so many exam slots for capitated patients.

Many doctors convey the attitude to the patient that "you get what you pay for." Although this is true, it is also true that all patients feel they are paying for competent care delivered in a pleasant fashion.

The doctor who cannot afford to deliver competent care in a pleasant fashion to a capitation plan should avoid the plan.

Write down your protocol for handling patients under each of your capitation plans here.

# Contenido

(Meds that can cause eye symptoms)

# Trastorno Acomodativo

## Definición
El trastorno acomodativo es una anomalía apresbiópica, no refractiva, sensoria y neuromuscular del sistema visual. Puede caracterizarse por precisión acomodativa inadecuada, facilidad y flexibilidad reducida, amplitud de acomodación reducida o por la inhabilidad de mantener acomodación.

## Síntomas
Los síntomas y signos asociados con una disfunción acomodativa están relacionados a las tareas prolongadas, de alta demanda visual, y centradas en la proximidad, incluyendo las siguientes:
1. Astenopía (fatiga ocular)
2. Visión borrosa transitoria
3. Fotofobia
4. Fatiga anormal
5. Dolores de cabeza
6. Dificultad para mantener la función visual cercana
7. Vértigo
8. Adaptación de postura anormal/distancia de trabajar anormal
9. Dolor orbital

## Factores diagnósticos
Las disfunciones acomodativas están caracterizadas por uno o más que uno de los siguientes hallazgos:
1. Amplitud acomodativa baja en relación a la edad
2. Facilidad acomomdativa reducida en visión cercana y/o distante
3. Rangos reducidos de acomodación relativa
4. Retraso anormal de acomodación
5. Descubrimientos acomodativos inestables
NOTA: Pueden ser apropiadas pruebas adicionales como parte del examen diagnóstico diferencial para la disfunción acomadativa para excluir otras condiciones médicas concurrentes y condiciones visuales asociadas.

## Consideraciones terapéuticas
### A. Manejo
El doctor de optometría determina las modalidades diagnósticas y terapéuticas apropiadas y la frecuencia de evaluación y el cuidado de seguimiento basadas en la urgencia y la naturaleza de la condición del paciente y de sus necesidades únicas. El manejo del caso y la duración del tratamiento son afectados por los siguientes factores:
1. La severidad de los síntomas y los factores diagnósticos, incluyendo el comienzo y la duración del problema
2. Las implicaciones a la salud general del paciente y la condición visual asociada
3. El alcance de las demandas visuales puestas en el individuo
4. Acatamiento por parte del paciente
5. Intervenciones previas

### B. Tratamiento
Un número de casos son tratados con éxito mediante el recetar de lentes terapéuticos y/o prismas. Sin embargo, las disfunciones acomodativas pueden también requerir terapia ortóptica o terapia de visión. La terapia optométrica de visión normalmente incorpora el recetar tratamientos específicos para lograr lo siguiente:
1. Normalizar la amplitud acomodativa relativa a la edad
2. Normalizar la habilidad de mantener la acomodación
3. Normalizar los rangos relativos de acomodación
4. Normalizar la facilidad acomodativa en relación a la edad
5. Normalizar relación acomodativa/de convergencia
6. Integrar la función acomodativa con el procesamiento de información

### Duración de Tratamiento
Los siguientes rangos de tratamiento están provistos como una guía para el procesamiento de reclamos (de seguros) de terceras partes y para el propósito de revisión. La duración del tratamiento dependerá de la condición particular del paciente y de las circunstancias asociadas. Cuando se requiere una duración de tratamiento más allá de estos rangos, puede ser justificable la documentación de la necesidad médica para los servicios de tratamiento adicionales.
1. La disfunción acomodativa hallada más comúnmente normalmente requiere de 24 a 32 horas de terapia en la oficina.
2. La disfunción acomodativa sin complicaciones, caracterizada por solamente una pérdida transitoria de función acomodativa, típicamente requiere hasta 8 horas de terapia en la oficina.

*Continued*

## Trastorno Acomodativo—cont'd

3. La disfunción acomodativa complicada por:
   a. Amplitud o facilidad reducida para la edad: hasta 12 horas adicionales de terapia en la oficina.
   b. Anormalidades acomodativas/de convergencia: hasta 16 horas adicionales de terapia en la oficina.
   c. Otras anomalías visuales diagnosticadas pueden requerir terapia adicional.
   d. Condiciones asociadas tales como la embolia cerebral, el trauma a la cabeza u otras enfermedades pueden requerir considerablemente más terapia en la oficina.

### Cuidado de seguimiento

A la conclusión del régimen de tratamiento activo, se deberán proveer evaluaciones periódicas de seguimiento a intervalos apropiados. Los lentes terapéuticos pueden recetarse a la conclusión de la terapia de visión para el mantenimiento de la estabilidad a largo plazo.

# Amblíopía

## Definición

La ambliopía describe la pérdida de la agudeza visual atribuible a un desarrollo visual anormal. Durante la niñez, se requiere de un estimulo visual apropiado para el buen desarrollo de la visión. La ambliopía tiene tres causas potenciales: la visión fuera de foco, ojos cruzados, y la deprivación visual. La visión fuera de foco suele ocurrir cuando uno o ambos ojos se encuentran con un grado sustancialmente avanzado de miopía, hiperopía, o astigmatismo. Cuando aparece una gran asimetría entre ambos ojos, el ojo menos enfocado puede desarrollar ambliopía. Cuando un ojo se voltea hacia adentro o hacia afuera, el cerebro suprimirá la visión en ese ojo a fin de evitar una doble visión. Sin embargo, el ojo volteado se vuelve amblíopico. Los anteojos, parches para los ojos, y las gotas dilatantes para los ojos, pueden reforzar el ojo amblíopico si es que han sido han sido recetadas tempranamente. Una causa menos común de la ambliopía es la deprivación visual la cual puede ser causada por una catarata congénita o un párpado caído congenital. La cirugía de cataratas o de párpados, en estos casos, puede minimizar la parición de la ambliopía.

## Síntomas

Los síntomas y signos asociados con la ambliopía incluyen los siguientes:

1. Agudeza reducida en el ojo afectado.
2. Percepción de la profundidad reducida.
3. Giro/inclinación de la cabeza
4. Falta de coordinación, capacidad reducida de dirigir y coordinar movimiento visual
5. Anisometropía
6. Estrabismo

## Factores pronóstico

La ambliopía está caracterizada por uno o más que uno de los siguientes resultados diagnósticos:

1. Agudeza reducida en el ojo afectado que no se normaliza con la receta optométrica para corregir la refracción, apropiada
2. Incapacidad de mantener una fijación foveal estable
3. Supresión de visión binocular.
4. Distorsión espacial.
5. Visión de profundidad reducida
6. Facilidad acomodativa reducida
7. Eficiencia motriz ocular inexacta
8. Asimetría en el funcionamiento de los dos ojos en las áreas relacionadas a la habilidad de procesar información ocular motriz y visual.

NOTA: Las pruebas adicionales pudiesen ser apropiadas como parte del diagnostico diferencial de la ambliopía a fin de excluir otras condiciones medicas concurrentes y diferenciar de otras condiciones visuales relacionadas.

## Consideraciones terapéuticas

### A. Manejo

Un oftalmólogo especialista en optometría establecerá las modalidades diagnósticas y terapéuticas apropiadas así como la frecuencia del proceso de evaluación y seguimiento en base al grado de urgencia y naturaleza de la condición del paciente y de sus necesidades especificas. El manejo del caso clínico y la duración del tratamiento pueden verse afectadas por los siguientes factores:

1. La gravedad de los síntomas y los factores pronósticos, incluyendo la aparición y la duración del problema.
2. Las implicaciones emergentes de la salud general del paciente y de sus condiciones visuales relacionadas.
3. La cantidad de demandas visuales ejercidas en un individuo.
4. El grado de seguimiento del tratamiento por parte del paciente.
5. Intervenciones quirúrgicas anteriores.
6. Otras anomalías relacionadas tales como la anisometropía o estrabismos.

### B. Tratamiento

Un pequeño porcentaje de casos pueden ser tratados exitosamente a través de una receta optometrica para lentes terapéuticos y/o prismas. Sin embargo, la mayoría de casos de ambliopía requiere terapia ortóptica / visual. La terapia ortóptica y visual usualmente incorpora tratamientos específicos con siguiente propósito:

1. Eliminar cualquier anisometropía.
2. Estabilizar la fijación foveal central
3. Normalizar la agudeza visual
4. Normalizar las destrezas monoculares, incluyendo las destrezas oculomotores y acomodativas y el tiempo de reacción
5. Minimizar la distorsión espacial
6. Eliminar la supresión de la vista
7. Eliminar cualquier tipo de estrabismo
8. Integrar la función visual con la respuesta motriz correcta y apropiada
9. Normalizar la función binocular

*Continued*

# Amblíopía—cont'd

### Duración de Tratamiento

Los siguientes límites de tiempo del tratamiento están proporcionados como una guía en relación al procesamiento de reclamos de seguros por terceras personas y como repaso de este material didáctico. La duración del tratamiento va a depender en las condiciones específicas del paciente y otras circunstancias conexas. Cuando la duración del tratamiento requiere que esta se extienda más allá de los límites abajo enumerados, la documentación sustentatoria correspondiente que justifica, desde un punto de vista medico, la necesidad de otorgar tratamientos adicionales puede ser requerida.

1. La ambliopía más frecuente diagnosticada usualmente requiere de 28 a 40 horas de terapia en el consultorio medico.
2. La ambliopía agravada por:
   a. Adaptaciones sensoriales conexas (por ejemplo, correspondencia retinal anómala, fijación excéntrica, distorsión espacial) requieren terapia adicional en la oficina.
   b. Anomalías visuales conexas (por ejemplo, estrabismo, nistagmo, catarata) requieren terapia adicional en el consultorio medico.
   c. Las condiciones relacionadas tales como defectos de nacimiento y cirugía para el estrabismo requieren un grado mayor de terapia en el consultorio medico.

## Seguimiento

A la conclusión del régimen de tratamiento activo, las pruebas periódicas que constituyen el seguimiento deben ser provistas en intervalos razonables. Los lentes terapéuticos pueden recetarse a la conclusión de la terapia de visión para el mantenimiento de la estabilidad a largo plazo. Algunos casos pueden requerir de terapia adicional debido a factores de descompensación ocular.

# La Rejilla de Amsler

La rejilla de Amsler fue desarrollada por Marc Amsler para permitir a los propios pacientes examinar el rendimiento de su propia visión central (de lectura) a fin de detectar signos tempranos de aquellas enfermedades de la retina que puedan ser tratables. La prueba consiste en una rejilla compuesta de líneas verticales y horizontales.

### Instrucciones de uso.

1. Mire a través de sus gafas (anteojos) de lectura o bifocales.
2. Sostenga la rejilla a una distancia aproximada de 12 pulgadas de su ojo.
3. Mantenga abiertos ambos ojos y observe fijamente el punto blanco situado en el centro de la rejilla.
4. Cubra su ojo izquierdo con una mano. Mientras observa el punto, responda a las siguientes preguntas: ¿Puede usted ver las cuatro esquinas de la rejilla? ¿Algunas de las líneas están desdibujadas, onduladas, deformadas, torcidas, se ven de color gris o simplemente no están?
5. Repita los pasos previos con su ojo derecho.
6. Si Usted nota cualquier cambio en su forma de ver la rejilla, llame a su oftalmólogo.
7. Le recomendamos usar la rejilla 2 ó 3 veces por semana.
8. Ponga usted la rejilla en algún lugar visible y accesible a fin de que usted se acuerde de usarla con regularidad (por ejemplo, en la puerta del refrigerador o en el espejo del cuarto del baño).

Usted puede usar la rejilla incluida en esta sección para hacer la prueba en la pantalla de su computadora. Baje la rejilla para usarla como un protector de pantalla. Caso contrario, descargue la versión en blanco y negro para su impresión.

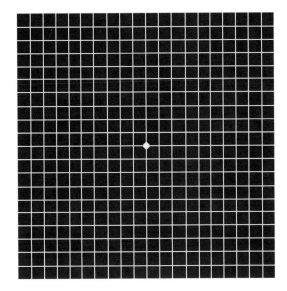

# Trastorno de Déficit de Hiperactividad y Visión

Algunos niños con dificultades de aprendizaje demuestran comportamientos específicos de impulsividad, hiperactividad, y distraibilidad. Un término comúnmente utilizado para describir aquellos niños que dan señales de este tipo de comportamiento, es trastorno déficit de hiperactividad y visión (ADHD).

Aquellos problemas de visión no detectados ni tratados pueden provocar algunos de los mismos signos y síntomas comúnmente atribuidos a ADHD. Debido a esta similitud, algunos niños con problemas de visón son erróneamente diagnosticados de padecer ADHD.

Una investigación reciente llevada a cabo por investigadores del Centro de Ojos para Niños (Children's Eye Center), de la Universidad de San Diego, ha descubierto una relación entre un trastorno común de visión, la insuficiencia de convergencia, y el ADHD. Dicha investigación "reveló que los niños con la insuficiencia de convergencia son tres veces más propensas a ser diagnosticados con ADHD que niños que no sufren de este trastorno". El doctor Granet del Centro de Ojos para Niños declaro que "no sabemos si la insuficiencia de convergencia agrava el ADHD o si la insuficiencia de convergencia es incorrectamente diagnosticada como ADHD. Lo que si sabemos es que es necesario investigar más profundamente este tema y que los pacientes diagnosticados con ADHD sean, también, evaluados con los exámenes de detección de insuficiencia de convergencia y para ser tratados de forma adecuada."

Estas nuevas investigaciones parecen apoyar lo que muchos médicos ya sabían de forma empírica por algún tiempo—un porcentaje significativo de niños con problemas de aprendizaje tienen algún tipo de problema de visión. Una investigación encontró que 13% de niños entre 9 y 13 años tiene insuficiencia de convergencia moderada hasta marcada, y hasta uno en cuatro, o un 25% de niños en edad escolar, podría tener un problema de visión que pueda afectar aprendizaje.

Los problemas de visión pueden tener un enorme impacto en la realización académica y el comportamiento en el salón de clases. Los padres que sospechan que un problema de visión pudiese estar contribuyendo a los problemas de aprendizaje o de comportamiento de su niño deberían solicitar una prueba completa de visión para su niño.

# Blefaritis

Las infecciones agudas del párpado—aquellas que estallan con o sin previo aviso—son irritantes y pueden afectar su visión. Usted puede presentar síntomas tales como ojos con picazón o ardor, visión difusa, sensaciones oculares arenosas o granulares o lágrimas grasosas. Estas condiciones se causan o por blefaritis, un término médico que significa inflamación de los párpados, o por meibomianitis, inflamación de las glándulas de los ojos que producen aceite.

La blefaritis es usualmente causada por la bacteria *Estafilococo* que florece en el excedente de aceite producido por las glándulas del párpado. La blefaritis a veces acompaña brotes de acné. La inflamación puede empeorar debido a la ingestión de té o alcohol y llegar a ser crónica. La esencia de la terapia correspondiente consiste en prevenir que la infección que es la causa de los síntomas crónicos o los problemas más severos.

Dependiente de la severidad de sus síntomas, podemos recetar alguna o todas las terapias descritas a continuación:

1. Compresas húmedas, tibias o calientes aplicadas al ojo.
2. Procedimientos de lavado del párpado. A pesar de que ni la limpieza ni las compresas curan la infección, dichas acciones pueden facilitar la eliminación de los detritos (mugre) que esta atrapado en las glándulas y las pestañas.
3. Extracción manual del excedente de aceite de las glándulas en las orillas de los párpados. La aplicación de compresas calientes previa a la extracción usualmente ayuda a que las glándulas fluyan más libremente y libera las bacterias atrapadas.
4. En los casos más severos podemos recetar gotas de ojo con antibiótico. Estos pueden o pueden no ser utilizados en combinación con un corticoesteroide, una droga antiinflamatoria. A veces, en lugar de gotas de ojo con antibiótico, se receta un ungüento antibiótico tópico, que debe ser aplicado a lo largo del las orillas de los párpados. Los antibióticos por vía oral pueden también ser utilizados (este es un tratamiento que esta normalmente reservado para casos especiales).

La blefaritis puede recurrir o persistir de forma crónica si no es completamente tratado. Los procedimientos de higiene ocular en el párpado son importantes para eliminar las bacterias que permanecen entrapadas en sus pestañas o en las áreas de sus párpados adyacentes a sus ojos.

## Instrucciones para aplicar compresas mojadas tibias a los

1. Lávese meticulosamente las manos.
2. Humedezca una toallita limpia con agua tibia.
3. Cierre los ojos y mantenga la toallita sobre el parpado durante aproximadamente 5 minutos.
4. Repita este procedimiento varias veces cada día.

## Instrucciones para el refregado del párpado

1. Lávese meticulosamente las manos.
2. Mezcle agua tibia con una cantidad pequeña de un tipo de champú que no irrite el ojo (por ejemplo, champú de bebé).*
3. Cierre un ojo y use una toallita limpia (una diferente para cada ojo) para refregar (masajear) la mezcla de champú de un lado a otro a lo largo de las pestañas y de la orilla del párpado.
4. Enjuague el área afectada con agua fresca y clara.
5. Repita el procedimiento con el otro ojo.

Si el ojo llega a enrojecerse o presentar dolor ocular, consulte inmediatamente a un oftalmólogo.

---

*Su doctor de optometría puede también recomendar aquellos refregados para los párpados comercialmente disponibles.

# Oclusión Ramal de la Vena de la Retina

La oclusión ramal de la vena de la retina (BRVO, siglas en inglés) es una causa de la pérdida de visión sin dolor en el campo superior, inferior o central de visión. También puede ocurrir sin ningún síntoma. La oclusión ocurre cuando el flujo de sangre en una vena se reduce o queda bloqueado.

Cuando ocurre BRVO, buscamos condiciones asociadas. Si la visión está afectada, el tratamiento con un láser puede mejorar la visión o reducir el riesgo de pérdida adicional de visión. En la mayoría de los casos, esperemos por un mejoramiento espontáneo. Si la visión es borrosa, el tratamiento está dirigido por técnicas que han sido probadas en investigaciones clínicas nacionales controladas.

En la BRVO, generalmente está presente una arteria que cruza sobre la vena de la retina en el punto de obstrucción. Esto puede pinchar la vena, como al pararse sobre una manguera, cortando así el flujo de sangre. El área de la retina drenaba a través de esta vena puede quedar congestionadas o hinchadas. Las áreas de la retina pueden sangrar o morir. A veces la obstrucción es reversible y a veces es irreversible.

La causa principal de visión borrosa en BRVO es la edema macular, en donde la hinchazón de la retina central es causada cuando la sangre no puede fluir a través de la vena bloqueada, permitiendo que agua se filtre dentro de la retina.

## Causas

La causa más común de BRVO es ninguna causa. Sin embargo, puede ser más probable de ocurrir en personas con antecedentes de hipertensión, diabetes, glaucoma, inflamación ocular o enfermedad de la arteria carótida. La BRVO puede ocurrir en síndromes de hiperviscosidad, en los cuales la sangre es demasiado espesa. Las condiciones asociadas con la BRVO son detectadas con exámenes oculares y generales completos y con análisis de laboratorio o de sangre. Si se encuentra una condición sistémica, el tratamiento reduce el riesgo para el otro ojo.

## Pérdida de Visión: Proliferación y Edema Macular

A su peor, la BRVO puede raramente causar el cierre de vasos sanguíneos en la mácula y falta de función. Las áreas de la retina con un flujo de sangre pobre a veces pueden permitir que crezcan nuevos vasos en la superficie de atrás del gel vítreo. Cuando estos vasos crecen, son frágiles y pueden romperse, sangrar y llenar el ojo con sangre. Puede haber síntomas de flotadores o telarañas.

La edema macular es la causa más común de la pérdida de visión en BRVO. Aparecen espacios quisteformos dentro de la retina, causando hinchazón y pérdida de visión potencialmente reversible.

## Tratamiento

Un láser es una luz enfocada hasta un tamaño de punta de alfiler. Puede secar tejidos retinales hinchados o quemar tejido retinal que tiene nuevos vasos sanguíneos. El tratamiento de láser para la edema macular es breve. Se usa un patrón de láser de rejilla si la visión es 20/40 o peor durante 2 a 3 meses con edema macular cistóideo. La terapia láser es un procedimiento ambulatorio simple llevada a cabo en la oficina. Ocasionalmente, el tratamiento tiene que repetirse si la hinchazón sigue presente 3 meses después del tratamiento láser inicial.

Un tratamiento alternativo para la edema macular en lugar de, o en adición al láser, es la inyección de triamcinolona en el vítreo. Este procedimiento también se lleva acabo en la oficina.

La cirugía en la vena obstruida y en la arteria superpuesta para aliviar el bloqueo con una vitrectomía demuestra alguna promesa.

Si crecen nuevos vasos sanguíneos, la fotocoagulación con láser disperso indirectamente trata estos vasos, reduciendo así el riesgo de sangrado.

## Pronóstico

Muchos casos de BRVO son asintomáticos. Si la visión está afectada, el tratamiento láser para la edema macular aumenta las posibilidades de mejoramiento de la visión por más de un 60%. Una inyección de un esteroide puede ayudar a los pacientes para los cuales el tratamiento láser por si mismo no ayuda. Si ocurre sangrado vítreo, el tratamiento de láser disperso reduce la posibilidad de pérdida severa de visión en más de un 85% de los pacientes. La sangre generalmente se despeja espontáneamente.

# Catarata

Una catarata es una película opaca u obnubilación que ocurre en el lente dentro del ojo. Puede consistir de opacidades y/o vacuolas de agua de tamaños variados. En general, es una alteración del tejido normal del lente que reduce su grado normal de alta transparencia. Esto, a su vez, interfiere con el grado y calidad de la luz que alcanza la retina.

## Síntomas

Los síntomas de catarata incluyen visión borrosa cercana y distante, visión nocturna pobre, sensibilidad al resplandor, la necesidad de más luz para ver adentro, luces distorsionadas al ver en la noche y aureolas alrededor de las luces.

## Factores de Riesgo

Los factores de riesgo incluyen la radiación (la luz solar y tratamientos), el fumar, el ingerir alcohol, los medicamentos y la genética. La causa primaria de catarata es la radiación de la luz solar. La luz solar "broncea" el lente dentro de nuestro ojo muy parecido a como broncea nuestra piel. Mientras que recibimos nuevas células de la piel en un promedio de cada 26 días, los lentes dentro de nuestros ojos tienen que durar por toda nuestra vida. La energía en la luz solar, particularmente la radiación ultravioleta, causa la formación de moléculas inestables que llamadas radicales libres. Estos radicales libres cambian el tejido del lente, causando distorsión y oscurecimiento.

Las cataratas pueden ser afectadas directa o indirectamente por medicamentos y enfermedades. Muchos medicamentos pueden causar que la abertura del ojo aumente, permitiendo que más luz dañina entre en el ojo. Ejemplos son antidepresivos, antihistamínicos, anfetaminas, nitroglicerina y bloqueadores beta. Otros medicamentos, tales como los esteroides y la tamoxifena, pueden causar cataratas. Algunos medicamentos, tales como los diuréticos (pastillas de agua), causan que el tejido sea fotosensibilice, lo cual resulta en un aumento en la sensibilidad a la luz solar. Las condiciones médicas como la diabetes, la hipertensión, la artritis reumatoide y otras enfermedades conectivas comúnmente están asociadas con las cataratas.

## Tratamiento

El tratamiento incluye gafas, lentes de contacto y cirugía. Las nuevas tecnologías en gafas y lentes de contacto permiten mejor visión. Los filtros de radiación ultravioleta, la tecnología antireflejo y la corrección de aberraciones de orden más alto con tecnología de frente de onda pueden resultar en mejor visión a través de los cambios de catarata. El mejor tratamiento preventivo para la progresión de cataratas consiste en lentes de sol polarizados con un recubrimiento antireflejos en las partes de atrás de los lentes.

Las cataratas generalmente no es extraen quirúrgicamente hasta que la visión no puede mejorarse a niveles razonables con gafas o lentes de contacto. La decisión de tener cirugía normalmente depende de si usted puede ver bastante bien para lo que quiere hacer. La facoemulsificación es una técnica quirúrgica usada para permitir pequeñas incisiones que a veces no necesitan suturas. Se implanta un lente artificial que puede proveer visión excelente sin la necesidad de gafas o lentes de contacto fuertes. El pronóstico para buena visión es excelente.

Las cataratas tienden a progresar a un ritmo lento y, como regla, pueden ser monitoreadas anualmente. En el momento apropiado podemos recomendar al mejor cirujano para su tipo particular de catarata.

Para el futuro cercano debemos controlar su estado de salud ocular y el desarrollo de sus cataratas con regularidad.

# Lentes Para Pacientes Con Cataratas Desarrolladas

Nuestros médicos y personal estamos contentos de poder proveerle la última tecnología en gafas. Resumido a continuación están nuevos adelantos en tecnología y los beneficios que están disponibles para usted.

Durante el curso de su examen descubrimos que usted presenta cambios de catarata. La tecnología de lentes de hoy nos permite recetarle gafas que retrasarán el desarrollo de sus cataratas a la vez que mejoran su visión restante. Usted puede recordar de la explicación dada por el médico que el lente dentro de su ojo tiende a volverse más nublado con la edad. Esto evita que el lente enfoque correctamente la luz en la retina en la parte de atrás del ojo, resultando en pérdida de visión. El nublar se produce como resultado de cambios químicos dentro del lente. La luz ultravioleta (UV) y la luz visible pueden causar que el lente se "broncee", muy parecido al broncear de su piel. Nosotros reemplazamos nuestras células de la piel cada 26 días, pero el lente dentro del ojo tiene que durar por toda nuestra vida.

## Lentes para Sol

La tecnología de lentes que le hemos recetado bloqueará 100% de la luz más dañina en la atmósfera. El tinte recomendado para usted bloqueará entre 60% a 80% de la luz visible necesaria para ver durante las horas diurnas. Algunos tintes se recetan para permitir la percepción normal del color y otros están diseñados para aumentar el contraste. El tinte apropiado depende de la extensión de sus cambios de catarata y sus necesidades personales. La nueva tecnología de lentes también reduce el resplandor de las superficies tales como las autopistas o de las reflexiones del agua.

Los lentes diseñados específicamente para inhibir la progresión de las cataratas están fabricados de polímeros de alta tecnología, los cuales son los menos probables de romperse en caso de accidente. El material del lente es el más liviano, más delgado y más seguro disponible.

## Lentes para Interiores

El nublar del lente del ojo causa que menos luz alcance la retina. Los nuevos lentes permiten que casi 10% más luz entre en el ojo. Los lentes más delgados también permiten que más luz alcance la retina. Los lentes más nuevos eliminan los reflejos irritantes y mejoran el contraste mediante tintes y recubrimientos de alta tecnología. La luz adicional, la pérdida de resplandor y la mejoría en contraste le permitirán leer más cómodamente y ver mejor al manejar de noche.

Estos lentes para interiores y de sol tienen propiedades que le proveerán con mejor visión a la vez que le protegen de los rayos de luz que contribuyen a las cataratas. Recuérdese de usar sus gafas de sol especiales durante todas las actividades al aire libre diurnas. Pruébelos en días nublados y usted podría descubrir que después de aproximadamente un minuto se adaptará y verá bien con los lentes de sol.

Nuestros médicos y personal continuarán monitoreando los cambios en la tecnología de lentes que le beneficiarán a usted. Con la tecnología de lentes de hoy y el seguimiento de la receta de su médico, usted puede esperar ver bien por el resto de su vida. Gracias por la oportunidad de proveerle con el cuidado de su visión. Esperamos volverle a ver en el futuro.

# Oclusión de la Vena Central de la Retina

La oclusión de la vena central de la retina (CRVO, siglas en inglés) es una causa de la pérdida de visión sin dolor a través del campo visual, frecuentemente peor en el centro. También puede ocurrir con síntomas mínimos. El flujo de sangre en la vena principal que drena la retina queda bloqueado o se reduce. Si la visión es pobre debido a la hinchazón de la retina central, podemos darle una inyección o llevar a cabo una cirugía para mejorar la visión. Si la visión está afectada severamente, a veces tenemos que llevar a cabo terapia láser para evitar glaucoma doloroso. Se han desarrollado guías de tratamiento, a través de ensayos clínicos nacionales controlados, para detener el crecimiento de venas malas en el ojo.

## Funcionamiento del Ojo

El ojo funciona como una cámara. El lente y la córnea enfocan los rayos de luz en la parte de atrás del ojo. La retina funciona como la película fotográfica en la cámara. La mácula es la parte central de la retina, con la cual vemos los detalles finos y el color.

Las arterias traen sangre a la retina. Las venas se llevan la sangre fuera de la retina. El vaso sanguíneo principal que va desde la retina, a través del nervio óptico hasta el corazón es la vena central de la retina.

## Obstrucción de la Vena Central de la Retina

En la CRVO generalmente está presente una obstrucción de la vena central de la retina en el nervio óptico. La vena puede quedar pinchada, como al pararse sobre una manguera, cortando el flujo. La retina puede sangrar, morir o quedar congestionada e hinchada. Una causa principal de la visión borrosa en la CRVO es la edema macular. En algunos casos tratamos esto para mejorar la visión, especialmente si la visión al momento de la presentación es pobre.

Si la visión se ha reducido a 20/200, hay una probabilidad de hasta 20% de mejorar a 20/100 o mejor sin tratamiento. Sólo un 6% mejora por tres líneas. Si la visión al comienzo es buena, frecuentemente permanece buena. Si la visión es regular, podría empeorar en un 47%.

## Causas de la Oclusión de la Vena Central de la Retina

La causa de CRVO generalmente se desconoce. Es más probable de ocurrir en personas con antecedentes de hipertensión, diabetes, glaucoma, inflamación ocular o enfermedad de la arteria carótida. También puede ocurrir en síndromes de hiperviscosidad, en los cuales la sangre es muy espesa. Las condiciones asociadas con la CRVO se detectan con exámenes oculares y generales completos y con análisis de laboratorio o de sangre. Su tratamiento puede reducir el riesgo de la oclusión de la vena en el otro ojo.

## Glaucoma Neovascular

La peor complicación de la CRVO es el crecimiento de nuevos vasos sanguíneos en el drenaje para líquido dentro del ojo o ángulo de la cámara anterior. Si la retina ha perdido flujo de sangre y la visión es bastante pobre, la retina produce un químico que provoca el crecimiento de nuevos vasos, lo cual puede causar glaucoma doloroso.

Los ojos con CRVO severa deberían monitorearse cada mes por 6 meses, luego cada 3 meses. Si se encuentran nuevos vasos sanguíneos, el tratamiento láser podría detener este crecimiento vascular, controlar la presión intraocular y evitar el dolor en el ojo.

## Neovascularización Retinal

Rara vez, los nuevos vasos sanguíneos crecen desde la superficie de la retina. Estos nuevos vasos pueden romperse, sangrar y llenar el ojo con sangre. El desprendimiento de la retina es una causa tardía de la pérdida de visión. El tratamiento láser con luz intensa y enfocada puede causar que los vasos sanguíneos desaparezcan y preservar así alguna visión. Si el ojo se llena de sangre, ocasionalmente se indica cirugía para restaurar alguna visión. Sin embargo, la visión para leer generalmente es pobre.

## Edema Macular

La hinchazón de la retina es una causa común de la pérdida de visión en la CRVO. En los ojos que aún tienen flujo sanguíneo a la mácula, los esteroides intravitreales puede llevar a mejoría visual, pero no en todos los casos. Más de una inyección podría ser necesaria. En otros, se puede indicar la vitrectomía con neurotomía radical óptica. No todos aquellos con CRVO y edema macular son candidatos para el tratamiento con inyección intravitreal de esteroides o para la neurotomía radical óptica. Pregúntele a su médico para más detalles.

## Conclusión

La CRVO es una causa significativa de la pérdida de visión e incomodidad. A menudo son necesarias visitas de seguimiento frecuentes. Nosotros somos capaces de mejorar la visión en algunos ojos, y el tratamiento láser apropiado podría prevenir el glaucoma severo.

# Corioretinopatía Central Serosa

La corioretinopatía central serosa (CSC, siglas en inglés) es una causa de la pérdida de visión sin dolor en el campo visual central en los hombres jóvenes. Pueden estar presente distorsión, un punto ciego o gris y cambios en la visión de color, y los objetos pueden verse más pequeños. En algunas personas el comienzo de los síntomas puede estar acompañado o precedido por dolores de cabezas parecidos a las migrañas.

En la mayoría de los casos esperamos por una mejoría espontánea, con la mayoría de los pacientes (80% a 90%) regresando a una visión de 20/25 o mejor.

Los pacientes con CSC clásica tienen un riesgo de 40% a 50% de recurrencia en el mismo ojo. Si la visión está afectada, el tratamiento con láser puede mejorar la visión o reducir el riesgo de pérdida de visión adicional.

## Funcionamiento del Ojo

El ojo funciona como una cámara. El lente y la córnea enfocan los rayos de luz. La retina funciona como la película fotográfica en la cámara.

La retina es transparente. La capa debajo de ella, el epitelio pigmentario de la retina (RPE, siglas en inglés), le da el color anaranjado al interior del ojo. Debajo de esto están las coroides, una capa de vasos sanguíneos que se creen son la fuente del líquido debajo de la retina en CSC.

## Líquido debajo de la Retina Central

La marca distintiva de la CSC es la presencia de líquido debajo de la retina central. Esto se ve como una filtración desde una o más manchas en una angiografía de fluoresceína. Los desprendimientos del RPE y las múltiples manchas filtrando también pueden estar presentes. El otro ojo se verá afectado en hasta un 20% de los pacientes en algún punto.

## ¿Quién Padece de Corioretiopatía Central Serosa?

Tradicionalmente, la CSC ha sido considerada como una enfermedad que afecta a los hombres jóvenes de entre 20 y 45 años de edad. Recientemente ha sido diagnosticada con mayor frecuencia entre pacientes mayores de 50 años. En este grupo de edad, la proporción de hombres a mujeres se reduce a 2:1 desde la proporción de 10:1 observada en los pacientes más jóvenes. La CSC es poco común entre los afro americanos pero es frecuente entre las personas blancas, los hispanos y los asiáticos.

## Causas

La causa exacta de la CSC es altamente controversial. Parece haber un desequilibrio en la cantidad de líquido que entra el espacio subretinal y la habilidad del RPE de extraerlo. Esto resulta en una acumulación neta de líquido debajo de la retina.

Las asociaciones sistémicas de la CSC incluyen los transplantes de órganos, el uso de esteroides exógenos, el hipercortisolismo endógeno (síndrome de Cushing), la hipertensión sistémica, el lupus eritematoso sistémico, el embarazo y el uso de algunos medicamentos.

Finalmente, las personalidades tipo A y los eventos estresantes mayores pueden estar asociados con la CSC, probablemente debido a los niveles elevados de cortisol y epinefrina.

## Tratamiento Láser para la Corioretinopatía Central Serosa

La fotocoagulación láser es la aplicación de una luz intensa al área de la filtración para sellar la mancha filtrante hallada en la angiografía de fluoresceína. El tratamiento láser acorta el curso de la enfermedad y reduce el riesgo de recurrencia para la CSC, pero no parece mejorar el pronóstico visual final.

La fotocoagulación láser debería considerarse bajo las siguientes circunstancias:

1. Persistencia de un desprendimiento serio por más de 3 a 4 meses
2. Recurrencia en un ojo con un déficit visual debido a una CSC previa
3. Presencia de deficiencias visuales en el ojo opuesto debido a episodios previos de CSC
4. Necesidad ocupacional u otra necesidad del paciente que requiere una recuperación rápida de la visión, tal como en los oficiales de la policía o los pilotos

El tratamiento láser puede considerarse en los episodios recurrentes del desprendimiento seroso con una filtración ubicada a más de 300 μm del centro de la fóvea. Cada caso debe tratarse individualmente.

En raras ocasiones los pacientes desarrollan neovascularización coroidal en el lugar de la filtración y del tratamiento láser. Si se lleva a cabo el tratamiento láser cerca del centro de la visión, puede estar presente un punto ciego que generalmente se desvanece. A pesar del tratamiento y de la fijación de la retina, la visión podría no regresar a lo normal.

## Pronóstico

El pronóstico para la recuperación visual en la CSC es generalmente bueno. Las filtraciones generalmente se cierran espontáneamente y el desprendimiento se resuelve durante un periodo de semanas a meses. La mayoría de los pacientes (más de un 90%) retendrá una visión de 20/30 o mejor en el ojo afectado. Sin embargo, algunos pacientes podrían aún notar cambios leves en la visión, tales como una reducción en el contraste, distorsión leve y visión nocturna reducida.

# Chalaciones Y Orzuelos

Sus párpados son bastante importantes. Ellos protegen sus ojos de los objetos que se acercan y de las partículas irritantes en el aire. Cuando usted parpadea, sus párpados ayudan a eliminar objetos extraños y a distribuir las lágrimas, las cuales lubrican sus ojos. Pero a veces sus párpados pueden sufrir problemas y requieren cuidado. Dos condiciones comunes que afectan los párpados son las chalaciones y los orzuelos.

Una **chalación** resulta de un bloqueo de una o más de las pequeñas glándulas productoras de aceite (glándulas de Meibomio) que se encuentran en los párpados superiores e inferiores. Estos bloqueos atrapan el aceite producido por las glándulas y causan un bulto en el párpado que generalmente es aproximadamente del tamaño de un guisante.

Los mismos generalmente no producen dolor, aunque en algunos casos puede parecer que usted tiene un ojo morado. Si la chalación se infecta, el párpado puede hincharse, inflamarse y volverse más doloroso.

Los **orzuelos** frecuentemente son confundidos con las chalaciones. Los orzuelos son infecciones o abscesos de una glándula del párpado cerca de la raíz o el folículo de una pestaña. Estos generalmente ocurren más cerca del borde, o del margen, del párpado que las chalaciones, donde forman un bulto rojo y doloroso, similar a un forúnculo o a una ampolla.

En algunos casos, tanto las chalaciones como los orzuelos pueden llegar a un punto crítico y drenar por su cuenta sin ningún tratamiento. Sin embargo, en la mayoría de los casos no lo hacen.

Una chalación puede tratarse mediante la aplicación de compresas calientes y/o gotas antibióticas.* En algunos casos, pueden inyectarse medicamentos esteroides en o adyacente al lugar de la chalación. También puede tratarse una chalación a través de una incisión quirúrgica y drenaje cuando sea necesario. A veces se recetan medicamentos orales.

Los orzuelos también pueden tratarse con compresas calientes.* Frecuentemente, pueden ser necesarias las gotas o los ung,entos antibióticos y/o esteroides.

Las chalaciones y orzuelos frecuentemente responden bien al tratamiento. Si se dejan sin tratar, sin embargo, pueden ser incómodos y poco atractivos y pueden llevar a otros problemas. Las chalaciones y los orzuelos pueden recurrir. Si ocurre muy frecuentemente, su médico de optometría podría recomendar pruebas adicionales para determinar si otros problemas de salud pudieran estar contribuyendo a su desarrollo.

## Direcciones para la Aplicación de Compresas Calientes
1. Lávese las manos completamente.
2. Humedezca una toalla pequeña limpia con agua caliente.*
3. Cierre sus ojos y coloque la toalla sobre el párpado por aproximadamente 10 a 15 minutos.
4. Rehumedezca la toalla según sea necesario para mantenerla caliente.
5. Repita al menos cuatro veces al día.

---

Precaución: Tenga cuidado de que el agua caliente no le cause quemaduras.

# Lentes Para Computadora

Más de 100 millones de americanos usan computadoras todos los días en su trabajo y un 70% de ellos tienen problemas de visión. El uso de computadoras coloca una gran demanda sobre sus ojos. El médico ha completado un examen diseñado para revelar problemas que pueden limitar su desempeño cuando usa una computadora. Él ha determinado que usted puede beneficiarse del uso lentes diseñados específicamente para el uso de computadoras.

## Enfocado para la Computadora

Los lentes diseñados para la computadora tienen muchos rasgos especiales. La receta enfocará sus ojos para permitir el mínimo esfuerzo al tratar de ver las distancias de computadora. El enfocar sus ojos para la computadora le permite a los músculos dentro de su ojo relajarse, reduciendo la posibilidad de fatiga ocular y fatiga.

## Lentes Antireflejos

Los lentes que le fueron recetados son lentes antireflejos. El reflejo es una causa constante de disturbio visual al usar computadoras. Los reflejos de las superficies de sus lentes pueden resultar en la pérdida de casi un 10% de la luz. Esta pérdida en la luz que entra en su ojo reducirá el contraste de las figuras y las letras. La pérdida de contraste puede ser un problema en especial en aquellas personas que están desarrollando cataratas o degeneración macular. Los reflejos de la parte de atrás de los lentes de las gafas también pueden entrar directamente en el ojo, causando un resplandor irritante y degradación de las imágenes ópticas. Este reflejo es particularmente notable en los individuos muy cortos de vista (miopes). El lente antireflejo permite que más luz llegue a la retina y reduce estos reflejos.

## Material de Lente de Alta Tecnología

La tecnología de hoy permite que los lentes estén fabricados de muchos materiales diferentes. Sus lentes están compuestos por policarbonato, el mismo material utilizado en la industria aeroespacial y en los discos compactos. El beneficio de este material es que es casi indestructible. El policarbonato es el material para lentes más seguro y es conocido como el lente más irrompible que se ha fabricado. El lente viene con un recubrimiento de alta tecnología, resistente a los rayazos que le permite durar más que otros lentes.

## Delgado y Liviano

Además de ser resistentes a las fracturas, sus lentes también son los más delgados y más livianos disponibles. Este peso más liviano permite que sus gafas mantengan el ajuste apropiado de manera que todas las medidas permanezcan en el lugar correcto, permitiéndole así la mejor visión.

## Diseños de Lentes de Alta Tecnología

El médico recetó un diseño de lente que le permite el mayor uso de su visión mientras usa la computadora. El diseño puede tomar varias formas. La nueva tecnología ha provisto diseños específicos para los usuarios de computadoras. Estos nuevos diseños de alta tecnología permiten posturas de la cabeza más normales, lo cual relaja los músculos del cuello y de los hombros. Los síntomas musculoesquetales frecuentemente son el resultado de posturas de la cabeza no apropiadas causadas por diseños de lentes o medidas pobres. Los lentes para computadora fabricados para usted están diseñados para darle la máxima visión y comodidad.

Estas gafas han sido ajustadas a sus necesidades particulares. Nadie más probablemente recibirá los mismos beneficios de ellos que usted recibe. A medida que sus ojos cambian en el futuro, alteraremos sus lentes para computadora para asegurar que usted tenga comodidad y sea capaz de maximizar su desempeño. Su tiene alguna pregunta, por favor llámenos. Acuérdese que nuestro tema y nuestra misión son "proveerle con buena visión por el resto de su vida".

(Reimpreso de *Diagnosing and Treating Computer-Related Vision Problems*, Sheedy y Shaw-McMinn)

# Síndrome de Visión de Computadora

### Recesos Visuales

- Reenfoque sus ojos lejos del monitor hasta al otro lado de la habitación por 5 segundos cada 15 minutos de observación del monitor. Observe objetos que están a diversas distancias de su computadora.
- Parpadee rápidamente varias veces para rehumedecer y reenfocar durante este receso visual. La aplicación de lágrimas artificiales o gotas humectantes para los usuarios de lentes de contactos durante este tiempo sería beneficioso.

### Ajustes a la Estación de Trabajo

- Debería estar disponible luz ambiental. Evite cambios drásticos de luminosidad entre la computadora y la habitación.
- Minimice el reflejo de la pantalla reubicando el monitor de la computadora o la fuente de luz para evitar el resplandor y los reflejos de luz o considere una pantalla antireflejos.
- Coloque el monitor directamente en frente suyo y no hacia un lado. Ajuste la nitidez, el contraste (ajustar a la comodidad individual), la luminosidad (igual a la luminosidad de la habitación), la distancia (20 a 26 pulgadas) y el ángulo visual (aproximadamente 15 grados desde los ojos hasta el centro del monitor).
- Un monitor más grande con una mayor resolución y velocidad de refresco (70 Hz o más) que su monitor actual podría también ser útil.
- Ajuste su silla de manera que ambos pies toquen el suelo con las rodillas aproximadamente a 90 grados del piso y los codos a aproximadamente 90 grados del teclado. Permita apoyo cómodo de los muslos.
- Ejercítese mientras está sentado con varios estiramientos y con rotación de articulaciones. El ponerse de pie y moverse también puede ser útil en mantener su sangre en circulación.

---

*Si los síntomas no se alivian o empeoran, vea un médico para tratamiento adicional.

# Hoja de Tratamiento Para el Síndrome de Visión de Computadora

El síndrome de visión de computadora (CVS) es un trastorno óptico y musculoesquetal complejo relacionado al trabajo cercano durante el uso de computadoras. Los síntomas más comunes del CVS incluyen los siguientes:

- Dolor de cabeza
- Pérdida de enfoque, visión borrosa
- Visión doble
- Ojos resecos, cansados y con ardor
- Fatiga muscular
- Lágrimeo excesivas
- Fatiga general
- Parpadeo o entrecerrar de ojos excesivo
- Estrés en general
- Dolor o tensión en el cuello o los hombros

Algunos individuos reaccionan con más dificultad al enfocar en los caracteres en la pantalla de la computadora en lugar de al leer material impreso en papel.

El tratamiento es variado y complejo, con soluciones diferentes para necesidades diferentes. Para la comodidad y el funcionamiento óptimo del paciente, generalmente es necesaria una corrección para computadora específica. Su optometrista evaluará sus necesidades ópticas. Hay una amplia variedad de estilos de lentes disponibles, que varía desde lentes para computadora de visión sencilla hasta bifocales de adición progresiva, los cuales pueden ayudarle en lograr el enfoque apropiado. También están disponibles muchos materiales de lentes y tratamientos diferentes (por ejemplo, tintes y recubrimientos antireflejos) para ayudarle con la comodidad.

Su médico evaluará sus ojos para ayudarle a encontrar cuál solución funciona mejor para usted. Algunas de estas pruebas pueden incluir las siguientes:

- Refracción detallada: una medida de las necesidades de potencia de enfoque de su sistema visual.
- Prueba de visión binocular: una evaluación de la eficiencia de sus ojos funcionando juntos a diferentes distancias.
- Retinoscopía dinámica: una evaluación de la función de enfoque de sus ojos para tareas cercanas.
- Evaluación de lágrima: una evaluación de la cantidad y calidad de sus lágrimas.

Los estudios muestran que aproximadamente tres cuartas partes de los usuarios de computadoras tienen síntomas de CVS. Las buenas noticias son que el ojo y los síntomas visuales, al igual que otros problemas de CVS, generalmente pueden aliviarse con buen cuidado ocular y por cambios en el ambiente de trabajo.

El médico ha recetado los siguientes tratamientos para usted en este momento:

❑ Mejoramiento de las lágrimas
❑ Lágrimas artificiales (gotas o gel para los ojos)
❑ Gotas antiinflamatorias para los ojos
❑ Tapones puntuales
❑ Gafas para computadora (con lentes para computadora especiales)
❑ Terapia visual (ejercicios oculares específicos que mejoran el enfoque)
❑ Recesos visuales (vea la parte trasera de esta hoja para más información)
❑ Ajustes a la estación de trabajo (vea la parte trasera de esta hoja para más información)

**Medicamentos recetados**          **Dosis y Frecuencia**
_____    _____
_____    _____

## Su Visita de Seguimiento

Fecha: _____    Dr.: _____
Hora: _____    Teléfono: _____

# Conjuntivitis

La **Conjuntivitis** es una infección de la membrana fina que reviste el interior de los párpados y de la parte blanca del ojo. Los tres tipos más comunes de la conjuntivitis son la viral, la bacteriana y la alérgica. Cada una requiere tratamientos diferentes. Con la excepción del tipo alérgico, la conjuntivitis típicamente es contagiosa.

La de tipo viral frecuentemente está asociada con un resfriado o con el dolor de garganta. Bacterias tales como *Staphylococcus* y *Streptococcus* frecuentemente causan la conjuntivitis bacteriana. La de tipo alérgica ocurre más frecuentemente entre aquellos con condiciones alérgicas. Cuando está relacionada con las alergias, los síntomas frecuentemente son temporales. La conjuntivitis alérgica también puede ser causada por la intolerancia a sustancias tales como los cosméticos, los perfumes o los medicamentos.

## Síntomas
- Descarga acuosa
- Irritación o sensación arenosa
- Picazón
- Párpados hinchados
- Hinchazón de la conjuntiva
- Enrojecimiento
- Lagrimeo
- Descarga mucosa que puede causar que los párpados se queden pegados, especialmente después de dormir

## Diagnóstico
La conjuntivitis se diagnostica durante un examen ocular con un biomicroscopio. En algunos casos se pueden tomar cultivos para determinar el tipo de bacteria que causa la infección.

## Tratamiento
La conjuntivitis requiere atención médica. El tratamiento apropiado depende de la causa del problema. Se recetan gotas para los ojos en adición a medicamentos antiinflamatorios no esteroideos, antihistamínicos, compresas frías y lágrimas artificiales. A veces se usa un antibiótico oral o en ungüento para tratar la condición. Como con un resfriado, la conjuntivitis viral no tiene cura, sin embargo, los síntomas pueden aliviarse. La conjuntivitis viral generalmente se resuelve dentro de 3 semanas.

Para evitar propagación de la infección, tome los siguientes pasos simples:
- Desinfecte las superficies, tales como las perillas y los mostradores, con una solución de blanqueador diluido
- No nade (algunas bacterias pueden propagarse en el agua)
- Evite tocar su cara
- Lávese las manos frecuentemente
- No comparta las toallas ni las toallas para la cara
- No vuelva a usar los pañuelos (los pañuelos de papel son mejores)
- Evite dar la mano

# Conjuntivitis Alérgica

Su oftalmólogo le ha dado la siguiente receta: _____

Se han recetado gotas para los ojos para aliviar los síntomas de la conjuntivitis alérgica. Un alérgeno ha irritado la membrana mucosa transparente y fina que reviste el interior de sus párpados y la parte blanca de su ojo, llamada la *conjuntiva*. Los síntomas varían de persona a persona. Más de 22 millones de personas en los Estados Unidos sufren de la alergia ocular más común: conjuntivitis alérgica.

## ¿Qué es una Reacción Alérgica?

Una reacción alérgica es una reacción fuerte del sistema inmunológico del cuerpo hacia sustancias extrañas conocidas como alérgenos, los cuales el cuerpo percibe incorrectamente como una posible amenaza. Cuando el ojo entra en contracto con ciertos alérgenos, puede resultar en una reacción alérgica. Los pólenes de las plantas, la caspa de animales, los ácaros, las esporas de moho, las yerbas y ambrosías, los cosméticos y perfumes, los medicamentos para la piel y la contaminación del aire frecuentemente pueden causar alergias. Nuestros ojos tienen millones de células cebadas (mastocitos) que liberan químicos que causan los síntomas.

Los síntomas comunes de la conjuntivitis alérgica incluyen los siguientes:

- Ojos y párpados con picazón
- Ojos llorosos
- Vasos sanguíneos dilatados en la conjuntiva
- Sensación de ardor alrededor de los ojos
- Enrojecimiento alrededor de los ojos
- Párpados hinchados
- Visión borrosa
- Sensación de llenura en los ojos o en los párpados
- Sensación de un cuerpo extraño dentro del ojo
- Deseo de frotar los ojos
- Crispamiento del párpado
- Ojos resecos
- Tiras largas de mucosidad en las esquinas del ojo
- Partículas flotando en las lágrimas

Las gotas recetadas aliviaran los síntomas causados por la liberación de estos químicos y bloquearán la liberación adicional por las células cebadas.

Existen dos tipos de conjuntivitis alérgicas, las temporales y las perennes. Las primeras son las más comunes de los dos tipos y ocurren en la mayoría de las personas que tienen esta condición. Están asociadas con las alergias temporales que ocurren comúnmente durante los meses de primavera y verano, y generalmente son causadas por la exposición a alérgenos aéreos, tales como las yerbas y los pólenes de plantas. La conjuntivitis alérgica perenne persiste a través del año y generalmente es provocada por alérgenos internos tales como la caspa de animales, los ácaros y las esporas de moho.

Su médico evaluará el éxito de las gotas para los ojos y le aconsejará acerca de su uso futuro. Si los síntomas parecen empeorarse, llame a la oficina.

# Insuficiencia de Convergencia

## Definición

La insuficiencia de convergencia es una anomalía sensorial y neuromuscular del sistema de la visión binocular caracterizada por la inhabilidad de converger o mantener la convergencia.

## Síntomas

Los síntomas y signos asociados con la insuficiencia de convergencia están relacionados con tareas prolongadas de alta demanda visual, centradas en la proximidad, que incluyen los siguientes:

1. Diplopía (visión doble)
2. Astenopía (fatiga ocular)
3. Visión borrosa transitoria
4. Dificultad para mantener la función visual cercana
5. Fatiga anormal
6. Dolor de cabeza
7. Dolor orbital
8. Adaptación de postura anormal

## Factores Diagnósticos

La insuficiencia de convergencia está caracterizada por uno o más de los siguientes hallazgos:

1. Exoforia alta en la proximidad
2. Proporción acomodativa-convergencia/acomodación estrecha
3. Punto de convergencia cercano alejado
4. Rangos de vergencias fusionales y/o de facilidades bajos
5. Disparidad de exofijación con una pendiente forzada pronunciada

NOTA: Pueden ser apropiadas pruebas adicionales como parte del examen diagnóstico diferencial para la insuficiencia de convergencia para excluir otras condiciones médicas concurrentes y condiciones visuales asociadas.

## Consideraciones Terapéuticas

### A. Manejo

El médico de optometría determina las modalidades diagnósticas y terapéuticas apropiadas y la frecuencia de evaluación y el cuidado de seguimiento basadas en la urgencia y la naturaleza de la condición del paciente y de sus necesidades únicas. El manejo del caso y la duración del tratamiento son afectados por los siguientes factores:

1. La severidad de los síntomas y los factores diagnósticos, incluyendo el comienzo y la duración del problema
2. Las implicaciones a la salud general del paciente y las condiciones visuales asociadas
3. El alcance de las demandas visuales puestas en el individuo
4. Acatamiento por parte del paciente
5. Intervenciones previas

### B. Tratamiento

Un pequeño porcentaje de casos son manejados exitosamente por el recetar de prismas y lentes terapéuticos. Sin embargo, la mayoría de las insuficiencias de convergencia requieren terapia ortóptica y/o terapia de visión. La terapia optométrica de visión generalmente incorpora el recetar tratamientos específicos para lograr lo siguiente:

1. Normalizar el punto de convergencia cercano
2. Normalizar los rangos y la facilidad de vergencia fusional
3. Eliminar la supresión
4. Normalizar las deficiencias asociadas en el control motor y la acomodación ocular
5. Normalizar la relación acomodativa/de convergencia
6. Normalizar el discernimiento de profundidad y/o estereopsis
7. Integrar la función binocular con el procesamiento de información

#### Duración del Tratamiento

Los siguientes rangos de tratamiento están provistos como una guía para el procesamiento de reclamos (de seguros) de terceras partes y para el propósito de revisión. La duración del tratamiento dependerá de la condición particular del paciente y de las circunstancias asociadas. Cuando se requiere una duración de tratamiento más allá de estos rangos, puede ser justificable la documentación de la necesidad médica para los servicios de tratamiento adicionales.

1. La insuficiencia de convergencia hallada más comúnmente normalmente requiere de 24 a 32 horas de terapia en la oficina.
2. La insuficiencia de convergencia sin complicaciones, caracterizada por solamente un punto de convergencia cercana remoto, típicamente requiere hasta 12 horas de terapia en la oficina.

*Continued*

## Insuficiencia de Convergencia—cont'd

3. La insuficiencia de convergencia complicada por:
   a. Rangos fusiónales restringidos generalmente requieren hasta 12 horas adicionales de terapia en la oficina.
   b. La supresión generalmente requiere hasta 6 horas adicionales de terapia en la oficina.
   c. Un elemento acomodativo generalmente requiere hasta 12 horas adicionales de terapia en la oficina.
   d. Otras anomalías visuales diagnosticadas pueden requerir terapia adicional.
   e. Condiciones asociadas tales como la embolia cerebral, el trauma a la cabeza u otras enfermedades sistémicas pueden requerir considerablemente más terapia en la oficina.

### Cuidado de Seguimiento

A la conclusión del régimen de tratamiento activo, se deberán proveer evaluaciones periódicas de seguimiento a intervalos apropiados. Los lentes terapéuticos pueden recetarse a la conclusión de la terapia de visión para el mantenimiento de la estabilidad a largo plazo.

# Compresas Húmedas y Frescas

Las compresas húmedas y frescas son útiles para aliviar la picazón ocular, la hinchazón de párpados y la incomodidad causada por las reacciones alérgicas.

1. Use agua de grifo. Deje el agua correr por aproximadamente 2 minutos para evitar el agua estancada que podría contener sedimento de la tubería. Usted no necesita usar agua destilada o agua potable purificada.
2. Use agua de grifo fría (a temperatura ambiente). No debería usar agua helada del refrigerador.
3. Remoje una toalla pequeña y limpia en el agua. Cierre ambos ojos y coloque la toalla sobre ambos ojos cerrados o según se indica:_____
4. Deje la toalla sobre sus ojos hasta que se entibie, entonces remójela en el agua fría.
5. Intente mantener consistentemente una temperatura fresca al aplicar las compresas.
6. Aplique las compresas por un total de 5 minutos o según se indica:_____
7. Aplique las compresas tres veces al día o según se indica:_____

# Abrasión de la Córnea

Una abrasión de la córnea es una lesión a superficie frontal del ojo. La lesión puede ocurrir cuando un objeto extraño entra en el ojo, cuando la córnea se raya o aún de frotarse los ojos muy fuerte. La córnea es muy sensible. Dependiendo de la ubicación y la profundidad de la lesión, una abrasión puede ser bastante dolorosa e inclusive puede amenazar la vista, resultando en incapacidad visual permanente.

El tratamiento es importante para evitar la infección dentro de la córnea lesionada. El medicamento que el médico recete ayudará a sanar la córnea y evitar la infección. Asegúrese de seguir las instrucciones del médico para que la córnea sane correctamente.

Las abrasiones pequeñas pueden sanar dentro de 24 horas pero las abrasiones más severas pueden tomar hasta varias semanas para sanar. Esta lesión puede tratarse de varias maneras. El médico probablemente recetará gotas o ungüentos para los ojos. Puede que usted tenga que usar un lente de contacto especial durante la noche o por más tiempo para ayudar con la curación. A veces puede ser necesario usar un parche en el ojo durante la noche.

El médico le ha recetado el siguiente tratamiento:

**Medicamentos/Tratamientos Recetados     Dosis/Frecuencia**

Instrucciones especiales (siga las instrucciones que su médico ha marcado):

❑ Despache la receta hoy y comience el medicamento tan pronto como sea posible.

❑ Aplique gotas para los ojos, luego cierre su ojo. Con un dedo, aplique presión leve a la esquina interior del ojo. Mantenga la presión en esta área por 90 segundos. Esto ayudará a que la gota permanezca dentro del ojo.

❑ Manténgase bajo techo y descanse sus ojos durante las primeras 24 horas. La luz solar será irritante. Si tiene que salir al aire libre, use gafas de sol.

❑ Usted debería notar alguna mejoría en su condición dentro de 24 horas. Si la condición empeora, llame a la oficina de su médico inmediatamente a uno de los siguientes números telefónicos:

Oficina: _____ Emergencia después de las horas laborables: _____

## Instrucciones para los Usuarios de Lentes de Contacto

❑ Está bien usar sus lentes de contacto.

❑ No use sus lentes de contacto hasta _____

## Su Visita de Seguimiento

# Retinopatía Diabética

La diabetes es una condición que interfiere con la habilidad del cuerpo de usar y almacenar azúcar. La diabetes también puede, con el tiempo, debilitar y causar cambios en los vasos sanguíneos pequeños que nutren la retina sensible a la luz en la parte de atrás del ojo en donde se enfocan las imágenes. Cuando ocurre esta condición, se llama retinopatía diabética. Estos cambios pueden incluir filtración de sangre, desarrollo de ramas como cepillo en los vasos sanguíneos y el engrandecimiento de ciertas porciones de estos vasos. La retinopatía diabética puede afectar seriamente la visión y, si se deja sin tratar, causar ceguera.

Debido a que esta enfermedad puede causar ceguera, su diagnóstico temprano es esencial. Recomendamos que se haga un examen la vista al menos anualmente si es diabético o si tiene antecedentes familiares de diabetes.

Para detectar la retinopatía diabética, observaremos dentro de sus ojos con un instrumento llamado un oftalmoscopio, el cual ilumina y magnifica los vasos sanguíneos de la retina en sus ojos. El interior de sus ojos también puede fotografiarse para proveer más información.

Las etapas iniciales de la retinopatía diabética pueden causar falta de claridad en su visión central y periférica (lateral), o puede no producir ningún síntoma visual. Mayormente depende de si los cambios en los vasos sanguíneos ocurren dentro de la retina de su ojo. A medida que la retinopatía diabética progresa, usted puede notar una nubosidad en su visión, puntos ciegos o flotadores, los cuales generalmente son causados por la filtración de sangre desde los nuevos vasos sanguíneos anormales que le impiden a la luz llegar a la retina.

En las etapas avanzadas, se forma tejido cicatrizado conectivo en asociación con el crecimiento de nuevos vasos sanguíneos, causando distorsión adicional y falta de claridad. Con el tiempo, este tejido puede encogerse y desprender la retina halándola hacia el centro del ojo.

Una vez que se diagnostica la retinopatía diabética, pueden usarse tratamientos láser u otros tratamientos quirúrgicos para reducir el progreso de esta enfermedad y reducir el riesgo de pérdida de visión.

Si usted tiene pérdida de visión debido a la retinopatía diabética, podríamos recetarle ayudas visuales especiales para ayudarle a maximizar su visión. Algunas de las ayudas visuales disponibles incluyen lentes telescópicos para la visión a distancia, lentes microscópicos, lupas y lupas electrónicas para el trabajo cercano.

No cada paciente diabético desarrolla retinopatía, pero las probabilidades de padecerla aumentan después de tener diabetes por varios años. La evidencia también sugiere que factores tales como el embarazo, la hipertensión y el fumar pueden causar que se desarrolle o se empeore la enfermedad ocular diabética.

Como diabético o persona en riesgo para diabetes, usted debería tomar medidas para ayudar a prevenir el desarrollo de retinopatía diabética, incluyendo las siguientes:

- Tome sus medicamentos recetados según le fue indicado.
- Siga una dieta apropiada.
- Ejercítese regularmente.
- Hágase un examen de la vista regularmente.

Al seguir estas recomendaciones, las probabilidades son buenas para que usted pueda disfrutar una vida entera de buena visión y buena salud.

# Medicamentos Que Causan Problemas Con Los Ojos

Si usted está tomando cualquiera de los siguientes tipos de medicamentos, usted podría eventualmente tener problemas con sus ojos. Hable con su oftalmólogo acerca de las formas en las que usted puede evitar la pérdida de visión cuando esté tomando estos medicamentos. Estos medicamentos pueden contribuir al desarrollo de cataratas, degeneración macular y glaucoma, u ocasionar síntomas irritantes.

Antihistamínicos
Antidepresivos
Agentes inotrópicos o vasopresores
Anticonceptivos orales
Antibióticos
Antifúngicos
Antimalariales
Tranquilizantes
Medicamentos sulfatícos
Isotretinoína
Corticosteroides
Agentes diabéticos orales
Anti-inflamatorios no esteroideos
Alopurinol
Estatinas
Medicamentos para el cáncer
Agentes para disfunción eréctil
Tetraciclina
Anfetaminas
Agentes antipsicóticos
Estos medicamentos pueden producir daño al tejido.

El daño al tejido ocurre cuando los rayos de luz de alta energía son absorbidos por el cuerpo, los cuales cambian su estructura. En los casos más extremos, el ADN se altera y el tejido canceroso crece. El cambio más común en el tejido ocular es la catarata, que ocurre cuando el lente dentro del ojo absorbe los rayos del sol. Algunos medicamentos mencionados anteriormente hacen que las pupilas de los ojos se dilaten, resultando en un ingreso, de luz, al ojo mayor de lo normal y causan daño.

En individuos tomando estos medicamentos, son necesarios los lentes absorbentes de ultravioleta al cien por ciento para proteger los ojos tanto en espacios cerrados como en exteriores. La necesidad de protección durante o después de la variedad de medicamentos es crucial para mantener una buena visión. La luz visible también tiene energía y puede causar daño, por lo que los lentes de sol oscuros serán necesarios para proteger la visión. Los lentes de sol que están polarizados reducirán el reflejo incómodo que se percibe al conducir o los reflejos producidos por el agua. Los lentes que cambian en la luz del sol también proveerán protección, excepto cuando el parabrisas de un automóvil les impide oscurecerse. Los efectos de las cataratas y de la degeneración macular se incrementan debido a la necesidad de tiempo de ajuste de los lentes según las distintas condiciones de luz. La tecnología antireflejo puede utilizarse en la parte trasera de los lentes para impedir que los reflejos vayan directamente hacia los ojos.

### Consulte a su Oftalmólogo

Cuando esté tomando medicamentos, consulte a su oftalmólogo acerca de la mejor manera de proteger sus ojos. Su oftalmólogo es un profesional dedicado a proveerle buena visión durante el resto de su vida.

# Drusas

A través de la retina transparente, las drusas se ven como pequeños puntos amarillos. Son esencialmente producto del desecho del metabolismo retinal que están presentes debido a que ciertas estructuras alrededor de la retina han desarrollado una capacidad reducida de procesar residuo metabólico. Esto parece ser, por lo general, parte del proceso normal de envejecimiento.

Las drusas se desarrollan, por lo general, en años tardíos; sin embargo, existen las excepciones. Las drusas pueden o no estar relacionadas a un problema de visión. Sin embargo, han de monitorearse de cerca porque pueden estar relacionadas a una pérdida de visión.

El efecto visual, si existe, puede ser apreciado y demostrado a través de la Rejilla de Amsler ubicada en la parte posterior de esta hoja.

El primer indicio de que las drusas pueden constituir un problema es cuando usted nota una distorsión en el diseño de la rejilla. La rejilla debería aparecer perfecta, con todas las líneas rectas y paralelas. Si usted nota alguna distorsión, vacíos o líneas onduladas, notifíquenos inmediatamente.

Recuerde, las drusas constituyen, en su mayoría, un cambio normal del proceso de envejecimiento y probablemente no terminen siendo un problema. Sin embargo, por cautela, uno no debe dejar estos asuntos al azar.

## Utilizando la Rejilla de Amsler

1. Si normalmente utiliza lentes de lectura, utilícelos.
2. Pruebe un ojo a la vez, cerrando el otro.
3. Observe (fijamente) el punto central y fíjese en el patrón de la rejilla. Si el patrón parece estar perfecto, usted ha completado la prueba. Si no está perfecto, marque el área de imperfección y notifíquenos.

Este prueba diaria solo toma unos poco segundos en administrarse.

# Ojos Secos

Las lágrimas naturales que sus ojos producen se componen de tres capas: la capa oleosa externa, la capa acuosa central y la capa mucosa interna.

Ojo seco es el término utilizado para describir los ojos que no producen suficientes lágrimas sin la composición química adecuada en ninguna de estas capas. El ojo seco es con frecuencia el resultado del proceso natural de envejecimiento de los ojos. Los ojos de la mayoría de las personas tienden a volverse más secos a medida que envejecen, pero el grado de sequedad varía, algunas personas tienen más problemas que otras. Además de la edad, el ojo seco puede resultar por lo siguiente:

- Problemas con parpadeo normal
- Ciertos medicamentos como antihistamínicos, anticonceptivos orales y antidepresivos
- Factores ambientales como clima seco y exposición al viento
- Problemas de salud en general como artritis o mal de Sjögren
- Quemaduras químicas o térmicas en el ojo

Los síntomas del ojo seco son con frecuencia distintos en distintas personas, pero los siguientes indicios son experimentados, comúnmente, por aquellas personas cuya producción de lágrimas es inadecuada:

- Irritación, , sequedad o malestar en los ojos
- Ojos rojos
- Ardor
- Sensación de tener un cuerpo extraño en el ojo
- Visión borrosa
- Exceso de agua a medida que los ojos intentan reconfortar un ojo demasiado seco
- Ojos que aparentemente han perdido el lustre transparente y vidrioso normal

Al no tratarlo, el ojo seco puede constituir algo más que simple irritación y malestar. El ojo seco en exceso puede dañar el tejido del ojo y posiblemente herir la córnea, la cubierta transparente frontal del ojo, perjudicando la visión. El uso de lentes de contacto puede ser más difícil debido a la posibilidad de una mayor irritación y la posibilidad aún mayor de una infección en el ojo.

Si usted tiene los síntomas de ojo seco, su optometrista puede realizar pruebas de ojo seco con instrumentos de diagnóstico para dar una visión altamente amplificada y con tintas especiales para evaluar la calidad, cantidad y distribución de las lágrimas. Su optometrista también necesitará saber sobre su actividad diaria, salud en general, medicamentos que usted esté tomando y factores ambientales que puedan estar causándole los síntomas.

En la mayoría de los casos el ojo seco no tiene cura, pero la sensibilidad de sus ojos puede ser disminuida y con tratamiento prescripto como para que sus ojos permanezcan saludables y su visión no se vea afectada. Los posibles tratamientos incluyen:

- Parpadeo frecuente para distribuir las lágrimas en el ojo, especialmente cuando se focaliza constantemente en un punto por un periodo extendido
- Cambiar los factores ambientales, como el evitar viento y polvo y aumentar el nivel de humedad
- Utilizar soluciones de lágrimas artificiales
- Utilizar ungüentos humectantes, especialmente a la hora de acostarse
- Administrar gotas inmunomoduladoras de ciclosporina

Otros tipos de tratamiento incluyen lo siguiente:

- Introducción de pequeños mecanismos en los rincones de los ojos que aminoren el drenaje y la pérdida de lágrimas
- En casos poco frecuentes, cirugía

Cualquiera sea el tratamiento prescripto, usted debe seguir cuidadosamente las instrucciones de su médico optometrista. El ojo seco no desaparece, pero al trabajar juntos, usted y su médico pueden mantener sus ojos saludables y proteger su visión.

## Tratamiento

El médico ha prescripto el siguiente tratamiento para usted.

Lágrimas artificiales                          Dosis y frecuencia
Instrucciones especiales

Una vez aplicadas las gotas, cierre su ojo y, con un dedo, aplique una leve presión sobre el rincón interno del ojo. Mantenga la presión en esta zona durante noventa segundos. Esto ayudará a que la gota permanezca en el ojo.

## Tratamiento adicional

El médico está considerando los siguientes tratamientos adicionales, dependiendo de los resultados de las lágrimas artificiales.

[ ] Medicamentos          [ ] Suplementos nutricionales          [ ] Oclusión puntal
Su visita de seguimiento

# Ocho Razones Por Las Cuales Usted Debería Adquirir Sus Gafas (Anteojos) Con Nosotros

**1. Servicio expedito**

Tenemos nuestro propio laboratorio óptico y especialistas ópticos de tiempo completo para que sus gafas (anteojos) puedan hacerse rápidamente. La mayoría de las recetas están lisas en 2 días, y muchas pueden estar listas en el mismo día.

**2. Garantía por un año**

Todas las gafas (anteojos) vienen con 1 año de garantía contra roturas sin cargo adicional. Si sus gafas se rompen por alguna razón, devuelva las piezas rotas y serán reparadas o repuestas gratuitamente.

**3. Garantía de cambio de lentes por 15 días**

Una vez adquiridas sus nuevas gafas, si usted decide que no le gusta la montura, usted puede cambiarla por cualquier otra. Si se requieren nuevos lentes, será cobrado un pequeño monto de duplicación por el laboratorio. El costo de duplicación varía según el tipo de lente utilizado; verifique con la oficina de recepción.

**4. Amplia selección de modelos y diseños de monturas**

Nuestro dispensario contiene un surtido de más de 3000 armazones disponibles, más de seis veces el de una oficina promedio. Nuestros estilistas de monturas le ayudarán a encontrar el tamaño, la forma y el color perfectos dentro de su espectro de precios.

**5. Garantía de precios competitivos**

Si usted encuentra la misma montura a un precio más bajo dentro de los 90 días de su compra, tráiganos prueba por escrito y con gusto le devolveremos la diferencia.

**6. Todos los lentes orgánicos tienen una cobertura resistente a las rayaduras gratuita (o - sin costo adicional)**

Esta cobertura aplicada de fábrica, hace que los lentes orgánicos sean resistentes. Están garantizados de no rayarse por 1 año, o de lo contrario serán reemplazados gratuitamente. (Reemplazo de un par por año solamente. Esta cobertura tiene un cargo opcional extra para recetas VSP).

**7. Respaldamos la medición de los lentes**

Nuestros médicos están a disposición para revisar sus recetas sin cargo si usted tiene dificultades. Queremos que usted se enamore de sus gafas.

**8. Servicio de reparos de emergencia y ajustes de lentes gratuito**

Nuestra oficina está abierta 6 días a la semana para servir mejor a nuestros fieles clientes. Traiga sus gafas a reparar, o ajustarlas gratuitamente y a limpiarlas para mantener el buen aspecto y la comodidad de sus monturas.

# Membrana Epiretiniana

El doblez macular o membrana epiretiniana (ERM), es un trastorno común de la retina central que causa síntomas de distorsión y borrosidad central. Una ERM es un tejido de cicatrización excesivo sobre la superficie de la retina. La mayoría de los ojos con ERM no presentan síntomas.

## Cómo se desarrolla una membrana epiretiniana

La capa vítrea se encoje a medida que envejecemos y finalmente se separa de la retina. Cuando se desprende de la retina torna áspera la superficie de la mácula. La retina responde enviando células reparadoras para suavizar su superficie, como una cáscara formándose sobre la piel de una rodilla rasguñada. Sin embargo, el tejido de cicatrizal puede volverse una estructura permanente que no se puede quitar pelándola. Si afecta la retina central, afectará la visión central. La mayoría de los ojos no requieren cirugía. Si la visión es lo suficientemente pobre, una vitrectomía con pelado de membrana puede mejorar la visión en un setenta y cinco por ciento a un ochenta y cinco por ciento de los pacientes. La cirugía puede ser realizada cuando la visión es de 20/50 a 20/70 o peor.

La ERM puede parecer transparente o una placa blanca densa. Puede arrugar la retina o inducir hinchazón de la mácula o de la retina central. Puede realizarse una angiografía fluoresceína para evaluar las posibles causas de la membrana y para determinar las características específicas. Si se deja sin tratar una ERM no causa ceguera sin embargo, una vez que la visión central se ve considerablemente afectada, rara vez hay una mejora espontánea. La visión de lectura fina puede empeorar.

Si la ERM es el resultado de un previo desprendimiento de retina, la visión central puede verse limitada por un desprendimiento macular anterior. La degeneración macular, catarata o un trastorno ocular patológico pre-existente también puede restringir la agudeza visual final después de la cirugía.

## Vitrectomía de la membrana epiretinal

La vitrectomía es la extracción quirúrgica del gel en el ojo, o vítrea. Se utiliza una aguja doblada o pico para elevar el borde de la ERM y entonces unas micro-pinzas quitan el tejido pelándolo de la retina. El gel se reemplaza con solución salina transparente estéril. Este es un procedimiento de paciente externo, que por lo general lleva 35 a 60 minutos. La cirugía es frecuentemente realizada bajo anestesia local pero también puede realizarse bajo anestesia general. El paciente puede irse a su casa el mismo día de la cirugía.

Después de la vitrectomía, usted puede sentir los puntos realizados con hilos que se auto reabsorben auto-absorbentes durante aproximadamente 4 semanas. Puede que se le receten gafas 3 meses después de la cirugía para obtener la mejor agudeza visual posible. La vitrectomía con pelado de membrana puede llevar a una mejoría visual de un setenta y cinco a un noventa por ciento de los ojos con suficiente distorsión y borrosidad para justificar una cirugía. El promedio de agudeza post-operatoria se encuentra en la mitad entre la visión pre-operatoria y la visión 20/20. La visión mejora en aproximadamente 3 meses pero puede continuar durante un año después de la cirugía.

La visión post-operatoria puede no ser perfecta, pero un noventa por ciento de los ojos sometidos a esta cirugía tienen una disminución en distorsión. Los ojos que han tenido un desprendimiento de retina anterior en la mácula tienen menor probabilidad de volver a tener una visión fina.

## Complicaciones de la cirugía vítrea

Cada vez que se realiza una cirugía, pueden ocurrir complicaciones poco frecuentes. Los riesgos de esta cirugía incluyen sangrado, infección, desgarramiento de retina y desprendimiento de retina. Todas estas complicaciones son bastante infrecuentes y son señalados no para asustarlo disuadiéndolo de la cirugía, sino para hacerle saber que cada vez que realizamos cualquier cirugía existe la posibilidad de complicaciones.

Más comúnmente, las cataratas pueden avanzar a un paso más acelerado después de la vitrectomía. La visión puede mejorar 3 meses después de la vitrectomía, y después tornarse borrosa por la catarata. Esto lleva por lo general de varios meses hasta años y responderá a una cirugía.

# Gotas Para Ojos Y Ungüento

## Aplicación de gotas para los ojos

1. Lave sus manos minuciosamente.
2. Lea la etiqueta y asegúrese que usted esté infundiendo las gotas correctas.
3. Agite bien si está indicado. Algunos medicamentos están en suspensión y deben ser agitados para asegurar la dosis correcta.
4. Párese frente a un espejo, mirando directamente hacia delante con la cabeza inclinada levemente hacia atrás.
5. Con gentileza, tire del párpado inferior con una mano mientras se coloca 1 ó 2 gotas del frasco con la otra mano. Para evitar la contaminación, no permita que el cuentagotas tome contacto con el ojo o la cara. El dispensar las gotas hacia el rincón externo del ojo es por lo general más fácil.
6. Después de infundidas, cierre el ojo con gentileza durante 2 minutos o presione firmemente el rincón interno de los párpados inferior y superior durante 1 minuto. Cualquiera de estas técnicas realzará el resultado.

## Aplicación de ungüento a los márgenes de los párpados

1. Lave sus manos minuciosamente.
2. Controle la etiqueta para verificar que sea el medicamento correcto y las instrucciones.
3. Aplique ¼ a ½ pulgada de ungüento en la punta de su dedo índice. Con el ojo cerrado, aplique a lo largo de los márgenes de los párpados en la línea de las pestañas. Cubra tanto el párpado superior como el inferior desde el rincón interno hacia el externo.
4. Técnica alternativa: coloque ¼ a ½ pulgada de ungüento sobre un aplicador con punta de algodón. Mientras esté mirando directamente al espejo, aplique a lo largo de los márgenes de los párpados en la línea de las pestañas tanto en el párpado superior como en el inferior.

## Aplicación de ungüento al interior del párpado inferior

1. Lave sus manos minuciosamente.
2. Controle la etiqueta para verificar que sea el medicamento correcto y las instrucciones.
3. Mire directamente al espejo e incline levemente la cabeza hacia abajo. Con gentileza tire del párpado inferior y coloque aproximadamente ½ pulgada de ungüento dentro del párpado inferior. Retuerza el tubo para separar el ung¸ento del tubo. Debido al riesgo de contaminación, evite tocar el párpado o el ojo con el tubo.
4. Técnica alternativa: coloque ¼ a ½ pulgada de ungüento sobre su dedo índice y transfiéralo al interior del párpado inferior.

**Medicación recetada**          **Frecuencia y duración**

**Su visita de seguimiento**

**Problemas de los párpados**

El médico ha recetado el siguiente tratamiento para usted.

## Compresas calientes

1. Lave sus manos minuciosamente.
2. Humedezca con agua tibia un paño limpio, doblado o enrollado, o caliéntelo en el microondas a potencia media durante 20 segundos. Asegúrese que el paño esté tibio y no caliente.
3. Manteniendo los ojos cerrados y el paño doblado/enrollado, aplíquelo a uno o ambos párpados. El ejercer un poco de presión sobre los párpados superiores es aceptable durante este proceso.
4. Aplique_____ vez o veces al día.
5. Continúe durante    []2 semanas      []1 mes        []de continuo        []otro_____

## Exfoliador de párpados

1. Lave sus manos minuciosamente.
   [] Utilice almohadillas de limpieza de párpados preparadas comercialmente en paquetes cerrados.
   [] Mezcle una pequeña cantidad de champú de bebés con agua tibia y sature una almohadilla para quitar el maquillaje con la solución.
2. Cierre el párpado y pase la almohadilla de limpieza sobre las pestañas superiores y el borde del párpado (aproximadamente 15 veces). Frote el párpado inferior apartándolo del ojo. Evite que el limpiador entre en el ojo. Repita en el otro ojo con una almohadilla diferente.
3. Enjuague el exceso de solución con agua limpia.
4. Realice _____ vez o veces al día.
5. Continúe durante [] 2 semanas      [] 1 mes  [] de continuo      []otro_____

**Medicación recetada**          **Frecuencia y duración**

**Instrucciones especiales**

**Su visita de seguimiento**
Fecha:                          Dr.:
Hora:                           Teléfono:

# Problemas de Los Párpados: Hoja de Tratamiento

Los párpados realizan muchas funciones importantes, incluyendo la protección y lubricación del ojo, producción de secreciones oleosas y ayuda en el drenaje de lágrimas. Las siguientes enfermedades no son generalmente serias y con frecuencia pueden ser tratadas fácilmente. Sin embargo, si no se atienden pueden causar malestar, ser poco atractivas y pueden conducir a problemas más serios. Los problemas de párpados pueden afectar el párpado superior o el inferior en uno o ambos ojos. Su médico ha marcado en el espacio o los espacios que describen su enfermedad.

## Blefaritis

La blefaritis es una inflamación crónica o de largo plazo de los márgenes del párpado (los bordes de los párpados) frecuentemente causada por bacterias alrededor de las pestañas y los tejidos externos del ojo.

Los síntomas incluyen hinchazón del margen del párpado, irritación, sensibilidad a la luz, picazón, quemazón, enrojecimiento a lo largo del margen del párpado y enrojecimiento del propio globo ocular. Una costra o aspereza a lo largo del margen del párpado y posiblemente caspa en las pestañas están presentes. Esto puede ser peor por la mañana al despertarse. Los pacientes que usen lentes de contacto tendrán, con frecuencia, estos síntomas en mayor grado debido a que los lentes parecerán secos.

## Tratamiento

En la mayoría de los casos, una buena higiene de los párpados y limpieza diaria de los márgenes de los párpados controlará la blefaritis. La higiene de párpados es particularmente importante al despertarse porque las bacterias se acumulan durante la noche. En los casos más severos, la higiene de los párpados y la medicación pueden ser combinados para un buen control. En los casos en los que la conjuntiva (superficie frontal del ojo) se vea afectada, el médico puede recetarle un tratamiento adicional.

## Chalazia

La chalazia resulta de una obstrucción a una o más de las glándulas productoras de cebo (o buscar un termino medico mas apropiado) que se encuentran en los párpados superior e inferior. Los síntomas son inflamación e hinchazón en forma de un abultamiento redondeado dentro del párpado que puede o no ser doloroso. Si la chalazia se infectase, el párpado puede hincharse, inflamarse y tornarse más doloroso.

## Tratamiento

Una chalazia puede ser tratada aplicándole compresas tibias. A veces el trastorno puede requerir tratamientos adicionales que su médico recetará.

## Orzuelos

Un orzuelo es una infección bacterial en una de las glándulas vecinas a los márgenes del párpado en la base de las pestañas. Se forma un abultamiento rojo, similar a un forúnculo, causando dolor e inflamación.

## Tratamiento

Los orzuelos son normalmente tratados con compresas tibias. También pueden ser necesarios antibióticos y/o gotas para ojos o ungüentos.

El tratamiento específico que su médico le ha recetado está descrito en la parte de atrás de esta hoja.

# Masaje de Párpados

Durante su examen de hoy, su médico encontró un exceso de aceite en las glándulas segregadoras de aceite en sus párpados. El exceso de aceite trastorna el funcionamiento normal de la capa lacrimal, y dicho exceso de aceite puede volverse duro y bloquear las glándulas, causándole más problemas de ojos secos, además de posibles obstrucciones crónicas de las glándulas y su ensanchamiento (chalazia). Un masaje de los párpados puede ayudarlo a restaurar el flujo normal de aceite y puede ayudarle a prevenir el bloqueo de las glándulas.

1. Utilice un paño limpio doblado a la mitad.
2. Utilice agua tibia, no caliente. Deje el agua correr durante 2 minutos. No utilice agua estancada, que puede tener sedimento de la cañería. Usted no necesita utilizar agua destilada o agua para beber purificada.
3. Remoje el borde doblado del paño en el agua tibia y escurra el exceso. Después cierre sus ojos y coloque el paño en sus párpados durante aproximadamente 30 segundos. Después remoje nuevamente el paño para mantenerlo tibio. Remójelo durante aproximadamente 2 minutos.
4. Después de empaparse con el paño, de un masaje a sus párpados superiores con el borde del paño mientras sus ojos permanecen cerrados. Al dar el masaje, vaya de un lado a otro con el paño, contando cada ida y vuelta como una vez. Dé un masaje tanto al párpado inferior como al superior aproximadamente 20 veces cada uno. Evite la parte central de su ojo o cualquier otra parte mientras sus ojos estén abiertos.
5. Dé un masaje a sus párpados dos veces al día o cuantas veces le sea indicado.
6. Utilice lágrimas artificiales según se le recomiende:

    Por favor, contáctese con nosotros si tiene alguna pregunta o problema.

    Próxima visita:

# Exfoliadores de Párpados

Durante su examen de hoy, su médico encontró células descamadas (o un término más apropiado) en sus pestañas que deben ser extraídas. Si estas no son removidas, la bacteria en las puede irritar sus ojos. Puede causar infecciones crónicas (conjuntivitis, queratitis, blefaritis) o posiblemente una pérdida parcial de sus pestañas o dejar cicatrices en sus párpados.

1. Utilice bolas de algodón o un paño doblado a la mitad.
2. Haga una de las siguientes soluciones:
   a. ½ cucharita de sal con un cuarto de galón de agua, *o*
   b. Una mezcla de champú para bebés y agua en proporción 1:4
3. Utilice agua a temperatura ambiente. Deje el agua correr durante 2 minutos. No utilice agua estancada, que puede tener sedimento de la cañería. Usted no necesita utilizar agua destilada o agua para beber purificada.
4. Utilice una bola de algodón por ojo, remojando la bola en la solución, escurriendo el exceso, o remoje la parte doblada del paño en la solución.
5. Frote gentilmente los párpados y las pestañas superiores con sus ojos cerrados. Al frotar los párpados y pestañas inferiores, mire apenas hacia arriba antes de comenzar a frotar. Al frotar, vaya de un lado al otro ya sea con la bola de algodón o con el paño, contando cada ida y vuelta como una vez. Frote tanto el párpado inferior como el superior aproximadamente 20 veces cada uno. Evite frotar la parte central de su ojo o cualquier otra parte mientras sus ojos estén abiertos. Cualquiera de las soluciones puede arder si toma contacto con sus ojos.
6. Deseche la bola de algodón cuando haya finalizado con un ojo y utilice una nueva bola de algodón para el otro ojo. Si usted necesita utilizar una segunda bola en el mismo ojo, utilice una nueva. No remoje una bola ya utilizada en la misma solución, ni enjuague el paño y remoje al frotar los otros párpados Para evitar la contaminación a otras zonas
7. Una vez que haya finalizado con una sesión de frotamiento, deseche la solución, no la guarde. Haga una solución nueva cada vez que usted frote sus pestañas y párpados.
8. Frote sus párpados dos veces al día o como le sea indicado_____.
   Por favor, contáctenos si usted tiene alguna pregunta o problema.
   Próxima visita:

# Flotadores Y Destellos

## Flotadores

Estos pequeños puntos negros, "insectos" o nubes que usted puede ver a veces moviéndose en su campo visual son denominados flotadores. Con frecuencia son visibles al mirar un trasfondo simple, como una pared en blanco o el cielo azul. Este fenómeno visual ha sido descrito por siglos; los antiguos romanos lo llamaban *muscae voliantes* o "moscas voladoras" porque se parecen a pequeñas moscas moviéndose en el aire. Los flotadores son de hecho pequeños aglomerados de gel o residuo celular dentro del vítreo, el fluido transparente de tipo gelatinoso que rellena el interior de la cavidad del ojo. Aunque estos objetos parecen estar en la parte delantera del ojo, están en realidad flotando en el fluido adentro del ojo y hacen sombras en la retina (la capa interior del ojo sensible a la luz). Al mover los ojos hacia arriba y abajo una y otra vez se crean corrientes dentro del vítreo capaces de mover el flotador fuera de la línea de visión directa.

## Causas

El gel vítreo se degenera en la mediana edad, formando, con frecuencia, aglomerados o hebras microscópicas dentro del ojo. El encogimiento vítreo o condensación es denominado desprendimiento vítreo posterior y es una causa común de los flotadores. También ocurre con frecuencia a personas con miopía o a aquellos que han sido sometidos a operaciones de cataratas o cirugías láser YAG. Ocasionalmente los flotadores resultan de una inflamación dentro del ojo o de yacimientos del tipo de cristales que se forman en el gel vítreo. La aparición de flotadores, ya sea en forma de pequeños puntos, círculos, líneas, nubes o telas de araña, puede ser alarmante, especialmente si se desarrollan de repente. Sin embargo, no son generalmente algo de lo cual usted deba preocuparse y simplemente resultan de un proceso normal de envejecimiento.

## ¿La aparición de flotadores es grave?

El vítreo cubre la superficie de la retina. Ocasionalmente, la retina es desgarrada cuando el gel vítreo en degeneración se desprende. Esto causa una pequeña cantidad de sangrado en el ojo, lo cual puede parecerse a un nuevo grupo de flotadores. Una retina desgarrada puede ser algo serio si se vuelve un desprendimiento de retina. Cualquier aparición repentina de varios flotadores nuevos o de luces parpadeantes debería ser puntualmente evaluada por su oftalmólogo. Los síntomas adicionales, especialmente la pérdida de visión periférica o lateral, requieren repetir el examen oftálmico.

## Luces parpadeantes

Cuando el gel vítreo, el cual rellena la parte interna del ojo, frota o tira de la retina, a veces produce la ilusión de luces parpadeantes o rayos de luz. Puede que usted haya experimentado esto; en general no es un motivo de preocupación. En rara ocasión, sin embargo, las luces parpadeantes acompañan a un gran número de flotadores nuevos e incluso una pérdida parcial o sombreado en la visión lateral. Cuando esto sucede, es importante realizarse un examen con un oftalmólogo pronto para determinar si ha ocurrido un desgarramiento de la retina o un desprendimiento de la retina.

Las luces parpadeantes que aparecen como líneas dentadas u "olas de calor" que con frecuencia duran desde 10 a 20 minutos, presentes en ambos ojos, son probablemente migraña causada por un espasmo de los vasos sanguíneos en el cerebro. Si le sigue un dolor de cabeza, se le denomina un dolor de cabeza migraña. Sin embargo, estas líneas dentadas u "olas de calor" ocurren con frecuencia sin el dolor de cabeza subsiguiente. En este caso, las luces parpadeantes son denominadas migraña oftálmica o migraña sin dolor de cabeza.

*La separación completa del vítreo toma aproximadamente 6 a 8 semanas y representa el periodo de más alto riesgo. Por lo tanto, el estado de salud de sus retinas debería ser examinado nuevamente en 8 semanas. Mientras tanto, controle su campo visual todos los días y avísenos inmediatamente si usted nota alguna reducción en su visión periférica (lateral), debilitamiento de su visión frontal, o un aumento de luces parpadeantes o flotadores.

# Glaucoma

El glaucoma es una enfermedad del ojo en la cual los pasajes que permiten el drenaje del fluido del ojo se obstruyen o bloquean. Esto hace que la cantidad de fluido se acumule en el ojo, causando un aumento de la presión en el ojo. Este aumento de presión daña el nervio óptico, el cual conecta el ojo al cerebro. El nervio óptico es el principal transportador de información visual al cerebro. El daño resulta en una menor cantidad de información enviada al cerebro y la pérdida de la visión.

La causa exacta de glaucoma es desconocida y en la actualidad no puede prevenirse. Es una de las principales causas de la ceguera en los Estados Unidos. Sin embargo, si es detectado en una etapa temprana y tratada rápidamente, el glaucoma normalmente puede ser controlado con poca o sin más pérdida de visión. Los exámenes oftálmicos frecuentes son, por lo tanto, importantes. Las personas de todas las edades pueden desarrollar glaucoma, pero ocurre con mayor frecuencia en las siguientes personas:

- Aquellas mayores de 40 años
- Aquellas con historial familiar de glaucoma
- Aquellas con mucha miopía
- Diabéticos
- Personas de raza negra

De los distintos tipos de glaucoma, el glaucoma primario de ángulo abierto se desarrolla gradualmente y sin dolor, sin indicios de advertencia ni síntomas. Este tipo de glaucoma es más común en personas de raza negra que en blancos. Puede causar daño y llevar a la ceguera más rápidamente en personas negras, por lo que los exámenes de ojos, incluyendo las pruebas de glaucoma, son particularmente importantes para personas negras mayores de 35 años. Otro tipo de glaucoma, el glaucoma de ángulo agudo cerrado, puede verse acompañado de los siguientes síntomas:

- Visión borrosa
- Pérdida de la visión lateral
- Aparición de anillos de color alrededor de las luces
- Dolor o enrojecimiento en los ojos

El realizar exámenes de ojos regularmente es un medio importante para detectar el glaucoma en etapas iniciales e incluyen lo siguiente:

- Tonometría: una medición simple e indolora de la presión del ojo
- Oftalmoscopía: un examen de la parte trasera del ojo para observar el estado de salud del nervio óptico
- Prueba de campo visual: controlar el desarrollo de puntos ciegos anormales

Normalmente, el glaucoma se puede tratar efectivamente con gotas de ojos u otros medicamentos. En algunos casos, la cirugía puede ser necesaria. Desafortunadamente, cualquier pérdida de visión por glaucoma por lo general no puede ser reestablecida. Pero, una detección temprana, un tratamiento inmediato y el monitoreo frecuente pueden permitirle el continuar viviendo casi de la misma manera en la que usted siempre ha vivido.

Proteja la salud de sus ojos y su visión; y no dude en visitar a su médico optometrista con frecuencia.

# Los Dolores de Cabeza, Los Ojos, y la Vision

Los dolores de cabeza son un síntoma común asociado con los ojos y la visión. Pueden estar relacionados con las alergias, esfuerzo muscular, visión forzada, reflejos, migrañas y enfermedad del ojo.

## Alergias

Los ojos están rodeados por varias cavidades sinusales, las cuales pueden congestionarse de resfriados o alergias. El tejido que reviste los ojos es igual al que reviste los senos paranasales. Su médico podrá reconocer los signos de alergias en sus ojos. Las personas con dolores de cabeza causados por alergias a menudo se despiertan con ellos. Casi 50% de la población en general tiene alergias.

## Esfuerzo Muscular

Los ojos son controlados por seis músculos en el exterior y músculos adicionales en el interior. Los músculos exteriores controlan los movimientos del ojo y la coordinación. Dificultad usando los ojos juntos a menudo causa dolores de cabeza, particularmente durante trabajos que se hacen de cerca tales como los trabajos de la computadora. Los músculos dentro de los ojos son usados para enfocarse. Un usuario de computadora cambia el foco unas 10,000 veces calculadas durante un día de 6 horas. Nuestros ojos no fueron hechos para esto. Problemas focalizándose comúnmente resultan en dolores de cabeza y visión borrosa.

## Visión forzada

Muchos individuos pueden ver lo suficiente para subsistir pero podrían notar un leve borrón o una imagen que traslapa la imagen clara. Aun cantidades pequeñas de astigmatismo pueden resultar en visión forzada, haciendo la diferenciación entre los números 8, 3, y 5 difícil. Otras veces una persona puede simplemente estar intentando leer material impreso que es demasiado pequeño o de bajo contraste. El intentar descifrar letra cursiva de baja calidad puede resultar en dolores de cabeza. Entre más clara la imagen, más cómoda su visión será.

## Reflejos

Cuatro clases de reflejos hacen el ver cómodamente más difícil. Los reflejos incómodos son causados por luz brillante diaria—afuera aun en días nublados, adentro con luces fluorescentes del techo. El reflejo limitativo es causado por luz excesiva, como de una ventana en un día brillante. El reflejo cegador viene de superficies brillantes tales como las pantallas de computadoras, vidrio, metal, agua, nieve o concreto. El reflejo viene de los reflejos de gafas sin tecnología deslumbradora. Cada uno de estos puede causar bizquera, vista cansada y dolores de cabeza.

## Migrañas

Dolores de cabeza intensos a menudo son pensados ser migrañas por el público en general. Las migrañas verdaderas realmente son causadas por la dilatación de los vasos sanguíneos en el cerebro. Normalmente los vasos sanguíneos se estrechan primero, causando la parte de la visión del cerebro a obtener menos oxígeno y resultando en un fenómeno extraño de la visión. Después de aproximadamente 20 a 30 minutes, el cerebro exige más oxígeno, dilatando los vasos sanguíneos y causando el dolor de cabeza. Las migrañas corren el las familias.

## Enfermedades de los Ojos

Muchas enfermedades de los ojos pueden causar dolores de cabeza y malestar. Una clase de glaucoma, conjuntivitis, iritis y otras inflamaciones del ojo pueden resultar en dolores de cabeza. A menudo son relacionados con síntomas tales como visión borrosa, aureolas alrededor de las luces, gotas para los ojos y extrema sensibilidad a la luz.

Su oftalmólogo usará varias técnicas de la examinación para descartar la visión y los ojos como causa de sus dolores de cabeza. El tratamiento puede incluir lentes, gotas para los ojos, medicamentos orales, tecnología deslumbradora, ejercicios del ojo o cambios en el ambiente.

# Iritis

Iritis es inflamación localizada predominantemente en el iris, el cual es la parte pigmentada del ojo. El iris controla el tamaño de la pupila, la apertura que permite que la luz entre a la parte de atrás del ojo. Está localizado detrás de la córnea y justo en frente del lente que se enfoca del ojo.

## Síntomas

- Dolor
- Sensibilidad a la luz
- Enrojecimiento del ojo
- Lacrimación
- Visión borrosa
- Manchas
- Pupila pequeña

Iritis es a menudo relacionado con una infección o enfermedad de otra parte del cuerpo, incluyendo espondilitis anquilosante, artritis reactiva (Síndrome de Reiter), artritis de la psoriasis, enfermedad del colon irritable y enfermedad de Crohn, múltiple esclerosis múltiple (HLA B15), sarcoidosis, lupus eritematoso sistémico lupus, enfermedad de Lyme, artritis juvenil idiopático, enfermedad "rasguño de gato", toxoplasmosis, toxicaria, síndrome de presunta histoplasmosis ocular, enfermedad de Whipple, fiebre del valle, tuberculosis, leptospirosis, fiebre manchada de las Montañas Rocosas y otras. Los pacientes conocidos por tener estos trastornos deben ser examinados para iritis leve crónico regularmente.

## Diagnóstico

Iritis es diagnosticado durante un examen con un biomicroscopio. Porque la iritis está relacionada con otras enfermedades, análisis de sangre, análisis de la piel y exámenes de las radiografías pueden ser usados para determinar la causa de la inflamación.

Cuando el iris está inflamado, los glóbulos blancos son derramados hacia la cámara anterior del ojo donde pueden ser observados en un examen biomicroscópico estar flotando en las corrientes de convección del humor acuoso. Estas células pueden ser contadas y forman la base para clasificar el nivel de inflamación. Esto es medido en una escala de 1 a 4, con 4 siendo la mayoría de las células.

## Tratamiento

El tratamiento inicial es a través del uso de corticosteroides tópicos. Si la adhesión es anticipada, entonces se usa una gota de dilatación para relajar el cuerpo ciliar para prevenir que el iris se adhiera al lente en una posición cerrada. La iritis que es persistente, recurrente o crónica puede requerir tratamiento sistemático a través del uso de esteroides orales u otros medicamentos inmunomoduladores.

Algunas de las consecuencias a la carencia del tratamiento o al infratratamiento son la formación de una membrana epirretinianas, edema macular cistóideo, cataratas, glaucoma, desprendimiento de la retina, hemorragia vítrea y vascularización de la retina. La uveítis es la tercera causa principal de ceguera prevenible en el mundo desarrollado.

# Ejercicios Para Los Ojos

### Propósito
El propósito de este ejercicio es mejorar su capacidad de cambiar el foco de sus ojos (adaptación) sin dificultad y de forma rápida sobre una amplia gama de distancias. Este ejercicio también le ayudará a mejorar su convergencia.

### Equipo
Un sello postal con detalles muy definidos, una ventana y un reloj con una segunda mano.

### Organización
Colocar el sello postal en una ventana transparente. Seleccione un blanco distante con detalle muy definido que usted pueda ver claramente. Un rótulo callejero o una placa harán un buen blanco.

### Procedimiento 1
Párese tan cerca como usted pueda al sello postal, manteniendo todo su detalle claro y solo. Salte su mirada fija (fijación) del sello postal al blanco distante y consígalo claro y solo. Vuelva rápidamente su fijación de nuevo al sello postal y una vez más concéntrese en conseguirlo claro y solo. *No cambie su fijación hasta que el blanco que usted está mirando está perfectamente claro y solo.*

Observe el tiempo que le toma para hacer 20 ciclos de distancia a cercano (40 saltos de la fijación). Haga _____ sucesiones de 20 ciclos con un periodo de descanso corto entre cada uno. Anote su mejor esfuerzo diario y la distancia que usted estaba parado del sello postal.

Su meta es poder cambiar su foco de distancia a cercano y de regreso sin dificultad y de forma rápida mientras parándose tan cerca como sea posible al blanco cercano.

### Procedimiento 2
Repetir el procedimiento 1 a través de un par especial de gafas o lentes con prendedor que serán suministrados por su clínico. Anote su mejor esfuerzo diario y la distancia del blanco cercano como antes.

# Queratocono

El queratocono es el adelgazamiento progresivo de la córnea que, si no es tratado correctamente, resultará en pérdida considerable de la visión de la forma córnea irregular que esta condición puede causar. La perforación de la córnea y cicatrización pueden suceder. Lentes de gafas solamente pueden mejorar la visión ligeramente y no ofrecen ningún efecto terapéutico. En otras palabras, el queratocono continuará a progresar.

La modalidad más universalmente reconocida y aceptada de tratamiento para el queratocono es la receta de los lentes de contacto permeables al gas, rígidos. En el futuro previsible lentes de contacto suaves estarán disponibles para tratar el queratocono usando tecnología de frente de onda para corregir aberraciones de orden superior.

Los lentes de contacto rígidos tienden a cambiar la forma del queratocono a una forma más razonable o más normal, así permitiendo al paciente alcanzar visión normal o casi normal. Porque la córnea es tejido suave, este efecto se logra solamente mientras se usan los lentes de contacto, lo cual es la razón porque los lentes deben ser usados según lo recetado.

El queratocono representa uno de los desafíos más difíciles de la adaptación de los lentes de contacto. Este requiere mucha paciencia y perseverancia para el paciente y para el médico. Observación continua regularmente es esencial porque el quertocono requiere una vida de apoyo y atención. No debe ser tomado a la ligera. Usted debe ser visto por lo menos cada 6 meses para hacer cambios cuando sea necesario y para asegurar el mantenimiento de la salud córnea. Lentes de contacto ajustados correctamente tienden a reducir la progresión del cono y ofrecer un mayor nivel de comodidad.

La mayoría de los pacientes con queratocono pueden mantener su visión corregida con los lentes de contacto por toda la vida con niveles aceptables de comodidad.

La única otra alternativa es la del transplante córneo, el cual, por razones obvias, está reservado como un tratamiento de último recurso.

# Hoja de Tratamiento Del Queratocono

El queratocono (KC) es una condición de la córnea, la "ventana transparente" en la superficie delantera del ojo. La córnea normalmente es redonda o esférica. Con el KC, la córnea se sobresale, se distorsiona y asume una forma de cono, causando visión distorsionada o borrosa. El KC puede suceder en uno o ambos ojos.

En las etapas iniciales, las gafas normalmente son exitosas en corregir la visión. Sin embargo, a medida que la enfermedad avanza, la visión no es adecuadamente corregida y requiere lentes de contacto rígidos para ayudar a aplanar la superficie corneal y proporcionar la corrección visual óptima. Su médico es un especialista en diseñar un lente de contacto hecho por encargo que se ajusta a la forma de la córnea.

La adaptación de los lentes de contacto puede ser dificultosa en los pacientes con KC, requiriendo visitas de seguimiento para observar la salud corneal y para hacer ajustes al diseño de los lentes de contacto. La meta es ajustar los lentes para maximizar comodidad, visión y salud de los ojos. Para el mayor éxito, los pacientes también serán requeridos usar gotas para los ojos y adherirse a un horario de uso recetado por su médico.

Cuando la buena visión ya no puede ser alcanzada con lentes de contacto o cuando se desarrolla la intolerancia al lente de contacto, un transplante córneo puede ser recomendado. Esto es solamente necesario en aproximadamente 10% de los pacientes con KC y lleva un índice de éxito de mayor que 90%.

El médico le ha recetado el siguiente tratamiento a usted por ahora.

❑ Compresas frías, aplicadas diariamente.

❑ Gotas de lubricación para mojar la superficie de sus ojos.

❑ Medicación tópica (gotas para los ojos) para aliviar los síntomas de picazón.

❑ Administración terapéutica de los lentes de contacto para mejorar la calidad de la visión.

❑ Consultación con un cirujano córneo.

**Medicación Recetada**                    **Dosis y Frecuencia**

_____        _____

**Gotas de Lubricación Recetadas**        **Dosis y Frecuencia**

_____        _____

## Instrucciones Especiales

No frote sus ojos porque esto puede ser uno de los factores contribuyendo al empeoramiento de la condición.

**Su Visita de Seguimiento**

Fecha: _____     Dr.: _____

Tiempo: _____     Teléfono: _____

# Degeneración de la Periferia de la Retina

La degeneración de la periferia de la retina es una degeneración retiniana periférica común caracterizada por manchas ovales o lineales de adelgazamiento retiniano. Orificios retinianos atróficos y desgarramientos retinianos de tracción pueden complicar la degeneración de la periferia de la retina y aumentar el riesgo del desprendimiento de retina. Los pacientes con degeneración de la periferia de la retina típicamente son asintomáticos, y las lesiones normalmente son un hallazgo secundario del examen dilatado.

El inicio agudo de manchas, destellos de luz, pérdida del campo periférico o pécentral de la visión puede indicar la presencia de un desgarrón retiniano o de desprendimiento retiniano, los cuales son complicaciones de lesiones de la periferia de la retina. Los pacientes con degeneración de la periferia de la retina deben ser examinados anualmente.

El ojo funciona como una cámara. El lente y la córnea enfocan rayos de luz. La retina funciona como la película fotográfica en una cámara. El centro vacío del ojo está lleno con un gel llamado vítreo. Cuando éste se encoge, puede tirar y desgarrar de la retina.

La degeneración de la periferia está caracterizada por manchas ovales o lineales de retina atrófica con una base rojiza y normalmente está localizada dentro de la parte delantera de la retina. La visión fina está en la macula.

## Adelgazamiento de la Retina

Las lesiones pueden ser aisladas o multifocales, variables en dimensión y normalmente orientadas concéntricas o levemente oblicuas al borde delantero de la retina. Vítreo condensado en los márgenes de las lesiones de la periferia de la retina parecen como opacidades vítreas y representan regiones de la adherencia vitreoretinal creciente. El vítreo sobre la periferia de la retina es líquido. Vasos esclerosos aparecen como líneas entrecruzadas, finas y blancas que justifican el término degeneración de la periferia de la retina.

Las lesiones de la periferia de la retina parecen ser causadas por la pérdida de vasos capilares retinianos periféricos, la cual lleva al adelgazamiento de todas las capas retinianas. El adelgazamiento puede llegar a ser tan profundo que un agujero retiniano de máximo espesor se forma en la lesión de la periferia de la retina.

El mejor examen y el que se usa más a menudo para detectar la degeneración de la periferia de la retina es el oftalmoscopio indirecto que ejerce presión en el ojo o en la depresión esclerotical para verlo en el borde.

## ¿Quién tiene degeneración de la periferia de la retina?

La degeneración de la periferia de la retina afecta a aproximadamente 10% de la población, con 30% a 50% de esos afectados teniéndolo en ambos ojos. La prevalencia llega a la cima por la segunda década y es minimamente progresiva. Puede ser más común en algunas familias. Es más común en los ojos miopes y se correlaciona con longitud axial creciente, alcanzando 15% prevalencia en los ojos más largos. Ningunas diferencias divulgadas contagiosas, del trauma, del género, o raciales existen en la degeneración de la periferia de la retina.

## Curso clínico sobre degeneración de la periferia de la retina

Las lesiones de la periferia de la retina se creen desarrollar temprano en la duración de la vida. Características tales como los vasos escleróticos entrecruzantes, la pigmentación y los agujeros retinianos atróficos pueden desarrollar subsiguientemente sobre muchos años.

El desprendimiento de retina es una complicación rara de la degeneración de la periferia de la retina (menos de 1% de los pacientes con la periferia de la retina). Pero la la periferia de la retina está relacionada con tanto como 40% de todos los desprendimientos relacionados con desgarrones retinianos.

Un desprendimiento vítreo posterior agudo complicado por la formación de un desgarrón retiniano normalmente es indicado por el nuevo inicio de manchas y/o destellos. Los pacientes con estos síntomas constituyen una verdadera emergencia oftalmológica y necesitan un examen oftálmico urgente.

## Tratamiento con láser para la degeneración de la periferia de la retina

La presencia de la periferia de la retina poco complicada no interfiere con la función visual y no constituye un alto riesgo para el desarrollo futuro del desprendimiento de retinar. El tratamiento profiláctico se indica claramente solamente en el contexto de circunstancias específicas.

La degeneración de la periferia de la retina complicada por desgarrones de tracción como el resultado de un desprendimiento vítreo posterior agudo representa una situación de alto riesgo para el desprendimiento retiniano futuro y es una indicación urgente para retinopexia láser. Los agujeros de la periferia de la retina y atróficos complicados por fluido subretinal progresivamente aumentando representan una indicación adicional para la intervención quirúrgica. La presencia de lesiones de la periferia de la retina en el otro ojo de los pacientes quienes han sostenido un desprendimiento retiniano en el primer ojo pueden ser tratados profilácticamente. Desprendimientos retinianos subsiguientes también pueden suceder como consecuencia de lesiones desarrollándose en la retina sana, así que la protección no es absoluta. Si una catarata, implante de lente o antecedentes familiares fuertes de desprendimiento retiniano están presentes, tratamiento preventivo de láser puede reducir la posibilidad de desprendimiento retiniano. En la ausencia de las características anteriormente mencionadas, datos definitivos todavía no existen para indicar claramente el tratamiento profiláctico de láser de las lesiones de la periferia de la retina.

## Prognosis de la degeneración de la periferia de la retina

Los pacientes con lesiones significativas de la periferia de la retina, y esos quienes han tenido tratamientos profilácticos, siempre están a mayor riesgo comparado con la población en general para pérdida de la visión causada por desprendimiento retiniano. Estos pacientes deben tener exámenes rutinarios de seguimiento. Esté consciente de los signos y los síntomas de desprendimiento retiniano y vítreo y la necesidad de buscar cuidado oftálmico urgente cuando sea necesario.

# Degeneración Macular

La degeneración macular es la causa principal que lleva a la pérdida de la visión central entre las personas mayores. Ésta resulta debido a cambios a la mácula, la parte de la retina responsable por visión aguda, clara, que está localizada en la pared de la parte posterior del interior del ojo.

La mácula es muchas veces más sensitiva que el resto de la retina; sin una mácula sana, el ver detalles o colores vívidos no es posible. La degeneración macular tiene varias causas. En una clase, el tejido de la mácula llega a ser delgado y para de funcionar bien. Esta clase se piensa ser una parte del proceso natural del envejecimiento en algunas personas.

En otra, los fluidos de los vasos sanguíneos nuevamente formados derraman en el ojo y causan pérdida de visión. Si se detecta temprano, esta condición puede ser tratada con terapia de láser, pero la detección temprana y el tratamiento inmediato son esenciales en limitando el daño.

La degeneración macular se desarrolla di forma diferente en cada persona, así que los síntomas pueden variar. Algunos de los síntomas más comunes incluyen los siguientes:

- Una pérdida gradual de la capacidad de ver los objetos claramente
- Visión distorsionada; los objetos parecen ser el tamaño o la forma incorrecta, o líneas rectas parecen estar onduladas o torcidas
- Una pérdida gradual de visión de color clara
- Una área oscura o vacía apareciendo en el centro de la visión
- Estos síntomas también pueden indicar otros problemas de la salud de los ojos, así que si usted está experimentando cualquiera de estos, llame a su médico de optometria inmediatamente.

En un examen comprensivo del ojo, su médico llevará a cabo una variedad de exámenes para determinar si usted tiene degeneración macular u otra condición causando sus síntomas.

Desafortunadamente, la visión central dañada por la degeneración macular no puede ser restaurada. Sin embargo, porque la degeneración macular no daña la visión lateral, herramientas tales como los lentes especiales telescópicos y microscópicos, lupas y lentes de aumento electrónicos pueden ser recetados para trabajo cercano para maximizar la visión restante. Con la adapción, las personas con degeneración macular con frecuencia pueden enfrentarse bien y continuar a hacer la mayoría de las cosas que ellos estaban acostumbrados a hacer.

Recuerde: la detección temprana de la degeneración macular es el factor más importante en determinar si usted puede ser tratado eficazmente. Use el chequeo simple de la visión en la parte posterior de esta hoja y mantenga un horario regular de exámenes optométricos para ayudar a proteger su visión.

# Monovisión

La monovisión es una metodología de compromiso hacia las necesidades visuales. Ésta compromete, hasta algún nivel la distancia y la visión de cerca. Sin embargo, permite que uno subsista razonablemente bien para ambos lejos y cerca sin el uso de gafas. La monovisión parece funcionar mejor para las ocasiones sociales, situaciones en todas partes en general y para esos pacientes haciendo trabajo ligero de oficina.

Un área de preocupación es el manejar un vehículo de motor, especialmente en tiempos de niveles bajos de iluminación. Por ejemplo, si la luz de una luz delantera que se aproxima fuera a dar el ojo de la visión de la distancia de modo que fuera ocluido o parcialmente obstruido, podría comprometer la visión de distancia porque los vehículos que se aproximan serían mayormente vistos a través del ojo de visión de cerca. Por esto es que recomendamos que un par de gafas sea llevado con los lentes de contacto, permitiéndole tener visión binocular de distancia mientras maneja. Las gafas serían corregidas para que el ojo cercano ahora sea enfocado para distancia. Con ambos ojos ahora enfocados normalmente para la distancia, el comprometerse no es necesario.

Otra área de preocupación para esos pacientes quienes han estado haciendo bien por la mayor parte con la monovisión, pero que han tomado demandas visuales adicionales para el trabajo cercano, es la incomodidad y el estrés. Esta situación también puede ser solucionada, usando gafas que corrigen el ojo de la visión de la distancia, de ese modo enfocando ambos ojos para la visión de cerca.

# No Existe Par de Lentes Perfectos

Nuestra meta como profesionales del cuidado de los ojos es proporcionar a cada paciente con el par perfecto de lentes. Desafortunadamente, en el mundo de hoy, cuando usted mira la variedad de las necesidades de los pacientes, llega a estar rápidamente claro que ningún par de lentes puede ser ideal en todas partes, en todo tiempo.

Cada paciente individual necesita ver bien en muchas situaciones diferentes. Ellos necesitan buena visión en el sol brillante y mientras manejan en la noche. Ellos necesitan ver mientras juegan tenis, trabajan en la computadora y hacen punto de aguja. Los pacientes también desean mirarse lo mejor posible que puedan en estas situaciones y muchas otras.

Un modo de mirar estas necesidades es recordar que cambiamos nuestra ropa por lo menos una vez cada día, y cada vez elegimos una apariencia o función específica. Usted lleva un conjunto de ropa para limpiar la casa, otro para ir al trabajo y aun otro para jugar tenis o socializar. Usted puede pensar de su "vestuario de anteojos" como siendo su armario de ropa, completo con opciones para el trabajo, el tiempo libre y ocasiones sociales.

Los anteojos con frecuencia son requeridos para los siguientes:
* Protección de los rayos dañinos del sol
* Comodidad en la computadora
* Deportes
* Pasatiempos
* Funciones sociales
* Manejando seguro de noche
* Imagen particular

Cada par de lentes que el médico le receta tiene una función especial. Los lentes que usted usa para trabajar en la computadora no son apropiados para jugar deportes. Los lentes del sol que usted usa para manejar durante el día no deben ser usados para ver películas en un cine oscuro. Un armazón puede ser de una forma excelente para su cara y se mirará bien en la oficina, y otro podría ser un armazón de deportes perfecto para correr y jugar al tenis.

Hoy en día, la persona promedio requiere lentes para prevenir daño a los ojos del sol, lentes para ver adentro y en la noche y lentes para computadora. Muchos idealmente tendrían pares adicionales dependiendo en su apariencia deseada y sus necesidades recreativas.

## Consulte a su oftalmólogo y a su optometrista

Su oftalmólogo determinará que es lo mejor para mejorar la calidad de su vida, permitirle llevar a cabo el nivel más alto de trabajo y recreación y evitar la pérdida de la visión. Su optometrista le proporcionará una variedad de lentes que le harán verse y sentirse bien.

# Hipertensión Ocular

La hipertensión ocular es una condición en la cual la presión de fluidos dentro del ojo es más alta que el promedio. Cuando la presión dentro del ojo se eleva hasta un punto que interfiere con la fisiología normal del nervio óptico, resultando en daño al nervio óptico, es referido como "glaucoma."

Muchas personas pueden tolerar presión ocular más alta que lo normal sin ningún compromiso del nervio óptico. Sin embargo, la precaución dicta que uno no debe dejar tales asuntos a lo imprevisto y que debe observar la presión ocular considerada ser más alta que el promedio regularmente.

Varias pruebas son importantes para asegurar la salud del nervio óptico con relación a la presión elevada. Para asegurar la seguridad del tejido de su nervio óptico, quisiéramos verlo de nuevo en _____ meses para llevar a cabo los siguientes exámenes que han sido circulados.

1. Examen del campo visual
2. Examen del fondo dilatado
3. Imagen del nervio óptico (para evaluación comparativa a largo plazo)
4. Examen de la presión ocular (mañana/mediodía)
5. Análisis de la capa retiniana de la fibra del nervio
6. Paquimetría

# Ortoqueratología

La ortoqueratología (Ortho-K) es un método no quirúrgico para reducir la miopía. Una serie de lentes de contacto rígidos son usados para aplanar la curvatora córnea. Porque dos tercios del poder total del ojo pueden ser explicados por la curvatura córnea, se han hecho esfuerzos para modificar la córnea para cambiar el estado refractivo total. ¿Se puede alterar el tejido fino córneo permanentemente por tales medios no quirúrgicos? La Escuela de Optometría de la Universidad de California en Berkeley y la Escuela de Medicina de la Universidad de California en San Diego ambas acordaron, después de tiempo sustancial y esfuerzo pasado en el proyecto Ortho-K, que ninguna mejora permanente significativa fue observada con respecto a la reducción de la miopía.

La reducción de la miopía fue observada con el uso de lentes de retención por una porción significativa de tiempo. Sin embargo, con la discontinuación permanente del uso de los lentes de contacto este efecto pronto fue perdido. Muchos de nuestros pacientes han tenido buen éxito con Ortho-K, habiendo calificado para empleo que requiere mejora en su agudeza visual sin corregir o dedicándose a pasatiempos (e.g., montañismo requiriendo oxígeno) o deportes que hacen el usar lentes o lentes de contacto impráctico.

# Errores Refractivos

Cuando considera todos los variables que van en el proceso visual total es, de hecho, un milagro que vemos tan bien como nosotros vemos. El proceso visual es uno sumamente complejo involucrando aspectos cerebrales y perceptivos que son muy involucrados para describir en una página.

El poder refractivo del sistema visual es mayormente atribuible a la curvatura córnea, con la media transparente y la longitud del globo ocular justificando el resto. Si todos estos variables coincidan agradablemente de modo que toda la luz se enfoca considerablemente en la retina, uno es dicho tener visión perfecta para ver a distancia o emetropía. Esta definición no considera aspectos perceptivos, integradores, o binoculares de la visión que, si no están en armonía con el estado refractivo, pueden resultar en incomodidad, problemas perceptivos y dificultades con la lectura.

Si la luz se enfoca prematuramente en frente de la retina, la condición es referida como la miopía, o visión de corto alcance, porque objetos cercanos son vistos más claros que objetos distantes. La mayoría de los casos de miopía se desarrollan antes de la edad de 25 años.

Si la luz pasa a través del medio como si la retina no estuviera allí e hipotéticamente se enfoca detrás de la retina, la condición es referida como hipermetropía, o visión de largo alcance, porque la visión es más adaptable para ver a la distancia. Las personas con visión de largo alcance involuntariamente y continuamente mantienen un esfuerzo de enfoque para mantener la visión clara. Una persona con visión de largo alcance no necesariamente tendrá visión de distancia clara y la visión borrosa o poco clara de cerca porque estos factores pueden ser modificados por la capacidad de enfoque además del nivel o la magnitud de la visión de largo alcance.

Otra condición refractiva es referida como el astigmatismo. En esta condición, toda la luz no se enfoca en la retina. La porción que no lo hace puede enfocarse en frente de la retina o detrás de ella. El nivel de disparidad o la diferencia es relacionado a la cantidad de astigmatismo.

Aproximadamente 20% de lo que causa borrones en el ojo típico es de aberraciones de orden superior. Hasta hace poco tiempo estos no podían ser medidos y corregidos por lentes o lentes de contactos. Aun personas quienes no tienen ningún error refractivo (emétropes) pueden tener muchas aberraciones de orden superior. El efecto normalmente es visión de noche pobre, particularmente cuando maneja. Corrigiendo la aberración le da al individuo visión de "alta-definición" semejante a los televisores de alta-definición. La reducción en función es algo que es más apreciado o reconocido según envejecemos. En la juventud uno podría correr una milla en 4 minutos, pero cuando uno alcanza la edad de 40 años, una milla de 6 o 7 minutos es todo lo que podemos lograr. Un proceso semejante sucede en el proceso visual. Nos referimos a esta reducción en función o capacidad reducida para modificar o ajustar el sistema visual para visión clara como presbicia.

La astenopia de punto cercano es una condición que no está necesariamente relacionada a un error refractivo específico pero puede estar relacionado con cualquiera de ellos. Estos pacientes parecen tener dificultad manejando trabajos de vista cerca, tal como el leer y notan un nivel significativo de estrés. Porque esta condición no está relacionada a la presbicia y con frecuencia es administrada o tratada de manera semejante, una categoría diferente es requerida. Este problema es uno en el cual el balance entre el enfocamiento y el giro de los ojos no está en armonía perfecta. Lentes apropiados de lectura (como en presbicia) generalmente restauran el balance. Sin embargo, de vez en cuando los ojos pueden requerir ejercicios visuales del entrenamiento para restaurar armonía.

# Comparación de Lentes de Aumentos

Las personas tienen muchas alternativas diferentes cuando seleccionan como ellos quisieran sus recetas llenadas para leer y trabajar de cerca. Cada una de las opciones tiene ventajas y desventajas. Esta página compara cada opción para permitirle hacer una decisión informada para cumplir con sus necesidades personales.

## Lentes solo de lectura

Lentes de lectura están enfocados solamente para la distancia de la lectura o distancia cercana (de 6 a 20 pulgadas). Cuando use estos lentes para leer, hacer trabajo de cerca, maniobras, pasatiempos o su trabajo, las cosas estarán claras. La desventaja de esta clase de lentes es que en cualquier momento que usted tenga que mirar a una distancia de más de 20 pulgadas y ver claramente, usted debe quitarse los lentes. Usted tiene la inconveniencia de tener que ponérselos y quitárselos. Usted también necesita considerar un armazón fuerte porque recibirán mucho más maltrato que si se dejaran puestos continuamente.

## Lentes medios ojos

Esta clase de lentes tiene la misma receta que los lentes de lectura excepto que solamente son mitad la longitud vertical de los lentes normales. Esto permite que usted haga su trabajo de cerca pero aun todavía mirar sobre ellos para ver a distancias más largas. Una de las desventajas de este sistema es otra vez que necesita un armazón durable porque sus lentes son puestos y quitados con mucha frecuencia.

## Bifocales

Este es un sistema en el cual uno tiene dos focos: lejos y cerca. Esto le permite leer y hacer trabajo de cerca; y entonces cuando uno mira de lejos, uno puede mirar claramente sin tener que quitarse los lentes. La ventaja más grande de los lentes bifocales es la conveniencia de no tener que quitarse y ponerse los lentes con tanta frecuencia.

## Trifocales

Este sistema de lentes tiene tres focos. Lejos, para mirar algo como un reloj en una pared lejos; leer, para objetos de 6 a 12 pulgadas de distancia y la extensión intermedia o entre medio, tales como latas de sopa en un estante o en el tablero de su carro.

## Multifocales de progresión invisible

Este sistema de lentes es la próxima extensión más allá del trifocal. Tiene la ventaja de no tener ningunas líneas y tiene una extensión continua de visión clara le lejos a intermedio a cerca. Hemos imprimido información y vídeos en la oficina sobre los multifocales que hablan sobre las ventajas y las desventajas. También, tenemos algunas muestras de cada uno para que usted vea. Por favor tome su tiempo y decida cual sistema funciona mejor para usted.

## Lentes de contacto bifocales

Esta alternativa tiene mérito para individuos quienes llevan a cabo trabajo cercano mínimo, tales como las amas de casa o las cajeras, en el cual la persona no está pasando varias horas a la vez leyendo o estudiando, por ejemplo.

## Monovisión

Este sistema funciona con un ojo enfocado para la distancia y el otro ojo enfocado para lo cercano. Esto se puede hacer con cualquier clase de lente de contacto.

# Lectura Y Escritura

Todos debemos de visualizar lo que significan las palabras que leemos y escribimos. Algunas personas con dificultades de aprendizaje relacionadas a problemas de visión, pueden ver las palabras, pero no pueden comprender su significado. Si usted ha tenido este problema, ¿se le ha hecho fácil leer y escribir?

La lectura y la escritura son las tareas más comunes que las personas realizan en la escuela o en un trabajo de oficina. Cada vez que leemos de un libro, de una hoja suelta o del monitor de una computadora, estamos realizando una tarea visual.

### Cómo leemos

Mientras leemos, necesitamos dirigir simultáneamente y exactamente, los dos ojos al mismo punto, al igual que lo siguiente:
- Enfocar ambos ojos para que el material de lectura sea claro
- Continuar o mantener el enfoque claramente
- Mover los dos ojos continuamente (como un equipo coordinado) a lo largo de la línea impresa.

Este proceso continua cuando nosotros movemos nuestros ojos a la siguiente línea impresa.

### Lectura de comprensión

Para aumentar la comprensión durante el proceso de lectura, nosotros tomamos constantemente la información visual y la decodificamos de una palabra escrita a una

imagen mental. La memoria y la visualización son también utilizadas constantemente para relacionar la información a lo que ya es conocido y así ayudar a entender lo que se esta leyendo.

### Cómo escribimos

La escritura es similar a la lectura, pero casi funciona en un orden revertido. Nosotros comenzamos con una imagen en nuestras mentes y la codificamos en palabras. A la misma vez, nosotros controlamos el movimiento del lápiz, mientras continuamos trabajando para que el material escrito haga sentido. Durante esto, nosotros enfocamos nuestros ojos y los movemos tal y como lo hacemos en el proceso de lectura.

Los procedimientos visuales complicados están envueltos en la lectura y en la escritura. Un problema con una o todas las partes visuales de los procesos descritos tendrán dificultad de algún tipo con la lectura y/o la escritura.

Algunas veces es fácil reconocer una dificultad visual que afecte la lectura o la escritura, en otras ocasiones puede ser más sutil de detectar. Un médico COVD está capacitado para evaluar todas las partes del proceso visual y si fuera necesario, puede recetar lentes y terapia de visión para mejorar las destrezas de lectura y escritura.

# Desprendimiento de Retina

El desprendimiento de retina ocurre cuando las dos capas de la retina se separan una de la otra y de la pared del ojo. La retina es como una película fotográfica en una cámara. Las células nerviosas en la retina detectan la luz que entra en el ojo y la convierten en señales neuronales que son enviadas al cerebro.

Una vez las dos capas de la retina, la retina sensorial y el epitelio de pigmento retinal, pierden contacto entre cada uno, la retina deja de funcionar apropiadamente, porque los ojos no pueden procesar lo que ven. Esto causa la pérdida de visión en el área afectada de la retina. El desprendimiento de retina siempre resulta en algún tipo de pérdida de visión, incluyendo una pérdida severa o ceguera.

## Síntomas

El desprendimiento de retina puede ocurrir sin ninguna advertencia. Los síntomas incluyen los flotadores en su campo visual y destellos o chispas de luz cuando usted mueve sus ojos o su cabeza. Los flotadores o destellos no siempre indican desprendimiento de retina, pero pueden ser una señal de advertencia que debe ser evaluada. Si un destello de luz ocurre y no desaparece en varios minutos, usted debe ser examinada inmediatamente. La primera señal de un desprendimiento de retina puede ser una sombra o efecto de cortina a lo largo de la parte del campo visual que no desaparece o la pérdida de visión reciente y súbita que empeora con el tiempo.

El desprendimiento de retina afecta primero la visión periférica (lateral). La pérdida de visión tiende a empeorar con el tiempo mientras más desprendimiento de retina ocurra, a veces dentro de unas pocas horas o días. Una vez el desprendimiento de retina se propaga al centro de la retina, la pérdida de visión se vuelve severa o hasta total. La cirugía es necesaria para reparar el desprendimiento de retina para prevenir la pérdida de visión.

## Diagnóstico

El desprendimiento de retina es diagnosticado por el historial médico y un examen de los ojos. Si usted tiene los síntomas de desprendimiento de retina, su médico examinará su retina utilizando la oftalmoscopia. La oftalmoscopia es una prueba que permite al médico visualizar la parte posterior del ojo con un instrumento de magnificación con una fuente de luz. Esta prueba permite al médico visualizar las lágrimas, agujeros y el desprendimiento de retina. Se podría tomar fotografías para documentar la apariencia de la retina.

## Tratamiento

El desprendimiento de retina casi siempre demanda cuidado urgente. Sin tratamiento, la pérdida de visión debido al desprendimiento retina puede progresar de menor a severo o total en pocas horas o días. Si se descubre en 24 a 48 horas, comparativamente, la cirugía de láser simple puede restaurar la visión buena. Si se deja progresar, las técnicas quirúrgicas serían más difíciles y la recuperación tomaría más tiempo, con mayor probabilidad de una pérdida de visión.

# Retinitis Pigmentosa

La retitinitis pigmentosa (RP) es una de un grupo de enfermedades que afectan la retina del ojo. Aproximadamente 400,000 americanos son afectados por RP y otras formas similares de RP hereditarias de degeneración de retina.

Algunos de los síntomas más comunes de RP incluyen la ceguera nocturna y la pérdida de visión periférica (lateral).

Los síntomas de RP en ocasiones ocurren por primera vez durante la infancia o la adolescencia. Los tropiezos con objetos que aparentan estar en plena vista y la torpeza pueden ser las primeras indicaciones de un problema. Los síntomas de RP generalmente empeoran durante un periodo de años. A pesar de que algunos pacientes con RP y edad avanzada pueden volverse ciegos, la mayoría podrían retener por lo menos alguna visión y ser clasificados como ciegos legalmente. Cada caso individual es difiere.

La RP se desarrolla en el interior de la capa pigmentada de la retina. La retina es una capa delicada de células que actúa como la película fotográfica de una cámara. Esta recoge la fotografía y la transmite al cerebro, donde la visualización de verdad ocurre. Los dos tipos de células en la retina que participan en el envío de mensajes visuales al cerebro son los conos y bastones. Las células de forma de bastón son mayormente utilizadas para ayudarle a usted a ver a través de la esquina de los ojos (visión periférica) y durante la noche. Las células de forma cónica le permiten a usted distinguir los colores, ver durante el día y ayudarlo a usted con la visión central.

Cuando RP comienza, las células de forma de bastón comienzan a perder la habilidad de funcionar. Como resultado, las personas con esta condición frecuentemente tienen problemas con la visión durante la noche o en áreas de luz tenue. La visión nocturna disminuida o empobrecida por si sola no es necesariamente un indicador de RP.

La visión "túnel" es otro síntoma de RP. Los campos de visión gradualmente se estrechan produciendo el efecto de mirar a través de un túnel constantemente.

Según RP progresa a una etapa avanzada, usted puede tener dificultad con la lectura, la distinción de colores y la visualización clara de objetos distantes. Esto es causado por una deterioración de las células de forma cónica.

Su optometrista puede ayudarle a maximizar la visión restante recetándole aditamentos especiales para poca visión. Algunos de los aditamentos ópticos disponibles incluyen los lentes telescópicos para la visión de distancia, lentes microscópicos, anteojos magnificadores, magnificadores electrónicos, alcances de visión nocturna, filtros especiales y engrandecimientos de campo.

Desafortunadamente, a pesar de que se esté conduciendo investigación extensiva, no hay tratamientos disponibles para revertir el curso de RP. Sin embargo, la consejería temprana de su optometrista puede ayudarlo a usted a ajustar exitosamente su estilo de vida y sus metas profesionales a esta discapacidad visual. Los problemas potenciales también pueden ser identificados y prevenidos al determinar los aditamentos apropiados, entrenamiento y otras modificaciones de trabajo en su campo profesional escogido. Usted puede tomar mayor ventaja de una guía profesional o educativa cuando RP es diagnosticada tempranamente.

# Estrabismo Y Ambliopía

El estrabismo es una condición en la cual la persona no es capaz de alinear ambos ojos simultáneamente bajo condiciones visuales normales (en ocasiones pareciendo como "ojos cruzados"). La fovea de cada ojo es utilizada para la visión distinta. Un ojo "gira" en relación al otro cuando estos no apuntan hacia un objeto al mismo tiempo. Este giro puede ser hacia adentro, hacia afuera, hacia arriba, hacia abajo o en cualquier combinación de direcciones. Este giro también puede ser constante, en el cual un ojo gira todo el tiempo o puede estar intermitente. Esto también puede alternar ocasionando que cada ojo gire. Además del giro obvio del ojo, el individuo tiene una reducción de la función binocular y de la esteropsis (percepción de profundidad) y puede desarrollar una visión reducida en un ojo (ambliopía).

El estrabismo tiene muchas causas diferentes. El tratamiento específico depende del tipo específico y de la causa. El estrabismo puede ser tratado a cualquier edad. Algunos factores favorecen a pacientes jóvenes y la conformidad y la motivación son más favorables con los adultos. El tratamiento típicamente consiste en lentes recetados, prismas y un programa de terapia de visión. En ciertos pacientes, la cirugía puede ser recomendada en conjunto con la terapia de visión. La cirugía puede enderezar cosméticamente los ojos, pero típicamente no mejora la función visual. El pronóstico para un resultado óptimo en estos casos es un aumento a través de la terapia de visión pre-quirúrgicamente y post-quirúrgicamente. El estrabismo, ya sea constante o intermitente, siempre requiere tratamiento. Raramente desaparece por su cuenta, y los niños no lo eliminan durante el crecimiento.

La ambliopía, comúnmente conocido como el "ojo vago", es una condición manifestada por visión reducida, no corregible por anteojos o lentes de contactos. No es atribuible a ninguna condición estructural o patológica aparente. Puede estar relaciona al estrabismo porque un ojo virado generalmente pierde visión hasta cierto punto por la falta de uso. Muchos pacientes con ambliopía no pueden tener conocimiento de la condición hasta que realizan un screening de visión o un examen comprensivo de visión. La ambliopía tiene muchas causas y el tratamiento depende de la causa. En general, el tratamiento consiste del uso de lentes y prismas en conjunto con un programa de terapia de visión. Un parcho sobre el ojo no ambliópico es de valor limitado, a menos de que sea parte de un programa activo de terapia de visión.

Por muchos años se pensó que la ambliopía era dócil a tratamiento durante el periodo crítico, hasta la edad de 7 ú 8 años. Las investigaciones recientes han demostrado conclusivamente que el tratamiento efectivo se puede llevar acabo a cualquier edad, pero la duración del periodo de tratamiento aumenta dramáticamente mientras más tiempo haya existido la condición antes del tratamiento. Las investigaciones han demostrado que los pacientes con ambliopía están más propensos a incurrir en lesiones que resulten en la pérdida del buen ojo, que los individuos que tienen dos ojos buenos. Por lo tanto, los exámenes a temprana edad son esenciales.

# Estrabismo

### Definición
El estrabismo es una anomalía sensorial y neuromuscular de la integración binocular resultando en el fracaso de mantener un alineamiento bifoveal manifestándose en una desviación divergente (exotropía) o convergente (esotropía) del ojo no fijo.

### Síntomas
Los síntomas y las señales asociados con el estrabismo incluyen lo siguiente:
1. Viraje ocasional o constante del ojo
2. Diplopía
3. Juicio pobre de profundidad
4. Cabeza inclinada/virada
5. Cerrar o cubrir un ojo

### Factores de diagnóstico
El estrabismo está caracterizado por uno o más de los siguientes descubrimientos diagnósticos:
1. Manifiesta un ángulo de desviación del ojo
2. Deficiencia de las habilidades de vergencia, rangos de fusión reducidos con pobre percepción/estereopsis de profundidad
3. Diplopía
4. Adaptaciones sensoriales (Por ejemplo, supresión, ambliopía y correspondencia anormal de la retina).

    NOTA: Exámenes adicionales pueden ser apropiados como parte del trabajo del diagnóstico diferencial para el estrabismo, para eliminar otras condiciones médicas concurrentes y diferenciar condiciones visuales asociadas.

### Consideraciones Terapéuticas
#### A. Manejo
El doctor de optometría determina el diagnóstico apropiado, las modalidades terapéuticas, la frecuencia de evaluación, el seguimiento en base a la urgencia y la naturaleza de la condición del paciente y sus necesidades únicas. El manejo del caso y la duración del tratamiento estarían afectados por los siguientes factores:
1. La severidad de los síntomas y los factores de diagnóstico, incluyendo el inicio y la duración del problema
2. Las implicaciones de la salud general del paciente y los condiciones visuales asociadas
3. Extensión de las demandas visuales impuesta en el individuo
4. La conformidad del paciente
5. Intervenciones previas

#### B. Tratamiento
Un pequeño porcentaje de los casos son manejados exitosamente por las recetas de lentes terapéuticos o prismas. Sin embargo, la mayoría de los pacientes con estrabismo requieren terapia de visión ortóptica y/o terapia de visión. La terapia de visión optométrica generalmente incorpora la receta de tratamientos específicos para lograr lo siguiente:
1. Normalizar el control motor ocular
2. Normalizar las habilidades de localización espacial
3. Normalizar las habilidades de acomodación
4. Eliminar las adaptaciones sensoriales
5. Establecer una respuesta de fusión a todas las distancias y en todos los campos de movimiento
6. Normalizar la relación de acomodación/convergencia.
7. Integrar la función oculomotora con el procesamiento de información

#### Duración del tratamiento
Los siguientes rangos de tratamiento son proveídos como guía para el procesamiento de reclamos de terceras personas y de propósitos de revisión. La duración del tratamiento dependerá de la condición particular del paciente y de circunstancias asociadas. Cuando la duración del tratamiento más allá de estos rangos es requerida, documentación de la necesidad médica para servicios de tratamiento adicional, pueden ser otorgados.

### Exotropía
1. La exotropía intermitente más comúnmente encontrada, generalmente requiere 36 a 48 horas de terapia en la oficina.
2. La exotropía constante mas comúnmente encontrada generalmente requiere 50 a 64 horas de terapia en la oficina.
3. La exotropía puede ser complicada por:
    a. Adaptaciones visuales asociadas (por ejemplo, la ambliopía y la correspondencia anormal de la retina) requieren terapia adicional en la oficina.
    b. Anomalías visuales asociadas (por ejemplo, la ciclotropía, hipertropía) requieren terapia adicional en la oficina.
    c. Condiciones asociadas, tales como embolia cerebral, trauma de la cabeza y la cirugía para el estrabismo requieren sustancialmente más terapia en la oficina.

# Estrabismo—cont'd

## Esotropia

1. La esotropía intermitente más comúnmente encontrada generalmente requiere 40 a 52 horas de terapia en la oficina.
2. La esotropía constante más comúnmente encontrada generalmente requiere 60 a 75 horas de terapia en la oficina.
3. La esotropía puede complicarse por:
   a. Adaptaciones visuales asociadas (por ejemplo, la supresión, la ambliopía y la correspondencia anormal de la retina) requieren terapia adicional en la oficina.
   b. Anomalías visuales asociadas (por ejemplo, la ciclotropía, hipertropía) requieren terapia adicional en la oficina.
   c. Condiciones asociadas, tales como la embolia cerebral, el trauma de la cabeza y la cirugía para el estrabismo requieren sustancialmente más terapia en la oficina.

## Atención de seguimiento

Al finalizar el régimen de tratamiento activo, evaluaciones periódicas de seguimiento deben ser proveídas a intervalos apropiados. Los lentes terapéuticos pueden ser recetados al concluir la terapia de visión para el mantenimiento de la estabilidad a largo plazo. Algunos casos pueden requerir terapia adicional debido a descompensaciones.

# Hemorragia Subconjuntival

Una hemorragia subconjuntival ocurre en la superficie del ojo. Es causada por una ruptura de un vaso sanguíneo pequeño debajo de la conjuntiva, la capa protectora transparente más externa del ojo. Esto permite que la sangre se propague debajo de este tejido, causando frecuentemente una presentación dramática. Sin embargo, en la mayoría de los pacientes no tiene ninguna consecuencia, pero puede tomar varias semanas para completamente resolverse o ser reabsorbida por el sistema vascular.

Generalmente, el ejercicio físico, hacer fuerza, toser o estornudar pueden ser responsables de la ruptura de un vaso sanguíneo pequeño debajo del área subconjuntival; sin embargo, frecuentemente ninguna causa puede ser identificada.

El tratamiento estándar recomendado consiste en aplicar compresas frías varias veces al día por 2 días para reducir cualquier flujo sanguíneo adicional al área, seguido por compresas tibias para facilitar la reabsorción.

Si las hemorragias subconjuntivales vuelven a ocurrir dos o más veces en un año, la posibilidad de enfermedad del sistema vascular debe de ser eliminada.

# Las Enfermedades Sístemicas Y Sus Ojos

Muchas enfermedades en otras partes del cuerpo pueden resultar en problemas con sus ojos. Los pacientes con ciertas enfermedades sistémicas deben de visitar al oftalmólogo regularmente para asegurar que no ocurra ninguna pérdida de visión. De la misma manera, durante el curso de un examen de ojo, el oftalmólogo puede frecuentemente detectar cambios en la estructura de sus ojos que indiquen una posible enfermedad sistémica. El oftalmólogo puede típicamente detectar señales de 400 enfermedades que ocurren en otras partes del cuerpo, incluyendo las siguientes:

| | |
|---|---|
| Diabetes | Anemia |
| Alta presión | Esclerosis múltiple |
| Colesterol elevado | Enfermedades auto inmunes |
| Enfermedades del corazón | Artritis |
| Arteriosclerosis | Toxoplasmosis |
| Leucemia | Histoplasmosis |
| Embolia cerebral | Rosácea |
| Miastenia gravis | Cáncer |

Debido a que la mayoría de las enfermedades del ojo no producen dolor y cambian gradualmente, usted no tendrá conocimiento de ellas, hasta que ocurra la pérdida de visión. En este punto podría ser muy tarde para recuperar la visión perdida. Un ejemplo es glaucoma o degeneración macular.

El oftalmólogo puede ver señales de enfermedad sistémica de muchas formas al examinar sus ojos. Al mirar la retina dentro sus ojos, él o ella puede observar la formación de nuevos vasos sanguíneos frágiles, como en diabetes. En alta presión, las arterias primero se estrechan, luego producen hemorragias y liqueos llamados exudados que eventualmente se desarrolla en un edema del nervio óptico, lo que puede indicar que una persona está próxima a morir. Las enfermedades del corazón pueden causar una hemorragia única llamada punto Roth. Las placas en la arteria retinal pueden señalar un aumento del riesgo de embolia cerebral. Las cicatrices en la retina pueden indicar una enfermedad fungal o parasítica. Casi cualquier enfermedad que pueda afectar los vasos sanguíneos puede ser observada dentro del ojo. El interior del ojo es el lugar donde el médico puede observar los pequeños vasos sanguíneos magnificados varias veces sin requerir una incisión de la piel.

La artritis puede estar asociada con la inflamación de la parte blanca del ojo, la esclera, o la parte colorida, el iris. El colesterol elevado puede ser detectado al observar un anillo blanco en la parte posterior de los lentes claros en la parte anterior del ojo, la córnea, o por depósitos amarillentos de colesterol en la piel del párpado, llamado xantilasma. El oftalmólogo puede observar los pequeños vasos sanguíneos dentro del ojo llenándose de colesterol. Si se están llenando, usted corre el riesgo de obstrucción de los vasos coronarios, ocasionando un ataque al corazón, u obstrucción de las arterias carótidas ocasionando una embolia cerebral.

Desórdenes neuronales, tales como esclerosis múltiple, pueden afectar el nervio óptico o los nervios dirigidos a los músculos oculares, los párpados y la cara. La rosácea puede afectar la lágrima y la parte anterior del ojo causando irritación. El melanoma y otros tipos de cáncer pueden metatizarse del ojo o al ojo.

Los exámenes regulares del ojo con el oftalmólogo pueden minimizar la pérdida de visión causada por enfermedades sistémicas. Su oftalmólogo también puede detectar señales de enfermedades que usted no tenía conocimiento.

# Terapia de Visión Para Adultos

Muchas personas creen que la terapia de visión es solamente para los niños. Esto no puede estar más lejos de la verdad. Los adultos tienen tanta necesidad de este tipo de cuidado de la visión como los niños. La terapia de visión es frecuentemente más efectiva para los adultos porque ellos generalmente están más motivados a mejorar sus habilidades visuales, mientras los niños puedan no comprender que tengan un problema o cómo ese problema puede afectar sus intereses o futuro.

Muchas personas tienen problemas visuales aguantando trabajo cercanos-centrados (lectura, escritura y uso de la computadora), y no son limitados en los niños que están en la escuela. Cuando las personas tienen problemas usando ambos ojos a la vez o que no pueden enfocar por largos periodos de tiempo, no tienden a salir de estos problemas. Los niños con problemas visuales frecuentemente se convierten en adultos con problemas visuales.

Los adultos pueden determinar varias maneras de compensar por sus problemas visuales, para poder continuar con cualquier trabajo visual extenuoso que tengan que realizar. Frecuentemente, los adultos llegan de trabajar extremadamente cansados cuando solamente lo que hicieron fue sentarse en un escritorio y realizar trabajos con documentos. ¡Algunas personas podrían sentirse como si acabaron de correr un maratón de 10K! Los niños, de otra manera, tienden a evitar tareas que son difíciles o que los hagan sentir inadecuados.

El médico correcto puede ayudar a reducir la tensión del trabajo cercano al igual que el trabajo con cualquier otro tipo de problema visual. Los lentes apropiados en conjunto con la terapia de visión logran una diferencia enorme en la habilidad del adulto para funcionar en el trabajo o en el juego, como los niños que están en la escuela.

# Compresas Calientes

Las compresas calientes ayudan a solucionar infecciones del ojo al acelerar el suministro de sangre al área afectada.

1. Use agua de la llave. Deje correr el agua por aproximadamente 2 minutos para evitar el agua estancada que podría contener sedimentos de las tuberías. No necesita usar agua destilada o purificada.

2. Use agua tibia, no caliente. El agua caliente puede causar daños a la piel delicada de los párpados.

3. Empape un paño limpio en el agua tibia corriendo. Cierre ambos ojos y coloque el paño sobre ambos ojos o como sea indicado:

   _____.

4. Deje el paño sobre sus ojos hasta que se enfríe o deje de estar tibio. Luego rehumedezca éste en el agua nuevamente. Usted probablemente necesitará rehumedecer el paño cada 30 segundos.

5. Trate de mantener una temperatura tibia consistente cuando humedezca el paño.

6. Humedezca el paño por un total de 5 minutos o como sea indicado:

   _____.

   Humedezca 3 veces al día o como sea indicado:

   _____.

# Terapia de Visión

La terapia de visión es definida como lo siguiente:
- Un programa progresivo de "ejercicios" o procedimientos de visión
- Se realiza bajo supervisión médica.
- Individualizado para cubrir las necesidades visuales de cada paciente
- Generalmente realizado en la oficina, en una o dos sesiones a la semana de 30 minutos a una hora
- Algunas veces suplementado con procedimientos realizados en el hogar entre los visitas a la oficina ("asignación')
- Recetado para ayudar a los pacientes a desarrollar o mejorar las habilidades fundamentales visuales
- Recetado para mejorar el comodidad, facilidad y eficiencia visual
- Recetado para cambiar como un paciente procesa o interpreta la información visual.

## No solamente ejercicios de los ojos

Diferentes a otras formas de ejercicios, la meta de la terapia de visión no es fortalecer los músculos oculares. Sus músculos oculares ya están increíblemente fortalecidos. La terapia de visión no debe ser confundida con cualquier programa de ejercicios oculares dirigidos por usted mismo que han sido mercadeados al público. La terapia de visión es supervisada por profesionales del cuidado de la salud y muchos tipos de equipo médico especializado pueden ser usados, tales como:
- Lentes terapéuticos (equipo médico regulado)
- Prismas (equipo médico regulado)
- Filtros
- Oclusores o parches.
- Objetivo electrónico con mecanismos de tiempo.
- Programas de computadora
- Tabla de balance

El primer paso en cualquier programa de terapia de visión es un examen comprensivo de la visión. Luego de una evaluación detallada, un profesional cualificado del cuidado de la visión puede aconsejarle con respecto acerca de que si eres un buen candidato para la terapia de visión y si la terapia de visión es un tratamiento adecuado para usted.

La terapia de visión es algunas veces referida como una terapia o entrenamiento de visión.

# Historial Medico Familiar Y Riesgo

Si usted o un familiar tiene historial de los siguientes desórdenes, usted está en riesgo de perder la vista. Consulte con su oftalmólogo acerca de como usted puede prevenir la pérdida de visión causada por otras condiciones médicas.

## Enfermedades médicas y oculares: un historial personal y familiar

En el historial médico, preguntas específicas acerca de enfermedades personales actuales o previas, médicas u oftálmicas pueden ser también de valor para recetar aumentos adecuados en los lentes que ayuden a promover la salud de la vista. El historial familiar es una extensión de esto. En un individuo con un historial familiar significativo de desórdenes oculares que amenacen la visión (por ejemplo, cataratas y degeneración macular), cuidado especial debe realizarse para minimizar el riesgo a que el paciente desarrolle problemas similares. Esta misma precaución se mantiene verdadera para pacientes que están comenzando con cataratas o aquellos con anormalidades de la retina, tales como drusas, que pueden progresar una degeneración macular mas seria. También es importante en el historial médico otras enfermedades que puedan tener implicaciones oculares tales como diabetes, desórdenes auto inmunes, cáncer y enfermedades circulatorias. Detección temprana y tratamiento cuando sea indicado son esenciales para mantener tanto una buena salud y una buena vista por toda una vida.

Usted corre un mayor riesgo de pérdida de visión, si usted o algún familiar tiene:

| | |
|---|---|
| Diabetes | Eczema o soriasis |
| Alta presión | Enfermedad de la tiroides |
| Leucemia | Hipoglicemia |
| Anemia | Enfermedades auto inmunes |
| Esclerosis múltiple | Glaucoma |
| Artritis | Cataratas |
| Migrañas | Degeneración macular |
| Enfermedades del corazón | Ambliopía |
| Colesterol elevado | Enfermedades de músculos oculares |
| Epilepsia | Alergias o asma |

## Protegiendo sus ojos

- Use gafas de sol que le protejan de la radiación ultravioleta.
- Use un sombrero de ala ancha para reducir los rayos solares directos.
- Coma una dieta rica en frutas y vegetales verdes.
- Monitoree la presión sanguínea y limite las grasas saturadas y el colesterol.
- Limite el consumo de alcohol.
- Y el más importante, **deje de fumar**.

# Index

# Índice